T0296657

GRAINGER & ALLISON'S DIAGNOSTIC RADIOLOGY

SIXTH EDITION

Oncological Imaging

GRAINGER & ALLISON'S DIAGNOSTIC RADIOLOGY

SIXTH EDITION

Oncological Imaging

EDITED BY

Vicky Goh, MA, MBBChir, MD, MRCP, FRCR

Andreas Adam, CBE, MB, BS(Hons), PhD, FRCP, FRCR, FRCS, FFRRCSI(Hon), FRANZCR(Hon), FACR(Hon), FMedSci

ELSEVIER

London   New York   Oxford   Philadelphia   St Louis   Sydney   Toronto

ELSEVIER

© 2016, Elsevier Ltd. All rights reserved.

The right of Andreas Adam, Adrian K. Dixon, Jonathan H. Gillard and Cornelia M. Schaefer-Prokop to be identified as editors of this work has been asserted by them in accordance with the Copyright, Designs and Patents Act 1988.

No part of this publication may be reproduced or transmitted in any form or by any means, electronic or mechanical, including photocopying, recording, or any information storage and retrieval system, without permission in writing from the publisher. Details on how to seek permission, further information about the Publisher's permissions policies and our arrangements with organizations such as the Copyright Clearance Center and the Copyright Licensing Agency, can be found at our website: www.elsevier.com/permissions.

This book and the individual contributions contained in it are protected under copyright by the Publisher (other than as may be noted herein).

> ## Notices
>
> Knowledge and best practice in this field are constantly changing. As new research and experience broaden our understanding, changes in research methods, professional practices, or medical treatment may become necessary.
>
> Practitioners and researchers must always rely on their own experience and knowledge in evaluating and using any information, methods, compounds, or experiments described herein. In using such information or methods they should be mindful of their own safety and the safety of others, including parties for whom they have a professional responsibility.
>
> With respect to any drug or pharmaceutical products identified, readers are advised to check the most current information provided (i) on procedures featured or (ii) by the manufacturer of each product to be administered, to verify the recommended dose or formula, the method and duration of administration, and contraindications. It is the responsibility of practitioners, relying on their own experience and knowledge of their patients, to make diagnoses, to determine dosages and the best treatment for each individual patient, and to take all appropriate safety precautions.
>
> To the fullest extent of the law, neither the Publisher nor the authors, contributors, or editors, assume any liability for any injury and/or damage to persons or property as a matter of products liability, negligence or otherwise, or from any use or operation of any methods, products, instructions, or ideas contained in the material herein.

ISBN: 978-0-7020-6935-2

Executive Content Strategist: Michael Houston
Content Development Specialist: Louise Cook
Project Manager: Andrew Riley
Design: Christian Bilbow
Marketing Manager: Rachael Pignotti

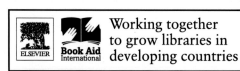

Working together to grow libraries in developing countries

www.elsevier.com • www.bookaid.org

CONTENTS

PREFACE, vi
LIST OF CONTRIBUTORS, vii

1 PRINCIPLES OF ONCOLOGICAL IMAGING, 1
David MacVicar • Vicky Goh

2 THE BREAST, 15
Jonathan J. James • A. Robin M. Wilson • Andrew J. Evans

3 RETICULOENDOTHELIAL DISORDERS: LYMPHOMA, 42
Sarah J. Vinnicombe • Norbert Avril • Rodney H. Reznek

4 BONE MARROW DISORDERS: HAEMATOLOGICAL NEOPLASMS, 71
Asif Saifuddin

5 BONE MARROW DISORDERS: MISCELLANEOUS, 82
Asif Saifuddin

6 IMAGING FOR RADIOTHERAPY PLANNING, 91
Peter Hoskin • Roberto Alonzi

7 FUNCTIONAL AND MOLECULAR IMAGING FOR PERSONALISED MEDICINE IN ONCOLOGY, 110
Ferdia A. Gallagher • Avnesh S. Thakor • Eva M. Serrao • Vicky Goh

INDEX, 127

PREFACE

The 7 chapters in this book have been selected from the contents of the Oncological Imaging section in *Grainger & Allison's Diagnostic Radiology, Sixth Edition*. These chapters provide a succinct up-to-date overview of current imaging techniques and their clinical applications in daily practice and it is hoped that with this concise format the user will quickly grasp the fundamentals they need to know. Throughout these chapters, the relative merits of different imaging investigations are described, variations are discussed and recent imaging advances are detailed. Please note that the following chapters represent a portion of the oncological imaging aspects in the comprehensive 6th edition of *Grainger's & Allison's Diagnostic Radiology* (for example, abdominal tumours are considered in section C 'Abdominal Imaging').

Grainger & Allison's Diagnostic Radiology has long been recognized as the standard general reference work in the field, and it is hoped that this book, utilizing the content from the latest sixth edition of this classic reference work, will provide radiology trainees and practitioners with ready access to the most current information, written by internationally recognized experts, on what is new and important in the radiological diagnosis of cancer.

LIST OF CONTRIBUTORS

Roberto Alonzi, BSc, MBBS, MRCP, FRCR, MD
Consultant in Clinical Oncology, Mount Vernon
Cancer Centre, Northwood; Senior Lecturer,
The Cancer Institute, University College London,
London, UK

Norbert Avril, MD
Professor and Research Scholar, Department of
Radiology, Case Western Reserve University,
University Hospitals Case Medical Center,
Cleveland, OH, USA

Andrew J. Evans, MRCP, FRCR
Professor of Breast Imaging, University of Dundee,
Hon Consultant Radiologist, NHS Tayside,
Ninewells Hospital and Medical School,
Dundee, UK

Ferdia A. Gallagher, MA, PhD, MRCP, FRCR
Cancer Research UK Clinician Scientist Fellow, CRUK
Cambridge Research Institute; Honorary Consultant
Radiologist, Addenbrooke's Hospital, Cambridge, UK

Vicky Goh, MA, MBBChir, MD, MRCP, FRCR
Chair of Clinical Cancer Imaging, Division of Imaging
Sciences and Biomedical Engineering, King's College
London; Honorary Consultant Radiologist, Guy's
and St Thomas' Hospitals, London, UK

Peter Hoskin, MD, FRCP, FRCR
Consultant in Clinical Oncology, Mount Vernon
Cancer Centre, Northwood; Professor in Clinical
Oncology, University College London, London, UK

Jonathan J. James, BMBS, FRCR
Consultant Radiologist, Nottingham Breast Institute,
City Hospital, Nottingham, UK

David MacVicar, MA, FRCP, FRCR, FBIR
Consultant Radiologist, Department of Diagnostic
Radiology, Royal Marsden Hospital, Sutton,
Surrey UK

**Rodney H. Reznek, MA, FRANZCR(Hon),
FFRRCSI(Hon), FRCP, FRCR**
Emeritus Professor of Cancer Imaging, Cancer
Institute, Queen Mary's University London,
St Bartholomew's Hospital, West Smithfield,
London, UK

Asif Saifuddin, BSc(Hons), MB ChB, MRCP, FRCR
Consultant Musculoskeletal Radiologist, Imaging
Department, The Royal National Orthopaedic
Hospital, Stanmore, Middlesex, UK

Eva M. Serrao, MD
Marie Curie Fellow, Cancer Research UK Cambridge
Research Institute, University of Cambridge, Li Ka
Shing Centre, Cambridge, UK

**Avnesh S. Thakor, BA, MA, MSc, MD, PhD,
MB BChir, FHEA, FRCR**
Fellow in Interventional Radiology, University of
Cambridge, UK; Visiting Scholar, Molecular Imaging
Program, Stanford University, CA, USA

Sarah J. Vinnicombe, BSc(Hons), MRCP, FRCR
Clinical Senior Lecturer, Cancer Imaging; Honorary
Consultant Radiologist, Division of Imaging and
Technology, Medical Research Institute, Ninewells
Hospital Medical School, Dundee, UK

A. Robin M. Wilson, FRCR, FRCP(E)
Consultant Radiologist, Department of Clinical
Radiology, The Royal Marsden Hospital, Sutton, UK

CHAPTER 1

PRINCIPLES OF ONCOLOGICAL IMAGING

David MacVicar • Vicky Goh

CHAPTER OUTLINE

INTRODUCTION

DIAGNOSIS

STAGING

PRINCIPLES OF STAGING INVESTIGATIONS

ASSESSMENT OF TREATMENT RESPONSE

SURVEILLANCE AND RESTAGING

CONCLUSION

INTRODUCTION

Cancer is one of the major causes of death in the Western world, costing an estimated US$125 billion in 2010. There were 1.6 million projected new cancer cases and 577,190 cancer deaths in the USA alone in 2012.[1] The incidence of cancer is also increasing in developing countries, related to factors such as smoking, and shifts towards a more Western lifestyle. The commonest cancers include lung, bowel, breast and prostate cancers. In recent years there have been major advances in the approach to the assessment and treatment of cancer: for example, the introduction of screening, genomic testing and multimodality treatment, including:

- Conventional chemotherapy and novel targeted drugs, e.g. antiangiogenic drugs, such as bevacizumab, an anti-vascular endothelial growth factor agent;
- Radiotherapy, including 3D conformal radiotherapy, intensity-modulated radiotherapy, stereotactic radiosurgery (cyberknife, gamma knife) and proton therapy; and
- Surgery, with the emphasis on maintaining a good quality of life and reducing morbidity.

The subspeciality of oncological imaging has evolved in tandem with this. Oncological imaging now forms a significant proportion of the workload of a radiology department.[2] Imaging plays a major role at different stages along the patient pathway. Cross-sectional imaging is used widely for diagnosis, staging, assessment of treatment response and surveillance. A variety of anatomical and functional imaging techniques are available in clinical practice currently. High-resolution cross-sectional imaging techniques such as computed tomography (CT) and magnetic resonance imaging (MRI), which allow the whole body to be imaged with high accuracy, remain the mainstay of imaging practice. However, physiologically based functional imaging techniques that assess different aspects of tumour biology such as diffusion-weighted MRI (water diffusion; a surrogate of tissue cellularity)

and dynamic contrast-enhanced CT or MRI (tumour perfusion and vascular leakage; a surrogate of angiogenesis) have been applied increasingly in clinical practice to improve tumour detection, staging and response assessment.

Molecular imaging techniques such as positron emission tomography (PET) provide more targeted imaging of tumour physiology and biology, with excellent anatomical localisation as hybrid imaging modalities (PET/CT and PET/MRI). While ^{18}F-fluorodeoxyglucose (FDG), an analogue of glucose, remains the commonest radio-labelled tracer in clinical use, allowing assessment of glucose metabolism, other tracers including ^{18}F-fluorothymidine (FLT), ^{11}C-choline, ^{18}F-misonidazole (FMISO), ^{18}F-FAZA, [61]C- or ^{64}Cu-ATSM and ^{11}C-acetate provide relevant information on tumour proliferation, hypoxia and lipogenesis, respectively. Each imaging modality has advantages and disadvantages (Table 1-1) and the 'best' imaging strategy will depend on the tumour type, tumour site, clinical indication (diagnosis, staging, treatment response assessment or surveillance), and availability and cost of the imaging technique.

A consequence of these advances in assessment and treatment has been improvements in patient outcome: this is especially so for early-stage disease, although survival for patients with advanced disease remains relatively poor. Another has been the recognition of the need for local, regional and national changes in the organisational aspects of cancer care. Typically in the United Kingdom, all new presentations of cancer are now assessed at a multidisciplinary meeting, and managed by a multidisciplinary team of specialists (including doctors (surgeons, medical and clinical oncologists, physicians, radiologists, pathologists), nurses, dieticians and physiotherapists) that are experienced in their cancer type in order to optimise clinical management. For a radiologist, this provides the opportunity to ensure the most suitable investigations are performed in a timely fashion at diagnosis, during treatment and in subsequent follow-up. This chapter will introduce key concepts in the imaging of patients with

TABLE 1-1   **The Different Imaging Techniques Available for Clinical Cancer Imaging**

Technique	Mechanism	Advantages	Disadvantages
Anatomical			
Plain film	Attenuation of X-rays by tissue structures	Availability Low cost	Limited resolution
Ultrasound	Attenuation of sound waves by tissue structures	Availability Low cost No radiation burden	Dependent on observer expertise
Computed tomography	Attenuation of X-rays by tissue structures	Availability Cross-sectional ability High spatial resolution	Radiation burden Relatively low contrast resolution
Magnetic resonance imaging	Absorption of radiowaves by atomic nuclei (most commonly hydrogen)	Cross-sectional ability High spatial and contrast resolution No radiation burden	Magnetic field effects and heating (particularly with high field systems)
Functional			
Diffusion-weighted MRI	Diffusion of water molecules	High spatial and contrast resolution No radiation burden Surrogate marker of tumour cellularity	Magnetic field effects and heating
Dynamic contrast-enhanced MRI	Kinetic modelling of gadolinium-based contrast agent to quantify vascular leakage	High spatial and contrast resolution No contrast burden Surrogate marker of angiogenesis	Magnetic field effects and heating
Blood oxygen level-dependent MRI	Paramagnetic effect of deoxyhaemoglobin	Surrogate marker of hypoxia (hypoxic blood volume)	Magnetic field effects and heating
Dynamic contrast-enhanced CT	Kinetic modelling of iodine-based contrast agent to quantify perfusion and vascular leakage	High spatial resolution Surrogate marker of angiogenesis and hypoxia	Radiation burden
Fluorodeoxyglucose (FDG) positron emission tomography	Uptake of ^{18}F-FDG, analogue of endogenous glucose	Cross-sectional ability May be combined with CT or MRI Quantification of tumour metabolic activity possible	Radiation burden Spatial resolution poorer than that of CT or MRI Relatively high cost

cancer. The role of imaging in diagnosis, staging, response assessment and surveillance will be described.

DIAGNOSIS

Primary Diagnosis

In the majority of cases, a patient will present with symptoms and signs related to the cancer, and appropriate investigations will be arranged, including imaging. Usually there are only a few diagnoses that can be made with confidence from imaging characteristics: for example, an ovarian dermoid, or other fat-containing tumours, and lesions that are obviously cystic. In most cases there is a differential diagnosis, requiring pathological confirmation of the diagnosis.

Confirmation of Diagnosis

Confirmation of a diagnosis may be undertaken using a variety of techniques, including cytological examination of fine needle aspiration samples, tumour specimens from automatic cutting needles and surgical biopsies (Figs. 1-1 and 1-2). Core biopsies yield a higher tumour volume than fine needle aspiration, and may be more suited for tumour biomarker analysis, often required by clinical trials.

Certain principles should be followed when needle aspiration or percutaneous core biopsy is being planned:

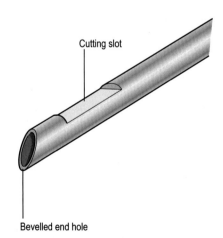

FIGURE 1-1 ■ **Diagram of Westcott-type needle.** This is used for aspiration of cytology samples. There is an end hole and a cutting side hole. Vacuum is applied when a central trocar is withdrawn following satisfactory placement of needle.

- The chosen technique should acquire sufficient tissue for a pathological diagnosis.
- The technique should be safe: for example, patient coagulation parameters should be checked and appropriate measures taken to minimise the risk of haemorrhage.
- For cytological specimens, a cytologist should be present to ensure enough material is present and to stain and interpret the cytology samples immediately.

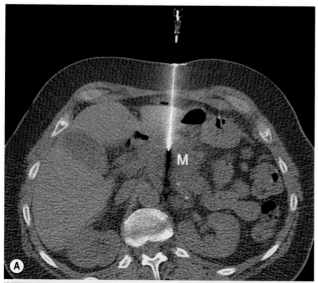

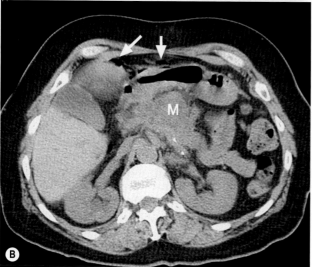

FIGURE 1-2 ■ **Coaxial system for biopsy.** (A) A coaxial needle has been introduced into a pancreatic mass (M) through the gastric antrum. Dense artefact is present at the tip of the trocar. Once the trocar is withdrawn, an automatic cutting needle of appropriate length is introduced through the cannula left in situ, and multiple biopsies can be obtained by angling in a variety of directions. (B) Once the system is withdrawn, limited free gas is present outside the stomach (arrows). No clinical symptoms developed and the patient was discharged 6 hours after the procedure.

- For core biopsies, specimen preparation should be discussed with the examining pathologist. Most specimens can be placed in formalin but others may require preparation for special staining techniques.
- If image-assisted tissue diagnosis is inconclusive, consideration of further percutaneous attempts or of open surgical biopsy should take into account the reason for diagnostic failure. For example, some tumours such as pancreatic carcinoma may have few malignant cells. The degree of risk involved in repeat biopsy, the technical ease with which the specimen was obtained and the likelihood of achieving positive tissue diagnosis on the second attempt should all be considered.

Several types of cutting needles may be used for core biopsy. The Tru-Cut needle has a central trocar that makes the initial movement forward, exposing a slot. The sheath is then advanced over the slot, cutting a piece of tissue into the slot, and the entire apparatus is withdrawn, with a core specimen contained in the slot. Coaxial systems enable multiple tumour cores to be obtained via a single puncture site. The principle involves placement of a needle from which the sharpened trocar is removed to leave a hollow unsharpened cannula in the mass for biopsy. An automatic cutting needle can then be placed down the cannula. Several cores can then be obtained, and different parts of the lesion may be sampled by angling the cannula slightly in a variety of directions. Since only one puncture is made of the skin and intervening tissue planes, more tissue is obtained without increasing the risk of track seeding. In some circumstances percutaneous needle techniques should not be used to avoid malignant seeding of the percutaneous biopsy track.

STAGING

Once the diagnosis of cancer has been confirmed, it is important for the subsequent management of a patient to stage the tumour, i.e. to assess the locoregional extent of the tumour as well as the presence/absence of distant metastatic disease.

The aims of a staging system are:
- To allow rational selection of primary therapy and assessment of the necessity for (neo)adjuvant treatment;
- To give some indication of the likely prognosis;
- To assist in the evaluation of results of treatment;
- To enable exchange of information between cancer treatment centres; and
- To contribute to the continuing investigation of human cancer.

Staging systems describe the anatomical extent of a tumour, and provide highly relevant information to guide appropriate therapy at diagnosis, although decision-making will be influenced also by other factors, including the histological grade of the tumour, its expected biological behaviour and the age and general fitness of a patient.[3] While clinical examination continues to have a significant role in the initial assessment of patients, imaging has a major role to play in the staging of cancer.

Staging Systems

An ideal staging system should be simple, precise, consistent and applicable to all clinical circumstances in oncology, and convey some prognostic information to facilitate best practice. Over the years, many staging systems have borne the name of eminent doctors (e.g. the Robson staging classification of renal tumours or Dukes' staging classification of colorectal cancer), institutions (e.g. the Royal Marsden Hospital staging classification for testicular germ cell tumours) or organisations (e.g. the Fédération Internationale de Gynécologie et d'Obstétrique (FIGO) classification systems for cervical, uterine and other gynaecological neoplasms). More recently, the tumour–node–metastasis (TNM system), espoused by the American Joint Committee on Cancer (AJCC) and the Union Internationale Contre le Cancer (UICC), has been adopted widely.

The TNM classification of malignant tumours and the AJCC cancer staging handbook are now in their seventh editions.[4] The system was originally devised by Pierre Denoix in the 1940s and has been modified over the subsequent decades. The 'T' category entails evaluation of local tumour extent. The 'N' category entails evaluation of nodal involvement. The 'M' category entails evaluation of disease at distant sites. The 'T' category, which may have the prefix 'c' to indicate 'clinical' staging, although this is frequently omitted, has several standard forms of notation: Tx indicates that primary tumour cannot be assessed; Tis indicates in situ disease with no evidence of invasion; T0 indicates no visible evidence of primary tumour; T1–T4 indicates increasing degrees of local tumour extent. These divisions may be adapted with the addition of subdivisions indicated by letters (e.g. 'a' or 'b') for greater flexibility in different tumour types. Although staging of the primary from T1 to T4 follows broad principles and there are some similarities between tumour types, refinements and adaptations for individual tumours are needed usually.

The 'N' category has similar notation. Direct spread of the primary tumour into an adjacent lymph node is classified as nodal spread. Nx is where regional lymph nodes cannot be assessed, N0 is where no regional lymph node metastases are present and N1, N2 and N3 indicate increasing involvement of regional lymph nodes. Likewise, these divisions may include subdivisions indicated by letters (e.g. 'a' or 'b'). The 'M' category assesses distant metastasis where Mx indicates that distant metastasis cannot be assessed, M0 indicates there are no distant metastases and M1 indicates the presence of distant metastasis. The category M1 may be further specified indicating which organs are involved. For example, PUL indicates pulmonary metastases, OSS indicates osseous metastases and HEP indicates hepatic metastases. Again, subdivisions may be indicated by letters (e.g. 'a' or 'b').

All tumours must be confirmed pathologically. A number of general rules apply when using the clinical TNM staging system. Clinical stage is assigned by physical examination, imaging and other relevant investigations, but may be amended as pathological information becomes available, and given the prefix pTNM stage where microscopic extent of disease is known. If there is doubt what stage should be assigned, the lower category should be used. Therefore, an imaging investigation that is suspicious but not diagnostic of spread to the pelvic sidewall will be disregarded unless supplemented by further imaging or confirmation by histopathology.

Once assigned, the pre-treatment TNM stage is recorded in the patient's records and remains unchanged through subsequent treatment. For multiple synchronous primary tumours, the tumour with the highest 'T' category is used for staging purposes. For synchronous primary tumours arising in paired organs, each tumour should be assigned a separate TNM stage. In modern usage the TNM system has the advantages of clarity of communication, but is complex. This has led to a further system of stage grouping, which is published within the AJCC system. Stage groups of 0–4 are assigned as tumour becomes more extensive and widespread.

National bodies, such as the Royal College of Radiologists in the United Kingdom, have published recommendations or guidelines on the choice of staging investigation (CT, MRI or PET/CT), recognising that local availability of advanced imaging techniques and the preference and experience of individual radiologists are important considerations.[5] A potential effect of advances in imaging technology over time is stage migration, e.g. via improvements in tumour detection, resulting in upstaging, and artefactual improvement in subgroup prognosis, although overall survival will remain stable unless more effective treatment is given.

PRINCIPLES OF STAGING INVESTIGATIONS

Primary Tumour Staging

The principles of staging are illustrated in this section, with the following examples of some of the most common cancers.

Rectal Cancer

Rectal cancer is a good example of a tumour in which a staging system has evolved and changed over a period of more than 70 years, and technical refinement of surgery over the past 20 years has gone hand-in-hand with increasingly sophisticated imaging of the primary tumour such that imaging is now central to decision-making. It remains true that the vast majority of patients with rectal cancer should be offered surgery, as local symptoms due to growth within the pelvis are associated with severe pain that can be difficult to palliate. However, the timing of surgery and the role of neoadjuvant chemotherapy and radiotherapy depend on the local tumour stage at the time of diagnosis.

In 1932, Dukes highlighted the importance of extramural spread in the prediction of local recurrence and survival. He also observed that lymph node invasion was present in 14% of patients with tumours confined to the bowel wall and 43% of patients with tumours extending beyond the serosa.[6] A number of other prognostic indicators have subsequently been identified, including the pattern of local spread (a well-circumscribed margin implies a better prognosis than a widely infiltrated tumour with ill-defined borders). Spread beyond the peritoneal membrane results in a high incidence of both local recurrence and transcoelomic dissemination; invasion of extramural veins by tumour and extent and number of tumour-involved lymph nodes are all independent predictors of a poor prognosis.

For many years the preferred operation for rectal cancer was synchronous combined abdominoperineal excision of rectum (AP resection). However, total mesorectal excision has become the gold standard since its introduction in the 1970s.[7] In this technique, the surgeon dissects from above and finds the mesorectal plane. As

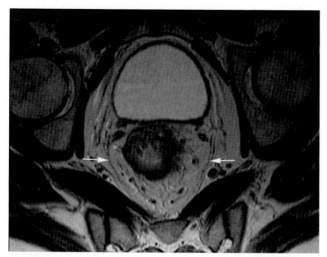

FIGURE 1-3 ■ **T2-weighted MRI of the rectum.** This axial image demonstrates a low signal adenocarcinoma predominantly involving the rectal wall to the left of the midline. There is evidence of spread into the mesorectum and extramural vascular invasion. The mesorectal fascia is clearly demonstrated (arrows). Neoadjuvant treatment with chemotherapy and radiotherapy may help to downstage the tumour prior to consideration of surgery.

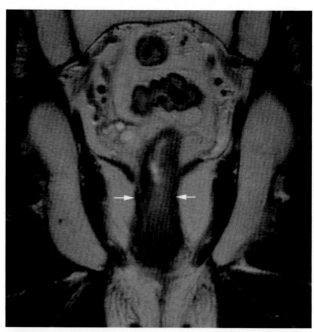

FIGURE 1-4 ■ **T2-weighted MRI of a low rectal tumour.** This coronal image demonstrates a tumour extending inferiorly to involve the anal sphincter complex (arrows). Sphincter-preserving surgery and re-anastomosis will not be technically possible.

the lymphatic vessels and nodes draining the tumour are located throughout the mesorectum, if this is divided or disrupted during surgical excision, spillage of malignant cells may occur and involved nodes may be left in situ. This increases the likelihood of local recurrence, and excision of the rectum is best achieved by dissection down the mesorectal fascia, allowing the mesorectum and rectum to be removed en bloc without disruption of the presacral fascia and the underlying venous plexus. The surgically excised specimen may then be sectioned transversely and the circumferential resection margin (CRM) examined for tumour involvement. The presence of tumour at the extremity of the resection margin is a major prognostic factor.[8]

In recent years, MRI has been shown to be the investigation of choice in demonstrating spread of tumour within the mesorectum and the mesorectal plane itself (Fig. 1-3). It is possible to demonstrate the relationship of the tumour to the anal canal, indicating the potential for sphincter-preserving surgery (Fig. 1-4). Criteria have been developed in pathologically correlated series for staging of the primary tumour and nodes within the mesorectum. Effectively, MRI can provide a 'road map' for the surgeon and studies have shown that the pathological status of the CRM can be predicted.[9,10] Other prognostic factors such as extramural venous invasion and peritoneal penetration can be demonstrated. If locally advanced disease with mural penetration is demonstrated, chemotherapy and radiation therapy may be employed to downstage the primary before an attempt at surgery, allowing a more tailored preoperative strategy.

Studies from the Royal Marsden Hospital have demonstrated that the incidence of tumour at the circumferential resection margin is only 2% in patients diagnosed by MRI as likely to have a safe resection margin for immediate surgery. Overall incidence of positive

resection margins in those patients seen by the MDT, including those who had undergone preoperative chemotherapy and radiotherapy for disease diagnosed by MRI to be locally advanced at initial presentation, was 8.5%. In a group of patients not assessed by the MDT, positive resection margins were present in 24%.[11] The implication is clear: all patients newly diagnosed with rectal cancer should be assessed by a multidisciplinary team, within the framework of a cancer network, to ensure that up-to-date investigation and treatment is available.

Non-Small Cell Lung Cancer

Lung cancer, the most common cause of cancer mortality worldwide, is a good example of a multimodality staging approach to optimise patient management. Plain radiographs, CT, MRI, endobronchial or endoluminal ultrasound (EBUS or EUS) and PET/CT are part of the diagnostic algorithm in patients with suspected lung cancer[12] (Fig. 1-5). For patients with an early-stage lung cancer, surgery offers the best chance of cure, provided co-morbidity and the patient's lung function do not preclude this. Accurate staging of locoregional and distant metastatic disease optimises the selection of patients for curative treatment and reduces futile thoracotomy rates compared to standard staging.[13,14]

Breast Cancer

Breast cancer is a good example of a disease where surgical techniques have undergone frequent revision, from the days of very radical surgery in the 1950s, to lumpectomy favoured in the 1970s and more recent regimens involving wide local excision or quadrantectomy followed by radiotherapy. Although many primary breast tumours can be staged by clinical examination, local management may benefit from imaging planning. When multifocal disease is suspected or tumour is diffuse, contrast-enhanced MRI has very high sensitivity for lesion detection (Fig. 1-6). However, specificity is lower as areas of

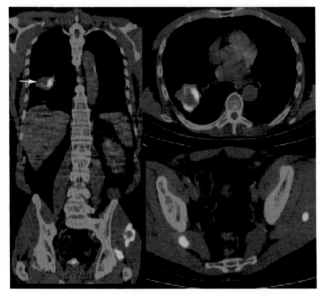

FIGURE 1-5 ■ ^{18}F-FDG PET/CT of a non-small cell lung cancer. This montage shows a right lung tumour with distant metastases within the gluteal muscles, precluding the patient from primary surgery.

gadolinium enhancement within the breast do not necessarily represent cancer. Ultrasound has the advantage of being able to stage the primary tumour, detecting abnormal lymph nodes in the axilla and facilitating fine-needle aspiration for cytology if abnormal nodes are detected.

The concept of sentinel-node detection prior to surgery also involves imaging. The principle is that the first lymph node in a nodal bed draining from a tumour will show metastatic disease if lymphatic spread has occurred. Absence of metastatic disease in a sentinel node in patients with breast cancer has been reported to have a negative predictive value for axillary nodal disease of 98%.[15] A combined technique using injected blue dye and an isotope, which is then localised by gamma camera imaging before surgery and with an intraoperative gamma probe during surgery, is usually recommended.

Prostate Cancer

Since the Radiologic Diagnostic Oncology Group (RDOG) demonstrated that both MRI and endorectal ultrasound show higher accuracy than clinical staging, and that MRI demonstrates higher sensitivity and specificity than endorectal ultrasound[16,17] for detection of extracapsular spread of prostate cancer, MRI assessment of prostate cancer has evolved. A multiparametric imaging approach, combining T1- and T2-weighted sequences with diffusion-weighted MRI, dynamic contrast-enhanced MRI and MRI spectroscopy, is utilised (Fig. 1-7). This has resulted in improvements in tumour detection and delineation of the extent of disease.[18,19] Nevertheless, it has been difficult to demonstrate a clear impact of using

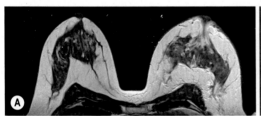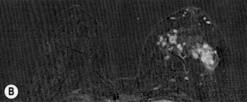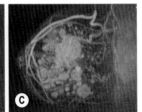

FIGURE 1-6 ■ MRI of a primary breast cancer. Axial T2-weighted (A), axial early subtracted dynamic contrast-enhanced T1-weighted MRI (B) and sagittal MIP image (C) of a left breast cancer showing an enhancing multifocal tumour.

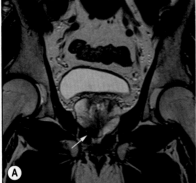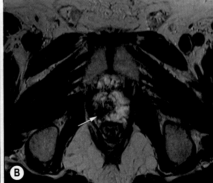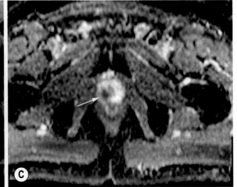

FIGURE 1-7 ■ MRI of a primary prostate cancer. T2-weighted coronal (A) and axial (B) images show there is low signal right apical peripheral zone tumour. The tumour extends to the capsular margin (arrow) but there is no confirmatory evidence of extracapsular spread indicating T2 disease. Diffusion-weighted imaging demonstrates restriction within this tumour, depicted as a low signal intensity area on the apparent diffusion coefficient map (C).

high-technology imaging on patient health. One of the reasons for this is that the natural history of the disease is heterogeneous and the optimal treatment of prostate cancer remains controversial.[20,21]

Staging Distant Metastatic Disease

Staging for distant metastatic disease remains an important facet in the management of cancer where a curative approach is being considered, e.g. surgery or radical radiotherapy. While CT remains the mainstay for staging distant metastatic disease, there is a role for other more sensitive modalities, i.e. ^{18}F-FDG PET/CT in certain cancer types, e.g. primary lung and oesophageal cancer.[13,22,23] The presence of metastatic disease does not necessarily contraindicate resection of the primary tumour, as local control will be necessary for symptomatic relief. Small-volume metastatic disease in liver and lungs may also be amenable to surgery ('metastectomy').

ASSESSMENT OF TREATMENT RESPONSE

The Role of Imaging

Imaging is used widely to demonstrate changes in tumour size with treatment but findings should be interpreted within the context of other response markers such as biochemical tumour markers, and the patient's clinical well-being on toxic therapy. In specialist cancer centres, the majority of patients are on clinical trials, which may stipulate the timing and technique of follow-up investigations. Nevertheless, even if the patient is not on a clinical trial, it is important to have some reproducible and objective technique that will allow directly comparable measurements to be made.

CT remains the most frequently used follow-up technique, although US, MRI and PET/CT can be used. It is important to ensure consistency at each attendance, i.e. that the same imaging protocol and sequences are used. The frequency of follow-up investigations depends on the perceived likelihood of response, and toxicity of treatment. The frequency may also be stipulated by clinical trials or physician preference: it is noticeable that some clinicians adopt shorter follow-up intervals for similar treatment regimens. There is also some pressure from the pharmaceutical industry to document reduction in tumour size: while overall survival rate remains the best objective parameter of efficacy of treatment, demonstration of some form of objective response earlier

in the course of disease encourages development of certain drugs.

Objective Response Assessment

Effective systemic chemotherapy and cross-sectional imaging developed side by side during the 1970s, and it became clear that a common language and definition of guidelines for the assessment of objective tumour response was necessary. The World Health Organisation (WHO) proposed a system that remains in limited use today.[24,25] Miller et al[25] recommended that a partial response should be designated when bi-dimensional measurement of a single lesion shows greater than 50% reduction in cross-sectional area (perpendicular diameters should be measured). Separate categories are available where one-dimensional measurements only are obtainable, but no consideration is given to calculation of tumour volumes. It also states that objective response can be determined clinically, radiologically, biochemically or by surgical/pathological restaging.

The WHO criteria have been superseded since by other criteria. The response evaluation criteria in solid tumours (RECIST) were proposed by the European Organisation for Research and Treatment of Cancer (EORTC) in collaboration with the National Cancer Institute in the USA and the National Cancer Institute of Canada Clinical Trials Group,[26] and were updated in 2010.[27] The RECIST criteria allow one-dimensional measurement of target lesions and the sum of these, rather than the product of two perpendicular linear measurements, is used. A partial response is defined of at least a 30% decrease in the sum of the longest diameter of target lesions, taking as a reference the baseline sum of longest diameters (Table 1-2 and Fig. 1-8).

The aim of the RECIST criteria was to simplify the way in which information was gathered and recorded, and not necessarily to increase precision. The fundamental problem of observer variability and subjectivity remains. It is still the responsibility of an investigator to select lesions for measurement, but one of the important recommendations of the RECIST Group was that results of trials claiming response by measurement should be validated by an independent review committee.

It remains important to assess size alterations within the context of the clinical state of the patient and the natural history of the disease. It is also important to be aware that anatomical measurement criteria will fail to take account of functional changes within tumours. Likewise, cyst formation and necrosis within tumours will not be assessed using size criteria alone. To this end, more

TABLE 1-2 RECIST Criteria for the Assessment of Therapeutic Response

Target Lesion*	Complete Response	Partial Response	Stable Disease	Progressive Disease
Up to 5 target lesions with a maximum of 2 lesions/organ	Resolution of all target lesions	At least 30% reduction in mean sum longest diameter target lesions	Response not fulfilling PR or PD category	At least 20% increase in mean sum longest diameter target lesions or new lesions

*Target lesion: Any measurable lesion within an organ that is >1 cm in longest dimension. For lymph nodes the measurement is the shortest dimension (short axis) and this should be >1.5 cm for the node to be considered as a target lesion.

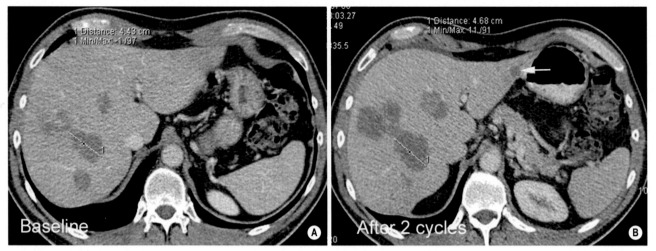

FIGURE 1-8 ■ **RECIST 1.1 assessment.** The target lesion chosen was a liver metastasis. Despite treatment there was disease progression with enlargement of existing metastases and development of a new metastasis (arrow).

recently criteria which take into account contrast enhancement change as well as size, as applied to gastrointestinal stromal tumours (Choi criteria)[28] and also to renal cell carcinoma[29,30] (modified Choi criteria), or which take areas of necrosis into account, as applied to non-small cell lung cancer, have been proposed.[31]

Imaging Residual Masses

A post-treatment residuum is frequently seen in several solid tumours, such as lung cancer, lymphoma and metastatic non-seminomatous germ cell tumours (NSGCT). Imaging techniques have been applied in an attempt to predict the likelihood of recurrence in these residual masses. Investigation has been most intensive in lymphoma. Enlargement of a residual lymphoma mass on CT is strong evidence of disease recurrence, but it is hoped that it will be possible to identify residual or recurrent disease earlier using functional techniques. There is good evidence of a high sensitivity for ^{18}F-FDG PET/CT in detection of residual disease. There are theoretical reasons for using ^{18}F-FDG PET/CT as a routine surveillance procedure following treatment. However, at the time of writing, there is no clear evidence to support this strategy.

MRI has also been evaluated in the investigation of residual lymphoma masses.[32] Reduction in signal intensity on T2-weighted images during treatment is taken as a sign of successful treatment, leaving a fibrotic residuum. However, MRI has not become a routine investigation because of high false-negative and false-positive rates. Imaging features suggestive of residual disease may help to select patients for repeat biopsy or further treatment, for example, with adjuvant radiotherapy. However, as treated cancer can leave abnormal tissue detectable by imaging, imaging alone is unreliable in predicting the pathological nature of the residuum.

Imaging of Treatment Toxicity

Radiotherapy and/or chemotherapy can affect all tissues of the body. Imaging features and the timing of their appearance vary from organ to organ. Radiotherapy causes acute change by a direct physical inflammatory process and later effects as a result of an ischaemic insult. Anticancer drugs have direct cytotoxic effects, but may also cause hypersensitivity reactions. Some organs are more susceptible to tissue damage than others, although observed imaging changes are not always of clinical importance. Interpretation is facilitated by knowledge of the type and timing of treatment.

Lung

A radiological diagnosis of radiation pneumonitis is made when there is evidence of acute radiotherapy change in the lungs, but this is always accompanied by clinical symptoms. Radiation pneumonitis usually appears 6–8 weeks after completion of treatment with 35–40 Gy, but is not generally seen at radiation doses below 30 Gy. It is almost always seen at doses over 40 Gy and will appear earlier than 6 weeks. It becomes most extensive 3–4 months after completion of radiotherapy. The histological appearance is of diffuse alveolar damage. At a later stage, an organising fibrosis develops, which becomes complete 9–12 months after termination of therapy. The histological appearances are non-specific, but the distinguishing feature on plain film radiography and CT is a straight edge corresponding to a radiation field. When there is significant volume loss, traction effects occur and there may be bronchiectatic changes.

Neoadjuvant cytotoxic chemotherapy enhances the effect of radiation, causing earlier radiation pneumonitis and more severe fibrosis. Drugs most commonly implicated include dactinomycin, doxorubicin, bleomycin, cyclophosphamide, mitomycin and vincristine. There is a growing list of cytotoxic drugs that are recognised to cause pulmonary parenchymal damage independent of radiation therapy. Bleomycin is used in the treatment of NSGCT, lymphoma and squamous cell carcinoma. The toxic effect is dose-dependent and exacerbated by the use of other agents in combination chemotherapy, adjuvant radiation therapy and oxygen therapy. Early radiographic abnormality is typically a reticular nodular pattern of interstitial disease, which is most severe in the basal segments. Lung damage may be progressive, leading to pulmonary fibrosis, which may be severe and cause traction pneumothorax and pneumomediastinum (Fig. 1-9).

Busulfan, which is used in haematological malignancy, causes interstitial lung damage. Methotrexate is responsible for a hypersensitivity reaction, which results in alveolar shadowing and sometimes in mediastinal adenopathy. If methotrexate therapy is prolonged, the lung damage may progress to fibrosis. Treatment-related lung toxicity can usually be seen on plain radiography, but CT is more sensitive.[33,34]

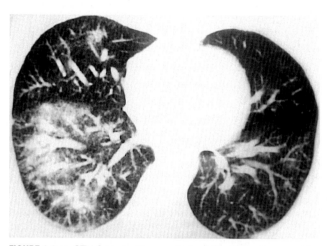

FIGURE 1-9 ■ **CT of acute bleomycin toxicity.** This shows widespread predominantly basal interstitial change.

Bone and Bone Marrow

Osseous changes in response to radiation were first described by Ewing as long ago as the 1920s. Local demineralisation and osteopenia are the earliest and often the only post-radiation changes noted on plain radiography. Later changes include mixed lytic and sclerotic areas and trabecular coarsening, which may develop 2 or more years after radiotherapy. Spontaneous fractures and aseptic necrosis can occur, but, in general, radiation damage to bone is becoming less common as a result of high-energy mega-voltage radiotherapy and more accurate dose distribution. However, the effect on bone marrow is frequently seen on MRI at relatively low doses, from 15 to 20 Gy. Haemopoietic bone marrow converts to fatty marrow, resulting in a high signal on T1-weighted sequences. Following treatment of metastatic bone disease or primary bone tumour with radiotherapy or chemotherapy, the marrow can take on a bizarre appearance on MRI that is virtually uninterpretable. For example, following treatment of lymphoma or neuroblastoma diffusely involving the bone marrow, the latter will usually alter its appearance, sometimes reverting to normal, but often leaving an array of mixed residual signal changes (Fig. 1-10).

Neurotoxicity

Therapeutic radiation to the brain induces an ischaemic insult, which is manifested as abnormality within the deep cerebral white matter. This is best demonstrated by MRI, where diffuse high signal is present on T2-weighted images or using the fluid attenuation inversion recovery

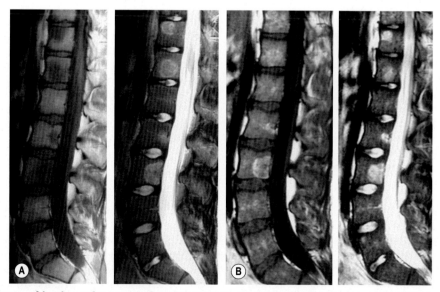

FIGURE 1-10 ■ **Lymphoma of lumbar spine pre- and post-treatment.** (A) Sagittal MRI of lumbar spine showing lymphoma in bone marrow. On T1-weighted sequence (left) low signal is returned from the marrow cavity of T11, 12, L2, 3 and 5. Corresponding focal areas of high signal are identified on the T2-weighted sequence (right). Uptake of ^{18}F-fluorodeoxyglucose (^{18}F-FDG) on PET was increased in these vertebrae. (B) Following chemotherapy, the T1-weighted sequence (left) shows a generalised increase of signal in the marrow cavities and focal high signal corresponding to previous tumour-involved areas. The signal is also increased on T2-weighted imaging (right) at these sites, although uptake of ^{18}F-FDG was normal. Although clearly abnormal, this MRI appearance was interpreted as successful treatment of lymphoma, and the patient remained disease-free 12 months after completion of therapy.

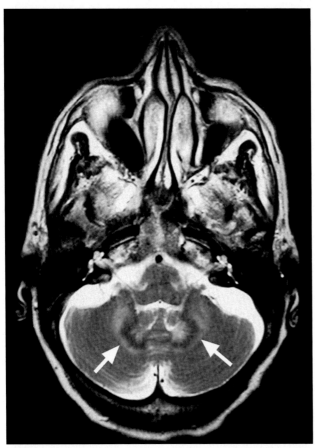

FIGURE 1-11 ■ T2-weighted MRI of posterior fossa. This shows diffuse high signal in cerebellum (arrows) following treatment with fluorouracil.

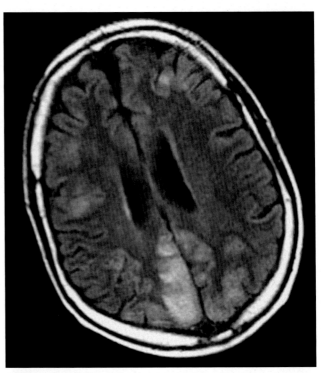

FIGURE 1-12 ■ MRI axial fluid attenuation inversion recovery sequence. This shows high signal in the parafalcine posterior grey and white matter with isolated areas of abnormal signal in both frontal lobes. This appearance is typical of the reversible posterior leukoencephalopathy syndrome seen following bone marrow transplantation, frequently attributed to toxicity from ciclosporin.

(FLAIR) sequence. Similar changes may be seen within the spinal cord as a result of radiation myelitis. White matter changes may also be identified with cytotoxic medications (Fig. 1-11), including fluorouracil, levamisole and intrathecal methotrexate. As with lung toxicity, a growing number of cytotoxic agents have been implicated in central neurotoxic events. Following bone marrow transplantation, immunosuppressive drugs, including ciclosporin, cause a reversible posterior leukoencephalopathy syndrome (RPLS), which has a characteristic distribution of grey and white matter change (Fig. 1-12).

Peripheral neuropathy is common with cytotoxic agents such as vincristine, but has no imaging features. However, radiation damage to the brachial plexus is occasionally encountered following treatment for breast cancer. This is due to an ischaemic insult to the vasa nervorum of the brachial plexus. Thickening of the elements of the brachial plexus within the radiation field is best demonstrated by MRI. This may be difficult to distinguish from the infiltrative forms of recurrent breast cancer. However, if there is no mass lesion, and if appropriate symptoms and clinical signs are present, MRI is an accurate way of diagnosing radiation-induced brachial plexopathy.[35]

Hepatic Toxicity

Many cytotoxic chemotherapy regimens induce abnormality of liver function. The change most frequently observed on imaging is hepatic steatosis. This may be reversible even if treatment is continued, which can be a source of confusion as contrast parameters within the liver in the presence of metastases can alter radically between examinations. It is, therefore, important to continue using the same imaging protocols throughout the treatment regimen.

Cardiotoxicity

Radiation to the thorax may cause acute and chronic pericarditis, cardiomyopathy and, in the long term, coronary artery disease and valvular dysfunction. A more frequent problem for the cancer patient is cardiotoxicity from cytotoxic agents; for example, doxorubicin is known to cause some degree of myocardial dysfunction in 50% of asymptomatic patients. In extreme cases, life-threatening congestive cardiac failure can develop. Circulatory problems may also develop due to fluid overload during hyper-hydration, which is necessary in a number of treatment regimens. Agents such as asparaginase can precipitate abnormalities of coagulation, resulting in venous thrombosis.

SURVEILLANCE AND RESTAGING

Surveillance of Asymptomatic Patients

Following the diagnosis and treatment of a primary tumour, decisions need to be made on how extensive the search for metastases should be, and how long imaging surveillance should continue. The approach differs between tumour types, and depends on the initial local (T) staging and tumour biology. Another factor to consider is whether there is a biochemical marker for the tumour, a rise in which would indicate the likelihood of a relapse that could subsequently be anatomically demonstrated by imaging. A good example of a tumour in which surveillance programmes are appropriate is NSGCT of the testis. Following orchidectomy, CT staging of chest, abdomen and pelvis is usually undertaken. Seventy per cent of patients will have no lymph node, pulmonary or other metastatic spread and will not relapse subsequently. However, 30% of patients with a normal CT study at the time of orchidectomy will relapse: 80% of this group will relapse within 1 year and 95% will relapse within 2 years. Two-thirds of these have a rise in tumour markers, but the remainder will be marker-negative. Cytotoxic chemotherapy for relapse is effective, with cure rates in excess of 90%. It is, therefore, justifiable to continue CT surveillance for 2 years; while some institutions practice a high-frequency surveillance programme, there is no definite evidence that a lower CT surveillance frequency at 6-monthly or even yearly intervals worsens prognosis. However, if large-volume disease is allowed to develop, this has an adverse prognostic significance, so shortening the inter-examination interval empirically makes sense.[36]

A further example where imaging is used to detect asymptomatic disease is colorectal carcinoma. Surgery in patients with resectable hepatic metastatic disease gives a 40% 5-year survival, compared with survival rates close to 0 in untreated patients.[37] Current strategies now aim to reduce the volume of hepatic metastatic disease so that previously non-resectable disease may undergo surgery with curative intent.[38] There is growing evidence that intensive follow-up that incorporates monitoring of carcinoembryonic antigen (CEA) and CT of chest, abdomen and pelvis contributes to detection of metastatic disease in patients who subsequently proceed to potentially curative resection.[39,40] CT has adequate sensitivity for detection of hepatic and pulmonary metastases, but ultrasound and MRI have a role in characterising liver lesions (Fig. 1-13).

^{18}F-FDG PET and ^{18}F-FDG PET/CT may prove to be valuable in early detection of metastatic disease, particularly in areas where CT alone lacks sensitivity such as the peritoneal cavity (Fig. 1-14). ^{18}F-FDG PET/CT is a valuable problem-solving technique when CEA is rising, and other imaging techniques fail to demonstrate the site of recurrence. The frequency and duration of imaging follow-up is controversial, but is influenced by factors such as the T stage of the colorectal primary, histology and factors that help to predict relapse, such as positive CRM and vascular invasion. These principles may be applied to any tumour type, and should be

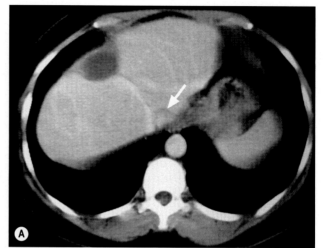

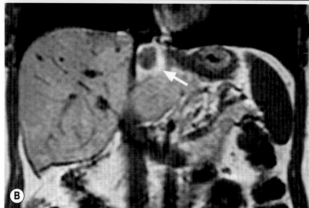

FIGURE 1-13 ■ CT and MRI of a patient following hepatic metastectomy. (A) Follow-up CT in a patient after hepatic metastectomy (low-attenuation post-surgical defect shown anteriorly). There is an intermediate attenuation abnormality in the upper liver close to the diaphragmatic surface (arrow). (B) Further investigation with mangafodipir trisodium (Mn-DPDP)-enhanced liver imaging shows perilesional enhancement on T1-weighted MRI 24 hours after administration of the contrast agent. This appearance is typical of a metastasis (arrow).

influenced by the likelihood of detection of metastatic disease.

Following treatment of primary breast cancer, there is considerable variation in practice. Some surgeons request chest radiography, liver ultrasound examination and radionuclide bone examination, whereas others request whole-body CT. In T1 and T2 primary tumours (less than 5 cm) the incidence of metastatic disease at the time of diagnosis is extremely low. In a series of almost 500 consecutive patients who were imaged at diagnosis with chest radiograph, liver ultrasound examination and radionuclide bone examination, no metastases were found in patients with T1 tumours. In patients with T4 tumours, the rate of detection of metastases was 18%. Overall, distant metastases were found at the time of primary diagnosis in 3.9% of patients.[41] However, there is limited evidence that detection of metastatic breast cancer in asymptomatic patients improves 5-year survival.[42,43] In testicular NSGCT, relapse is eminently treatable with cytotoxic chemotherapy. In colorectal cancer, surgery for

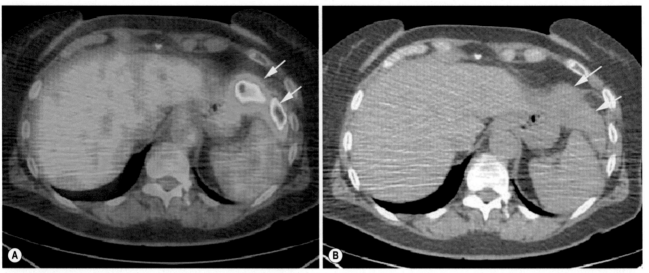

FIGURE 1-14 ■ **¹⁸F-FDG PET/CT in a patient with rising CEA a year after resection of a colonic carcinoma.** PET/CT demonstrates evidence of peritoneal disease within the left upper quadrant (arrow) lying anterior to the stomach.

metastatic disease is beneficial, but in breast cancer surveillance protocols are less useful, owing to the natural history of the disease. Such factors need to be considered for each individual tumour type before embarking on prolonged and costly investigation.

Restaging of Symptomatic Patients

Once a patient has been diagnosed with a malignancy it often becomes the most important element of their medical history. Any prolonged or persistent complaint will usually precipitate a search for recurrence. Lethargy, fatigue and weight loss are frequent symptoms, but imaging investigation is easier to direct when there are localising symptoms such as abdominal pain or distension, dyspnoea, bone pain or a neurological event. The choice of investigation should be directed appropriately; for example, patients with abdominal pain should first be investigated with an ultrasound examination of the abdomen. A knowledge of the pattern of disease spread will assist choice and interpretation of investigations. With a history of colorectal cancer, hepatic pain from metastatic disease is likely, whereas ovarian tumours are more likely to disseminate through the peritoneal cavity, causing poorly localised abdominal pain and ascites.

Acute bone pain can be investigated with plain radiography, but more frequently radionuclide bone examinations are used. Most tumours can metastasise to bone, but breast, prostate, lung, kidney and thyroid do so particularly frequently. However, some metastases are not detectable by radionuclide bone examination, because of their failure to excite sufficient osteoblastic response. For example, in breast cancer 7% of patients with a normal skeletal scintigram have metastatic bone disease on MRI (Fig. 1-15).[44]

A neurological presentation, such as a convulsion in a patient with a previous diagnosis of cancer, is best investigated with CT or MRI of the brain. The cause of dyspnoea may be diagnosed using chest radiography. There is a trend towards whole-body imaging to search

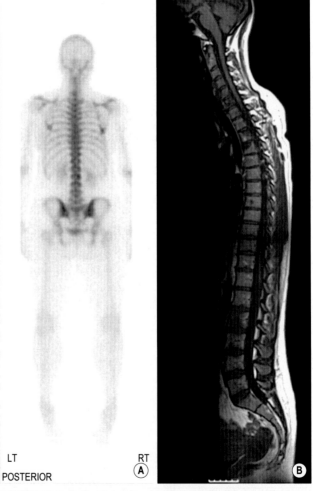

LT   RT
                     (A)
POSTERIOR

FIGURE 1-15 ■ **Patient previously diagnosed with breast cancer presenting with back pain.** (A) Skeletal scintigram. There are no focal areas of abnormal uptake in the skeleton. (B) T1-weighted sagittal MRI study of spine demonstrating multiple areas of low signal in the vertebral bodies consistent with bony metastases. Mechanical cord compression is threatened in the upper thoracic area. MRI was performed a week after scintigraphy.

for metastases, and CT of the thorax, abdomen and pelvis is often requested without any real attempt to investigate the presenting symptom. Whole-body CT is a widely available test, but some authors have suggested whole-body PET or whole-body MRI using the short tau inversion recovery (STIR) sequence.[45,46] Potentially, the greatest disadvantage of whole-body imaging techniques is that they will generate false-positive findings, or diagnose recurrence for which treatment is not possible or not necessary. It should always be borne in mind when investigating symptoms in a patient with a history of cancer that the diagnosis of metastatic disease is a major blow for the patient, and the diagnosis should only be made when there is a high degree of certainty. The imaging findings should be consistent with the known patterns of metastatic spread for the relevant tumour. If the imaging features are unconvincing or atypical, it is preferable to delay a positive finding of metastatic disease rather than to overdiagnose.

CONCLUSION

Oncological imaging is a rapidly evolving subspeciality of radiology, and forms a large proportion of imaging performed within a radiology department. It demands a sound knowledge of anatomy and understanding of patterns of spread and biological behaviour of individual tumour types. In these respects it is similar to other imaging specialities, but there are also many toxic effects of treatment and associated conditions, which must be discriminated from manifestations of the underlying malignancy. An accurate clinical history and a high level of multidisciplinary cooperation greatly enhance the practice of oncological imaging.

REFERENCES

1. Siegel R, Naishadham D, Jemal A. Cancer statistics, 2012. CA Cancer J Clin 2012;62:10–29.
2. Hopper KD, Singapuri K, Finkel A. Body CT and oncologic imaging. Radiology 2000;215:27–40.
3. Gospodarowicz MK, Henson DE, Hutter RVP, et al, editors. Union Internationale Contre le Cancer (UICC): Prognostic Factors in Cancer. 2nd ed. New York: Wiley; 2001.
4. Edge SB, Byrd DR, Compton CC, et al, editors. AJCC: Cancer Staging Manual. 7th ed. New York: Springer-Verlag; 2010.
5. iRefer. The Royal College of Radiologists Referral Guidelines, version 7; ISBN:978-1-905034-55-0.
6. Dukes CE. The classification of cancer of the rectum. J Path Bact 1932;35:323.
7. Heald RJ. Total mesorectal excision is optimal surgery for rectal cancer: a Scandinavian consensus. Br J Surg 1995;82:1297–9.
8. Quirke P, Durdey P, Dixon MF, et al. Local recurrence of rectal adenocarcinoma due to inadequate surgical resection. Histopathological study of lateral tumour spread and surgical excision. Lancet 1986;2:996–9.
9. Beets-Tan RG, Beets GL, Vliegen RF, et al. Accuracy of magnetic resonance imaging in prediction of tumour-free resection margin in rectal cancer surgery. Lancet 2001;357:497–504.
10. The MERCURY study group. Diagnostic accuracy of preoperative magnetic resonance imaging in predicting curative resection of rectal cancer: prospective observational study. BMJ 2006;333:779.
11. Burton S, Brown G, Daniels IR. MRI directed multidisciplinary team preoperative treatment strategy: the way to eliminate positive circumferential margins? Br J Cancer 2006;94:351–7.
12. NCCN website. http://www.nccn.org/professionals/physician_gls /f_guidelines.asp.
13. Lardinois D, Weder W, Hany TF, et al. Staging of non-small-cell lung cancer with integrated positron-emission tomography and computed tomography. N Engl J Med 2003;348:2500–7.
14. Fischer B, Lassen U, Mortensen J, et al. Preoperative staging of lung cancer with combined PET-CT. N Engl J Med 2009;361:32–9.
15. Turner RR, Ollila DW, Krasne DL, et al. Histopathologic validation of sentinel lymph node hypothesis for breast carcinoma. Ann Surg 1997;226:271–8.
16. Rifkin MD, Zerhouni EA, Gatsonis CA, et al. Comparison of magnetic resonance imaging and ultrasonography in staging of early prostate cancer. Results of a multi-institutional cooperative trial. N Engl J Med 1990;323:621–6.
17. Tempany CM, Zhou X, Zerhouni EA, et al. Staging of prostate cancer: results of Radiology Diagnostic Oncology Group project comparison of three MR imaging techniques. Radiology 1994;192:47–54.
18. Sciarra A, Barentsz J, Bjartell A, et al. Advances in magnetic resonance imaging: how are they changing the management of prostate cancer. Eur Urol 2012;59:962–77.
19. Turkbey B, Choyke PL. Multiparametric MRI and prostate cancer diagnosis and risk stratification. Curr Opin Urol 2012;22:310–15.
20. Sonnad SS, Langlotz CP, Schwartz JS. Accuracy of MR imaging for staging prostate cancer: a meta-analysis to examine the effect of technologic change. Acad Radiol 2001;8:149–57.
21. Engelbrecht MR, Jager GJ, Laheij RJ. Local staging of prostate cancer using magnetic resonance imaging: a meta-analysis. Eur Radiol 2002;12:2294–302.
22. Tangoku A, Yamamoto Y, Furukita Y, et al. The new era of staging as a key for an appropriate treatment for esophageal cancer. Ann Thorac Cardiovasc Surg 2012;18:190–9.
23. Barber TW, Duong CP, Leong T, et al. ^{18}F-FDG PET/CT has a high impact on patient management and provides powerful prognostic stratification in the primary staging of esophageal cancer: a prospective study with mature survival data. J Nucl Med 2012;53:864–71.
24. World Health Organization. WHO Handbook for Reporting Results of Cancer Treatment. Geneva, Switzerland: World Health Organization; 1979. p. 48.
25. Miller AB, Hoogstraten B, Staquet M, et al. Reporting results of cancer treatment. Cancer 1981;47:207–14.
26. Therasse P, Arbuck SG, Eisenhauer EA, et al. New guidelines to evaluate the response to treatment in solid tumors. European Organization for Research and Treatment of Cancer, National Cancer Institute of the United States, National Cancer Institute of Canada. Natl Cancer Inst 2000;92:205–16.
27. Eisenhauer EA, Therasse P, Bogaerts J, et al. New response evaluation criteria in solid tumors: revised RECIST guideline (version 1.1). Eur J Cancer 2009;45:228–47.
28. Choi H, Charnsangavej C, Faria SC, et al. Correlation of computed tomography and positron emission tomography in patients with metastatic gastrointestinal stromal tumor treated at a single institution with imatinib mesylate: proposal of new computed tomography response criteria. J Clin Oncol 2007;25:1753–9.
29. Nathan PD, Vinayan A, Stott D, et al. CT response assessment combining reduction in both size and arterial phase density correlates with time to progression in metastatic renal cancer patients treated with targeted therapies. Cancer Biol Ther 2010;9:15–19.
30. Van der Veldt AA, Meijerink MR, van den Eertwegh AJ, et al. Choi response criteria for early prediction of clinical outcome in patients with metastatic renal cell cancer treated with sunitinib. Br J Cancer 2010;102:803–9.
31. Crabb SJ, Patsios D, Sauerbrei E, et al. Tumor cavitation: impact on objective response evaluation in trials of angiogenesis inhibitors in non-small-cell lung cancer. J Clin Oncol 2009;27:404–10.
32. Hill M, Cunningham D, MacVicar D, et al. Role of magnetic resonance imaging in predicting relapse in residual masses after treatment of lymphoma. J Clin Oncol 1993;11:2273–8.
33. Torrisi JM, Schwartz LH, Gollub MJ, et al. CT findings of chemotherapy induced toxicity: what radiologists need to know about the clinical and radiologic manifestations of chemotherapy toxicity. Radiology 2011;258:41–56.
34. Libshitz HI, Shuman LS. Radiation-induced pulmonary change: CT findings. J Comput Assist Tomogr 1984;8:15–19.

35. Qayyum A, MacVicar AD, Padhani AR, et al. Symptomatic brachial plexopathy following treatment for breast cancer: utility of MR imaging with surface-coil techniques. Radiology 2000;214:837–42.

36. MacVicar D. Staging of testicular germ cell tumours. Clin Radiol 1993;47:149–58.

37. Choti MA, Sitzmann JV, Tiburi MF, et al. Trends in long-term survival following liver resection for hepatic colorectal metastases. Ann Surg 2002;235:759–66.

38. Shankar A, Leonard P, Renaut AJ, et al. Neo-adjuvant therapy improves resectability rates for colorectal liver metastases. Ann R Coll Surg Engl 2001;83:85–8.

39. Renehan AG, Egger M, Saunders MP, et al. Impact on survival of intensive follow up after curative resection for colorectal cancer: systematic review and meta-analysis of randomised trials. BMJ 2002;324:813.

40. Chau I, Allen MJ, Cunningham D, et al. The value of routine serum carcino-embryonic antigen measurement and computed tomography in the surveillance of patients after adjuvant chemotherapy for colorectal cancer. J Clin Oncol 2004;22:1420–9.

41. Schneider C, Fehr MK, Steiner RA, et al. Frequency and distribution pattern of distant metastases in breast cancer patients at the time of primary presentation. Arch Gynecol Obstet 2003;269: 9–12.

42. Yeh KA, Fortunato L, Ridge JA, et al. Routine bone scanning in patients with T1 and T2 breast cancer: a waste of money. Ann Surg Oncol 1995;2:319–24.

43. Miller KD, Weathers T, Haney LG, et al. Occult central nervous system involvement in patients with metastatic breast cancer: prevalence, predictive factors and impact on overall survival. Ann Oncol 2003;14:1072–7.

44. Jones AL, Williams MP, Powles TJ, et al. Magnetic resonance imaging in the detection of skeletal metastases in patients with breast cancer. Br J Cancer 1990;62:296–8.

45. Rostom AY, Powe J, Kandil A, et al. Positron emission tomography in breast cancer: a clinicopathological correlation of results. Br J Radiol 1999;72:1064–8.

46. Walker R, Kessar P, Blanchard R, et al. Turbo STIR magnetic resonance imaging as a whole-body screening tool for metastases in patients with breast carcinoma: preliminary clinical experience. J Magn Reson Imaging 2000;11:343–50.

CHAPTER 2

THE BREAST

Jonathan J. James • A. Robin M. Wilson • Andrew J. Evans

CHAPTER OUTLINE

METHODS OF EXAMINATION

NORMAL ANATOMY

BREAST PATHOLOGY

ADDITIONAL IMAGING TECHNOLOGIES

BREAST CANCER SCREENING

CONCLUSION

Breast cancer is the most common malignant tumour in the UK with over 48,000 diagnoses annually—80% of cases are in women over the age of 50. It accounts for over 12,000 deaths per annum. Imaging is essential for the early detection and accurate diagnosis of breast cancer. Population screening with mammography aims to reduce mortality by detecting the disease at an earlier stage, before it has spread beyond the breast. Mammography and ultrasound are the first-line imaging investigations in women with breast symptoms. Magnetic resonance imaging (MRI) is established as an adjunctive diagnostic tool because of its high sensitivity for invasive breast cancer. Percutaneous image-guided breast biopsy is used for the pathological assessment of breast lesions. The combination of imaging, clinical examination and needle biopsy—known as 'triple assessment'—is the expected standard for breast diagnosis.

METHODS OF EXAMINATION

Mammography

Mammography remains one of the principal imaging modalities for diagnosis, although its use is rarely indicated in women under the age of 35. The main indications for mammography are:

- evaluation of breast symptoms and signs, including masses, skin thickening, deformity, nipple retraction, nipple discharge and nipple eczema;
- breast cancer screening;
- follow-up of patients with previously treated breast cancer; and
- guidance for biopsy, or localisation of lesions not visible on ultrasound.

Mammography places stringent demands on equipment and image quality. The breast is composed predominantly of fatty tissue and has a relatively narrow range of inherent densities. Consequently, special X-ray tubes are required to produce the low-energy radiation necessary to achieve high tissue contrast, enabling the demonstration of small changes in breast density. High spatial resolution is required to identify tiny structures within the breast, such as microcalcifications measuring in the order of 100 μm; and short exposure times are necessary to limit movement unsharpness. Where the breasts are thicker or are composed of denser glandular tissue, higher energy radiation is required, although radiation dose must be kept to a minimum.

X-ray tubes produce a spectrum of radiation energies, which are determined by the target and filter combination and the peak kilovoltage (kVp). A molybdenum target is used because it produces a low-energy spectrum with peaks of 17.5 and 19.6 keV, providing high contrast. A tungsten target is less desirable because it produces higher energies (Fig. 2-1). The spectrum is refined further by adding a filter to reduce the proportion of radiation above and below the desired range. Commercially available target/filter combinations include molybdenum/molybdenum, molybdenum/rhodium, rhodium/rhodium, tungsten/molybdenum and tungsten/rhodium. Molybdenum/molybdenum is the most frequently used combination.

To achieve the required spatial resolution, mammography tubes must have an extremely small focal spot, 0.3 mm for routine mammography. For magnification mammography a smaller focal spot of 0.1 mm is required. Tube current should be as high as possible in order to keep exposure times short. Movement unsharpness may occur when exposure times exceed 1 second. Grids are used routinely for all mammographic studies. These reduce scattered radiation and so increase contrast, especially in the dense or thick breast. Modern mammography machines have a facility for automatic selection of target/filter combination, kVp and tube current according to the breast density and the thickness of the compressed breast. In addition, automatic exposure control devices detect the amount of radiation striking the detector and terminate the exposure at a preset level.

Standard Projections

There are two standard mammographic projections: a mediolateral oblique (MLO) view and a craniocaudal

(CC) view (Fig. 2-2). Correct positioning is crucial to avoid missing lesions situated at the margins of the breast. The MLO view is taken with the X-ray beam directed from superomedial to inferolateral, usually at an angle of 30–60°, with compression applied obliquely across the

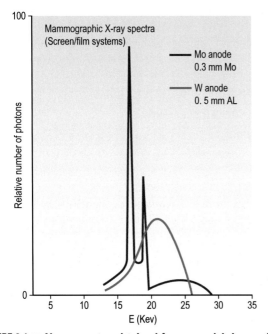

FIGURE 2-1 ■ **X-ray spectra obtained from a molybdenum (Mo) target tube set at 29 kVp and a tungsten (W) target tube set at 26 kVp.** (With permission from Haus A G, Metz C E, Chiles J T, Rossman K 1976 The effect of X-ray spectra from molybdenum and tungsten target tubes on image quality in mammography. Radiology 118: 705–709.)

chest wall, perpendicular to the long axis of the pectoralis major muscle (Fig. 2-3A). The MLO projection is the only projection in which all the breast tissue can be demonstrated on a single image. A well-positioned MLO view should demonstrate the inframammary angle, the nipple in profile, and the nipple positioned at the level of the lower border of the pectoralis major, with the muscle across the posterior border of the film at an angle of 25°–30° to the vertical (Fig. 2-2A).

For the CC view, the X-ray beam travels from superior to inferior. Positioning is achieved by pulling the breast up and forward away from the chest wall, with compression applied from above (Fig. 2-3B). A well-positioned CC view should demonstrate the nipple in profile. It should demonstrate virtually all of the medial tissue and most of the lateral tissue except the axillary tail of the breast. The pectoralis major is demonstrated at the centre of a CC film in approximately 30% of individuals and the depth of breast tissue demonstrated should be within 1 cm of the distance from the nipple to the pectoralis major on the MLO projection (Fig. 2-2B).

Additional Projections

Supplementary views may be taken to solve specific diagnostic problems.[1,2] For example, the CC view can be rotated to visualise either more of the lateral or medial aspect of the breast, compared to the standard CC projection. Localised compression or 'paddle views' can be performed. This involves the application of more vigorous compression to a localised area using a compression paddle (Fig. 2-4). These views are used to distinguish real lesions from superimposition of normal tissues and to define the margins of a mass. A true lateral view may be

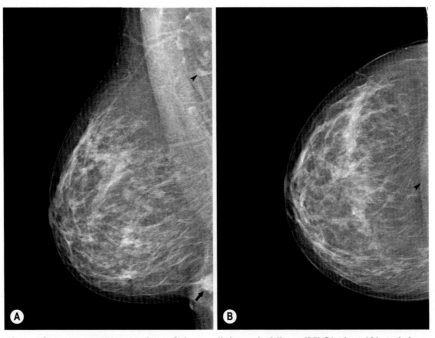

FIGURE 2-2 ■ **A standard set of mammograms consists of the mediolateral oblique (MLO) view (A) and the craniocaudal (CC) view (B).** (A) A cancer is seen in the inframammary area on the MLO view (arrow), illustrating the importance of correct positioning to avoid missing lesions. Normal lymph nodes (arrowhead) are frequently seen on the MLO projection. (B) The cancer is not demonstrated on this correctly positioned CC view, with pectoral muscle visualised at the back of the mammogram (arrowhead).

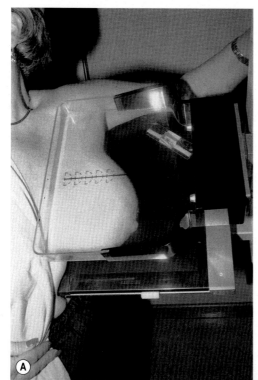

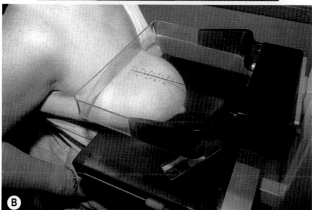

FIGURE 2-3 ■ **Breast positioning.** Positioning for the (A) mediolateral oblique and (B) craniocaudal views.

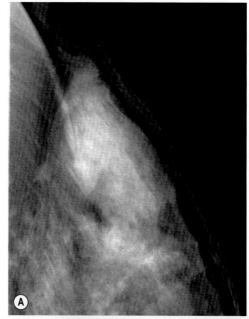

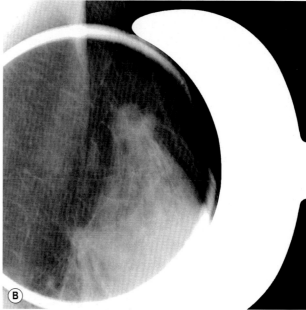

FIGURE 2-4 ■ **Additional mammographic views.** (A) An area of concern was identified in the lateral aspect of the left breast on initial mammography. (B) A 'paddle view' was performed and two suspicious spiculate mass lesions were demonstrated much more clearly. Both proved to be invasive carcinomas on subsequent biopsy.

used to provide a third imaging plane in order to distinguish superimposition of normal structures from real lesions or to increase the accuracy of wire localisations of non-palpable lesions. The true lateral view is performed with the mammography unit turned through 90° and a mediolateral or lateromedial X-ray beam.

Magnification views are most frequently performed to examine areas of microcalcifications within the breast, to characterise them and to establish their extent. Magnification views are typically performed in the craniocaudal and lateral projections. The magnified lateral view will demonstrate 'teacups' typical of benign microcalcifications, described later in the chapter. Mammographic technique may need to be modified in women with breast implants. Silicon and saline implants are radio-opaque and may obscure much of the breast tissue. Consequently, mammography is of limited diagnostic value in some

women. The Eklund technique can be employed to displace the implant posteriorly, behind the compression plate, maximising the volume of breast tissue that is compressed and imaged.[3] Mammography-induced implant rupture has not been reported to date.

Breast Compression

Compression of the breast is essential for good mammography, for the following reasons:
- It reduces geometric unsharpness by bringing the object closer to the film.

- It improves contrast by reducing scatter.
- It diminishes movement unsharpness by permitting shorter exposure times and immobilising the breast.
- It reduces radiation dose, as a lesser thickness of breast tissue needs to be penetrated and scatter is reduced.
- It achieves more uniform image density: a homogeneous breast thickness prevents overexposure of the thinner anterior breast tissues and underexposure of the thicker posterior breast tissues.
- It provides more accurate assessment of the density of masses. As cysts and normal glandular tissue are more easily compressed, the more rigid carcinomas are highlighted.
- It separates superimposed breast tissues so that lesions are better seen.

Radiation Dose

Mammography uses ionising radiation to image the breast. The risks of ionising radiation are well known and any exposure needs to be justified, with doses kept as low as possible. The radiation dose for a standard two-view examination of both breasts is approximately 4.5 mGy.[4] The average effective dose of radiation from mammography is equivalent to 61 days of average natural background radiation.[5]

Dose is more of an issue in a population screening programme, where women who may never develop breast cancer are being exposed to radiation. It has been estimated that the risk of inducing a breast cancer in women screened in the United Kingdom National Health Service Breast Screening Programme (NHSBSP) is 1 in 100,000 per mGy. A risk–benefit calculation has established that the benefits of screening far outweigh the risk of inducing a cancer, with the ratio of lives saved to lives lost calculated as approximately 100 : 1.[4]

Digital mammography systems have the potential to reduce patient dose without loss of image quality.

The Detector

Traditionally, the mammographic image has been recorded on film, but this has been superseded by digital technology. Manufacturers have developed a number of different approaches to producing a digital mammogram. The first type of digital system developed for mammography used photostimulable phosphor computed radiography (CR). This uses an imaging plate coated with a phosphor to replace the traditional screen/film mammography cassette. The imaging plate, stored in a conventional-looking cassette, is exposed in the usual fashion in a conventional (analog) mammography machine. A latent image is stored in the phosphor after exposure. The imaging plate is scanned by a laser beam in a plate reader and light is emitted in proportion to the absorbed X-rays. The emitted light is then detected by a photomultiplier system and the resulting electrical signal is digitised to produce the image.

More recently, full-field flat-panel detectors have been developed. One type of detector consists of a phosphor layer coated onto a light-sensitive thin-film transistor (TFT) array composed of amorphous silicon. Charge from the TFT array produced in response to the light emission from the phosphor is measured and digitised. The above digital systems require multiple conversion steps in the acquisition of the image: X-ray energy is converted into light energy, which is then converted into electrical energy. Multiple conversion steps are inefficient and have the potential to degrade image quality. Systems that avoid these conversion losses are described as being more 'direct'. Some manufacturers use amorphous selenium or silicon dioxide in the detector, allowing the energy of the X-ray photon to be directly converted into electrical energy.

Digital Mammography in Clinical Practice

There are clear logistical advantages to digital mammography, including the potential to improve patient throughput, as traditional screen/film mammography is labour intensive, with time taken in handling cassettes, loading/unloading film and processing. Digital mammography equipment interfaces directly with picture archiving and communication systems (PACS), leading to further increased efficiencies associated with image storage and display, with soft-copy reporting from high-resolution (5 megapixel) monitors.

It is important to establish whether an improvement in image quality can translate into an improvement in cancer detection. A powerful test of the potential of digital mammography to improve cancer detection rates is in a screening setting. Several early studies found that digital mammography was at least equivalent to screen/film mammography in terms of cancer detection rates.[6,7] The larger Oslo II study, which randomised over 25,000 women to either conventional or digital mammography, showed an increase in cancer detection in the women undergoing a digital mammogram, but this did not quite reach statistical significance ($p = 0.053$).[8]

To detect significant differences between the two techniques, the population size needs to be large, as the cancer detection rate in a screening population is around 6 per 1000 women screened. The North American Digital Mammographic Imaging Screening Trial (DMIST) enrolled 49,500 women.[9] This study found that overall the diagnostic accuracy of digital and conventional mammography was similar. However, there were some groups of women where digital mammography outperformed screen/film mammography, showing significantly improved diagnostic accuracy. These were women under the age of 50, those with dense breast parenchyma and women who were pre- or perimenopausal. Encouragingly, it is in these groups of women that conventional screen/film mammography had shown reduced sensitivity for detecting breast cancer.

Computer-Aided Detection

Computer-aided detection (CAD) is a software system that is designed to assist the film reader by placing prompts over areas of concern, to reduce observational oversights. CAD systems are highly sensitive for detecting cancers on screening mammograms. CAD will correctly prompt around 90% of all cancers, with 86–88% of all masses and 98% of microcalcifications correctly marked. Specificity is much more of a problem with a high rate of false-positive prompts. The number of false prompts will vary according to the level of sensitivity at which the system is set; typically, there are between two and four false prompts per standard set of mammogram images.[10–12]

The routine use of CAD remains controversial and there is no consensus in the literature as to whether CAD improves film reader performance; despite this, CAD is used in the interpretation of screening mammograms in around 75% of cases in the United States.[13] Some prospective studies of the use of CAD in the screening setting have shown a significant improvement in a single film reader's performance when CAD software is applied, whereas others have shown no effect on cancer detection rates.[12,14] A large multicentred retrospective review of the use of CAD in the interpretation of screening mammography in the United States found its use associated with a decrease in the specificity of screening, with an increase in recall rates for only a very minimal improvement in sensitivity, largely the result of a non-significant increase in the detection of ductal carcinoma in situ.[13]

It is difficult to extrapolate the findings of these studies to the UK breast screening programme (NHSBSP), where virtually all films are double read by two readers. Double reading is known to increase cancer detection rates by 4–14% compared to single reading, and so the question is whether one reader using CAD could produce results equivalent to double reading and whether CAD is a more cost-effective solution to recruitment problems than training non-medically qualified film readers. The Computer-Aided Detection Evaluation Trial (CADET II) was a large prospective trial of over 30,000 women that reported a comparable cancer detection rate for single reading with CAD to double reading but with a small but significant increase in recall rate.[15] A further sub-analysis has suggested that at the present time CAD is not a cost-effective alternative to double reading in the NHSBSP in view of the increase in recall rates.[16]

Digital Breast Tomosynthesis

One of the limitations of mammography is that it produces a two-dimensional (2D) radiographic view of a three-dimensional structure and, as a consequence, a cancer may not be detected due to overlapping normal glandular tissue obscuring the presence of a tumour. Lesions may be simulated by the superimposition of normal tissue, leading to unnecessary recalls following screening mammography. These factors result in a reduction in the sensitivity and specificity of mammography. Breast tomosynthesis is an emerging digital mammographic technique where thin slices through the breast are reconstructed from multiple low-dose projections acquired at different angles of the X-ray tube. The resulting thin sections can be scrolled through by the reporting radiologist, with the potential to alleviate the effects of tissue superimposition.

The role of tomosynthesis is still being defined, and there is debate surrounding its use as an adjunct or replacement for conventional 2D digital mammography. Its role in diagnosis and screening requires clarification. It has the potential to be an additional tool, for the work-up of screen-detected abnormalities replacing traditional 'paddle' views.[17] When used as a screening tool, studies show an improvement in specificity, with a reduction in recall rates of up to 11%; improvements in sensitivity over conventional 2D mammography are not so clear.[18]

Ultrasound

The main indications for ultrasound are:
- characterisation of palpable mass lesions;
- assessment of abnormalities detected on a mammogram;
- primary technique for the assessment of breast problems in younger patients; and
- guidance for biopsy and wire localisations.

Breast ultrasound requires high-quality, high-resolution grey-scale imaging, using linear probes with high frequencies typically between 7.5 and 15 MHz. Higher frequencies result in greater resolution, but as the frequency increases, the ability of the ultrasound beam to penetrate to deeper breast tissue decreases. Consequently, the frequency selected has to be appropriate for the size of the breast to be examined. Parameters such as harmonics and compounding are available on modern ultrasound machines and can be applied to enhance the displayed image. Their use is subject to operator preference. Techniques such as colour flow imaging (Doppler) and elastography may also have a role in lesion characterisation.

Elastography is an ultrasound technique that can provide additional information based on tissue stiffness or hardness. The concept that malignant lesions feel firmer or stiffer than the surrounding breast tissue is well recognised from clinical palpation. There are two methods of producing an elastography image or elastogram: strain elastography, where the operator gently manually compresses the breast tissue, and shear wave elastography, where pulses are generated by the transducer producing transverse shear wave propagation through the breast tissue. The main advantage of shear wave elastography is that the technique is quantitative and highly reproducible. Information regarding stiffness can be displayed as a black and white or colour overlay onto the grey-scale image (Fig. 2-5). Features on the elastogram that can be measured include quantitative elasticity (stiffness) in kPa and size ratios relative to conventional grey-scale imaging. In general, breast cancers tend to be stiff, with benign lesions or normal tissue appearing softer (elasticity <80 kPa). Invasive breast cancers often produce areas of stiffness that are larger than the grey-scale abnormality, likely due to changes in the tumour-associated stroma. Elastography has the potential to improve the specificity of breast ultrasound for differentiating benign from malignant masses, reducing the number of benign biopsies. In a recent study, the use of shear wave elastography resulted in a significant improvement in the specificity of breast mass assessment from 61.1 to 78.5%.[19]

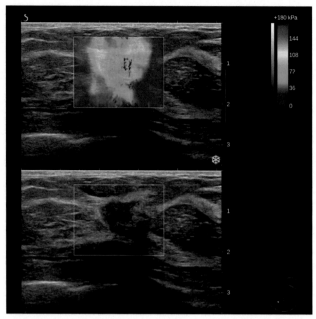

FIGURE 2-5 ■ **Elastography.** A hypoechoic mass is demonstrated in the left breast. Shear wave elastography is displayed simultaneously as a colour overlay. The colour scale is seen to the right and set to a maximum of 180 kPa. The zone of stiffness is larger, irregular and heterogeneously stiff, with elasticity values in the yellow to red end of the spectrum (108–180 kPa). All these features are suspicious of malignancy, with biopsy confirming an invasive ductal carcinoma.

Ultrasound Technique

The patient is examined in the supine position with the ipsilateral arm placed behind the patient's head. When imaging the outer portion of the breast it helps to turn the patient into a more oblique position. The aim is to flatten the breast tissue against the chest wall, reducing the thickness of breast tissue to be imaged. It is best to image the breast tissue in two planes perpendicular to each other. A transverse and a sagittal plane is a common combination, but some authors advocate examining the breast in a radial and anti-radial direction. The theory behind this method is that the ducts of the breast are positioned in a radial direction, running towards the nipple rather like the spokes of a bicycle wheel. Most breast cancers begin in the ducts and so tumours extending along the ductal system may be better visualised in this plane.[20]

NORMAL ANATOMY

The breast lies on the chest wall on the deep pectoral fascia with the superficial pectoral fascia enveloping the breast. Suspensory ligaments—called Cooper's ligaments—connect the two layers, providing a degree of support to the breast and giving the breast its shape (Fig. 2-6). Centrally, there is the nipple–areolar complex. Collecting ducts open onto the tip of the nipple. There are sebaceous glands within the nipple–areolar complex called Montgomery's glands. Small raised nodular

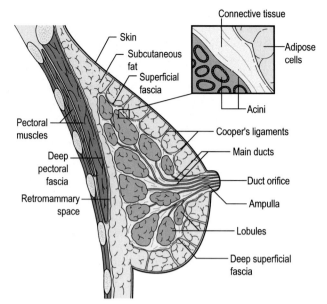

FIGURE 2-6 ■ **Gross anatomy of the breast.**

structures called Morgagni's tubercles are distributed over the areola, representing the openings of the ducts of Montgomery's glands onto the skin surface.[21] Deep to the nipple–areolar complex, the breast is divided into 15–25 lobes, each consisting of a branching duct system leading from the collecting ducts to the terminal duct lobular units (TDLUs), the site of milk production in the lactating breast.

The number of TDLUs per lobe varies according to age, lactation, parity and hormonal status. At the end of reproductive life there is an increase in the amount of adipose tissue and, although the main duct system is preserved, there is considerable loss of lobular units. These changes in breast composition are manifested by changes in the breast density on mammography.

Younger women tend to have denser glandular breast tissue. In older women, the mammographic density tends to decrease, with replacement of the glandular tissue by fatty tissue. Classification systems have been developed to describe the density of breast tissue on mammography. One of the best known is the Wolfe classification:[22]

- Wolfe N1 refers to a breast containing a high proportion of fat;
- Wolfe P1 refers to a predominantly fatty breast with <25% visible glandular tissue;
- Wolfe P2 refers to a breast with >25% visible glandular tissue; and
- Wolfe DY refers to extremely dense breast tissue.

Similarly, the American College of Radiology (ACR) breast imaging reporting and data system (BIRADS) lexicon defines four patterns of increasing density, where 1 is almost entirely fatty and 4 is extremely dense.[23]

Mammographic density is a risk factor for the development of breast cancer, with a dense background pattern associated with a higher than average risk of developing breast cancer and more aggressive tumour characteristics.[24] The mechanism through which increased density contributes to breast cancer risk remains unclear. In addition, dense breast tissue may hide abnormalities in the breast, making cancer detection more difficult. The sensitivity of mammography for detecting breast cancer is directly related to the density of the breast tissue. In general, mammography is more sensitive at detecting breast cancer in older, postmenopausal women because the breast tends to be composed of greater amounts of fatty tissue.

BREAST PATHOLOGY

Benign Mass Lesions

Cysts

Cysts are the most common cause of a discrete breast mass, although they are often multiple and bilateral. They are common between the ages of 20 and 50 years, with a peak incidence between 40 and 50 years. Simple cysts are not associated with an increased risk of malignancy and have no malignant potential.

On mammography they are seen as well-defined, round or oval masses (Fig. 2-7A). Sometimes a characteristic halo is visible on mammography. Ultrasound also demonstrates well-defined margins, with an oval or round shape. There is an absence of internal echoes indicating the presence of fluid. The area of breast tissue behind a cyst appears bright on ultrasound (posterior enhancement) due to improved transmission of the ultrasound beam through the cyst fluid (Fig. 2-7B). When these features are present, a cyst can be diagnosed with certainty. Aspiration is easily performed under ultrasound guidance to alleviate symptoms or when there is diagnostic uncertainty. Cytology on cyst fluid is not routinely performed unless there are atypical imaging features or the aspirate is bloodstained.

Fibroadenomas and Related Conditions

Fibroadenomas are the most common cause of a benign solid mass in the breast. They present clinically as smooth, well-demarcated, mobile lumps. They are most frequently encountered in younger women with a peak incidence in the third decade. With the advent of screening, many previously asymptomatic lesions are detected.

On mammography, fibroadenomas are seen as well-defined, rounded or oval masses (Fig. 2-8A). Coarse calcifications may develop within fibroadenomas, particularly in older women (Fig. 2-9).

Ultrasound features have been described that are characteristic of benign masses.[20] These include hyperechogenicity compared with fat, an oval or well-circumscribed lobulated or gently curving shape and the presence of a thin echogenic pseudocapsule. If these features are present with no features suggestive of malignancy, then a mass can be confidently classified as benign.

These features are demonstrated by fibroadenomas (Fig. 2-8B). Most fibroadenomas are isoechoic or mildly hypoechoic relative to fat, with an oval shape and

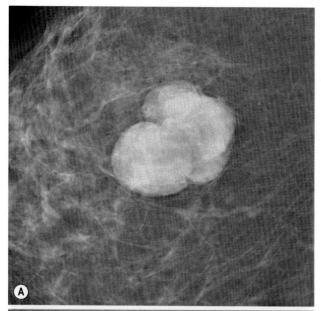

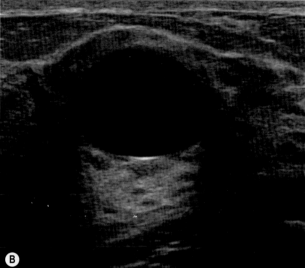

FIGURE 2-7 ■ Cyst. (A) A well-defined rounded mass, with an associated lucent halo typical of a cyst. (B) The absence of internal echoes and the posterior enhancement of the ultrasound beam are diagnostic of a cyst.

lobulated contour. A thin echogenic pseudocapsule may be seen. Percutaneous biopsy may be avoided in women under the age of 25, where the risks of any mass being malignant are very small;[20] however, in most cases, even though the mass appears benign, percutaneous biopsy is undertaken to confirm the diagnosis.

Fibroadenomas must be distinguished from well-circumscribed carcinomas; this is done by percutaneous biopsy. Phyllodes tumour can also have a similar appearance to fibroadenoma, leading to diagnostic difficulties (Fig. 2-10). The pathological characteristics can also be similar to those of large fibroadenomas. Most phyllodes tumours are benign, but some (less than 25%) are locally aggressive and may even metastasise.[21] When a diagnosis of phyllodes tumour is made, surgical excision must be

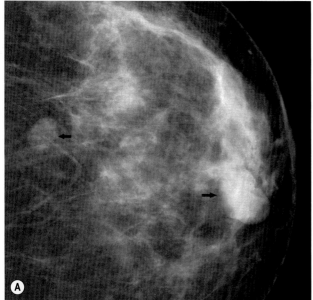

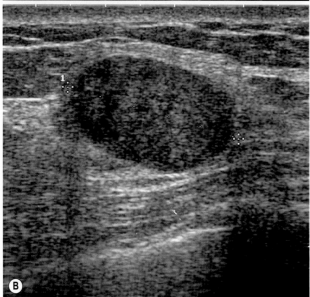

FIGURE 2-8 ■ **Fibroadenoma.** (A) Two well-defined masses on mammography (arrows). (B) Ultrasound of the lesion nearer the nipple showed a well-defined oval mass. Both lesions were confirmed as fibroadenomas on ultrasound-guided core biopsy.

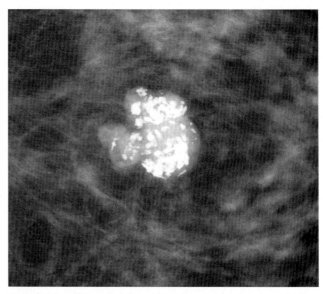

FIGURE 2-9 ■ **Fibroadenomas.** Fibroadenomas may develop coarse 'popcorn'-type calcifications.

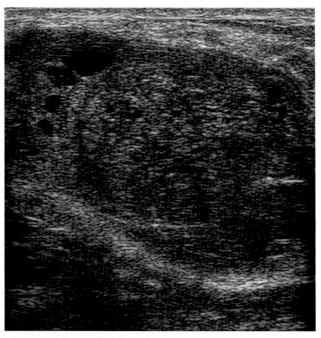

FIGURE 2-10 ■ **Phyllodes tumour.** The presence of several cystic spaces within this large, well-defined mass suggested the possibility of a phyllodes tumour. This was confirmed on core biopsy and surgical excision.

complete with clear margins to prevent the possibility of recurrence. Many larger fibroadenomas (over 3 cm) and those that show a rapid increase in size are excised in order to avoid missing a phyllodes tumour.

Papilloma

Papillomas are benign neoplasms, arising in a duct, either centrally or peripherally within the breast. Many papillomas secrete watery material, leading to a nipple discharge. As they are often friable and bleed easily, the discharge may be bloodstained.

On mammography, they may be seen as a well-defined mass, commonly in a retroareolar location (Fig. 2-11A).

Sometimes the mass is associated with microcalcifications. On ultrasound, they typically appear as a filling defect within a dilated duct or cyst (Fig. 2-11B). On aspiration, any cyst fluid may be bloodstained. As it is impossible to differentiate papillomas from papillary carcinomas on imaging criteria, percutaneous biopsy is required.

Papillomas are associated with an increased risk of malignancy, particularly if they are multiple or occur in a more peripheral location within the breast.

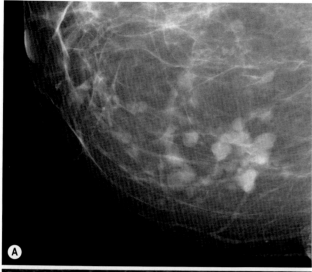

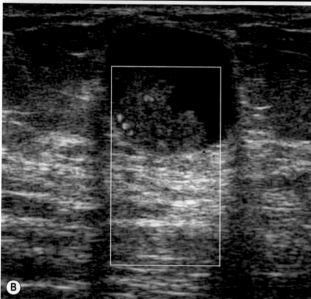

FIGURE 2-11 ■ **Multiple small papillomas.** (A) Papillomas are frequently well defined on mammography, although part of the mass may have an irregular or ill-defined contour. (B) On ultrasound, the presence of a filling defect within a cystic structure suggests the diagnosis. Colour Doppler can be useful for distinguishing debris within a cyst from a soft-tissue mass.

Consequently, excision of papillary lesions is desirable and may be therapeutic in cases of nipple discharge. In situations where percutaneous biopsy shows no evidence of cellular atypia, an alternative to surgical excision is piecemeal percutaneous excision using a vacuum-assisted biopsy device.

Lipoma

Lipomas are benign tumours composed of fat. They present clinically as soft, lobulated masses. Large lipomas may be visible on mammography as a radiolucent mass (Fig. 2-12A). On ultrasound their characteristic appearance is that of a well-defined lesion, hyperechoic compared with the adjacent fat (Fig. 2-12B).

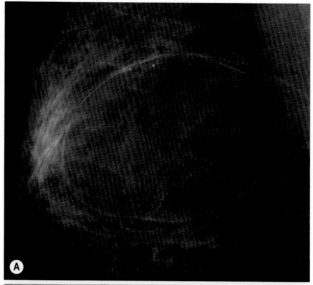

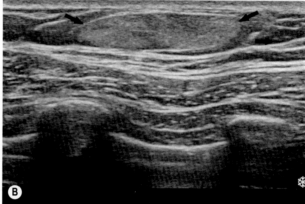

FIGURE 2-12 ■ **Lipoma.** (A) On mammography, a lipoma may be seen as a well-defined mass of fat density, contained within a thin capsule (arrowheads). (B) On ultrasound, a well-defined hyperechoic lesion characteristic of a lipoma is seen (arrows).

Hamartoma

Hamartomas are benign breast masses composed of lobular structures, stroma and adipose tissue—the components that make up normal breast tissue. They occur at any age. On imaging they may be indistinguishable from other benign masses, such as fibroadenomas. Sometimes large hamartomas are detected on screening mammograms and are impalpable (Fig. 2-13). On mammography they classically appear as large, well-circumscribed masses containing a mixture of dense and lucent areas, reflecting the different tissue components present. Diagnostic difficulty may be encountered because percutaneous biopsy specimens may be reported as normal breast tissue.

Invasive Carcinoma

Breast carcinomas originate in the epithelial cells that line the terminal duct lobular unit (TDLU). When malignant cells have extended across the basement membrane of the TDLU into the surrounding normal breast tissue, the carcinoma is invasive. Malignant cells contained by the basement membrane are termed non-invasive or in situ.

Classification of Invasive Breast Cancer

There is much confusion regarding the classification of breast cancer. Some tumours show distinct patterns of growth, allowing certain subtypes of breast cancer to be identified. Those with specific features are called invasive carcinoma of special type, while the remainder are considered to be of no special type (NST or ductal NST). Special-type tumours include lobular, medullary, tubular, tubular mixed, mucinous, cribriform and papillary. Different types of tumour have different clinical patterns of behaviour and prognosis. It should be understood that when a tumour is classified as of a special type this does not imply a specific cell of origin, but rather a recognisable morphological pattern.[21,25]

Histological grade has implications for tumour behaviour, imaging appearances and prognosis. The morphological features on which histological grade is based are tubule formation, nuclear pleomorphism and frequency of mitoses.[25] Low-grade tumours that are well differentiated are less likely to metastasise.

Imaging Appearance of Invasive Breast Cancer

Mammography. Carcinomas typically appear as ill-defined or spiculate masses on mammography (Figs. 2-14A, B). Lower-grade cancers tend to be seen as spiculate masses, due to the presence of an associated

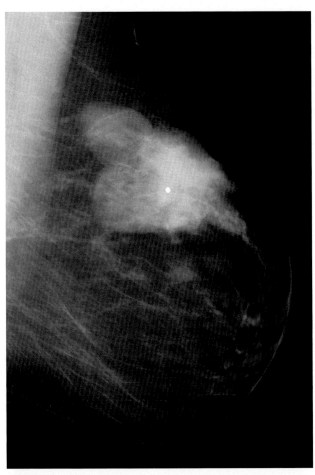

FIGURE 2-13 ■ **Hamartoma.** Hamartomas are frequently encountered on screening mammograms as large, lobulated masses with areas of varying density reflecting the presence of elements which are of fat and soft-tissue density.

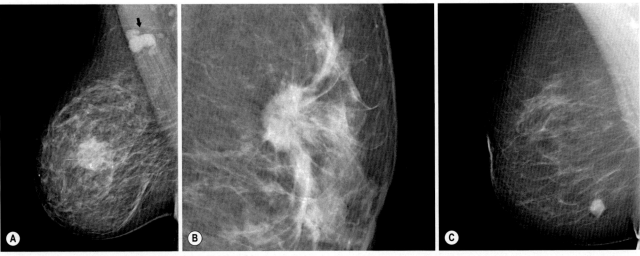

FIGURE 2-14 ■ **Mammographic appearances of invasive carcinoma.** Ill-defined and spiculate masses are typical of malignancy. (A) There is an ill-defined mass lying centrally in the right breast, containing some microcalcifications. Calcifications, representing DCIS, may be found in association with invasive carcinoma. There are also several enlarged lymph nodes in the axilla (arrow) which were proven to contain tumour on ultrasound-guided biopsy. (B) A spiculate mass that proved to be a ductal NST tumour of intermediate histological grade on ultrasound-guided biopsy. (C) Sometimes high grade tumours that exhibit rapid growth may appear well defined.

desmoplastic reaction in the adjacent stroma. Higher-grade tumours are usually seen as an ill-defined mass, but sometimes a rapidly growing tumour may appear relatively well defined, with similar appearances to a benign lesion such as a fibroadenoma (Fig. 2-14C).

Many breast cancers arise from areas of ductal carcinoma in situ (DCIS) and are associated with microcalcifications on mammography (Fig. 2-14A). This is particularly true for high-grade invasive ductal carcinomas that are often associated with high-grade DCIS.[26]

Special-type tumours can have particular mammographic characteristics:

- Lobular carcinomas can be difficult to perceive on a mammogram due to their tendency to diffusely infiltrate fatty tissue. Compared with ductal NST tumours, lobular cancers are more likely to be seen on only one mammographic view, are less likely to be associated with microcalcifications and are more often seen as an ill-defined mass or an area of asymmetrically dense breast tissue.[27]
- Tubular and cribriform cancers often present as architectural distortions or small spiculate masses.[28]
- Papillary, mucinous and medullary neoplasms may appear as new or enlarging multilobulated masses and may be well defined, simulating an apparently benign lesion.[29,30]

Sometimes the only clue to the presence of an invasive tumour may be abnormal trabecular markings, known as an architectural distortion, or the presence of microcalcifications, which tend to be visible even when the breast parenchyma is dense. The ability to perceive small or subtle cancers on a mammogram is improved by having the two standard mammographic views available and seeking out previous studies for comparison. An increase in the size of a mass or the presence of a new mass is suspicious of malignancy, whereas a lesion that remains unchanged over many years is invariably benign. Multiple masses in both breasts would favour a benign disease such as cysts or fibroadenomas.

Ultrasound. There are characteristic malignant features on ultrasound:[20]

- Carcinomas are seen as ill-defined masses and are markedly hypoechoic compared with the surrounding fat (Fig. 2-15).

- Carcinomas tend to be taller than they are wide (the anterior to posterior dimension is greater than the transverse diameter).
- There may be an ill-defined echogenic halo around the lesion, particularly around the lateral margins, and distortion of the adjacent breast tissue may be apparent, analogous to spiculation on the mammogram.
- Posterior acoustic shadowing is frequently observed, due to a reduction in the through transmission of the ultrasound beam in dense tumour tissue.

Poorly differentiated, high-grade tumours are more likely to be well defined, without acoustic shadowing (Fig. 2-15B); hence, the importance of carrying out a biopsy of solid masses even when the ultrasound appearances are benign. Microcalcifications are sometimes observed, associated with high-grade tumours arising in areas of DCIS, although this is less frequently encountered than with mammography (Fig. 2-15C). Lobular carcinomas can be difficult to demonstrate on ultrasound. They may produce vague abnormalities, such as subtle alterations in echotexture, or the ultrasound findings may even be normal.

Doppler imaging and elastography can help differentiate benign from malignant masses. Doppler may show abnormal vessels that are irregular and centrally penetrating in a malignant mass. Conversely, benign lesions such as fibroadenomas tend to show displacement of normal vessels around the edge of a lesion. Shear wave elastography of malignant lesions tends to demonstrate areas of increased elasticity, with the area of increased tissue stiffness larger than the grey-scale abnormality (Fig. 2-5).

Ultrasound is a useful tool in the local staging of breast cancer preoperatively. It tends to be a better predictor of tumour size than mammography and may detect intraductal tumour extension. Ultrasound may also detect small satellite tumour foci not visible on mammography (Fig. 2-16).

It has long been recognised that involvement of axillary lymph nodes is one of the most important prognostic factors for women with breast cancer. Traditionally, the axilla has been staged at the time of surgery by lymph node sampling procedures, sentinel node biopsy or clearance of the axillary lymph nodes. Surgical clearance of

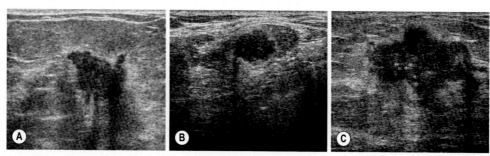

FIGURE 2-15 ■ **Ultrasound appearances of invasive carcinoma.** (A) This irregular hypoechoic mass with acoustic shadowing and an echogenic halo is typical of a carcinoma. (B) Occasionally, high-grade tumours may appear well defined, mimicking benign lesions. This shows the importance of performing a core biopsy even on apparently benign-appearing mass lesions. (C) Small echogenic foci of microcalcification associated with malignant lesions may be identified.

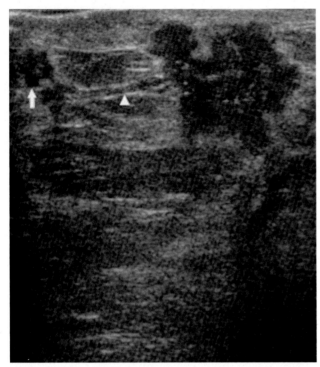

FIGURE 2-16 ■ **A small satellite tumour focus.** A small satellite tumour focus (arrow) is visible adjacent to the main tumour mass. A duct can be appreciated extending between the two lesions (arrowhead).

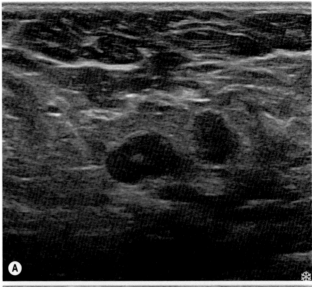

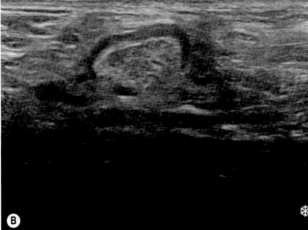

FIGURE 2-17 ■ **Axillary lymph nodes.** Axillary lymph nodes can be assessed on the basis of shape and the morphology of the cortex. (A) Nodes are likely to contain tumour if their longitudinal-to-transverse diameter ratio is less than 2 (the node appears round rather than oval). Nodes are more likely to contain tumour if the cortex is thickened to more than 2 mm. (B) This node has a normal shape, but the cortex has a thickness of 3 mm. Ultrasound-guided biopsy showed tumour containing lymph nodes in both cases.

axillary lymph nodes carries the risk of significant post-operative morbidity, with some women developing disabling lymphoedema in the arm. Ultrasound can identify abnormal nodes preoperatively that can then be biopsied percutaneously under ultrasound guidance (Fig. 2-17), allowing a preoperative diagnosis of lymph node involvement to be made in just over 40% of patients who are lymph node positive.[31] This enables the more radical axillary clearance to be targeted to those patients with a preoperative diagnosis of axillary disease, with the sampling or sentinel node procedures reserved for those patients with a much lower risk of axillary involvement.

The Differential Diagnosis of Malignancy

Many apparently suspicious findings seen on mammography or ultrasound can be caused by benign disease or even normal breast tissue. A surgical scar may result in a spiculate mass or an architectural distortion (Fig. 2-18). Radiographers should be encouraged to record the presence and position of any scars when performing a mammogram to aid image interpretation by the film reader.

Infection and inflammatory processes in the breast can be mistaken for malignancy on mammography and ultrasound. Breast abscesses are typically encountered in young lactating women. Treatment is with antibiotics and aspiration of the pus, frequently under ultrasound guidance. Inflammation in a non-lactating breast is a more worrying feature, although infections and more unusual inflammatory conditions such as granulomatous mastitis can occur. Skin erythema and oedema may be caused by

an underlying carcinoma, termed 'inflammatory carcinoma'. In this situation, skin thickening and oedema may be the only signs of malignancy recognised on the mammogram. In any case of unexplained inflammation, or when infection fails to resolve, percutaneous biopsy is required to make the diagnosis or exclude malignancy.

Radial scars, also called complex sclerosing lesions, can produce a spiculated lesion, indistinguishable from malignancy on both mammography and ultrasound (Fig. 2-19). Many of these lesions are asymptomatic and are encountered on screening mammography. Epithelial atypia, DCIS and invasive carcinoma are found in association with radial scars.

Superimposition of normal breast tissue may produce apparent masses, distortions or worrying asymmetric densities on mammography. These summation shadows

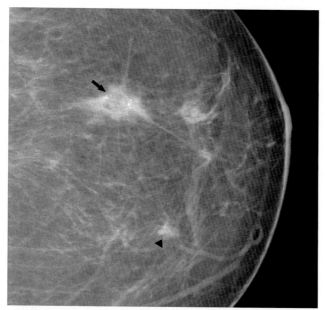

FIGURE 2-18 ■ **Postoperative scar.** A surveillance mammogram on a patient who has undergone a previous wide excision for a screen-detected cancer. The surgical scar (arrow) contains an area of lucency and coarse calcifications indicating associated fat necrosis. A small spiculate mass is demonstrated adjacent to the surgical scar (arrowhead); this was found to be recurrent tumour on ultrasound-guided biopsy.

are usually evaluated with additional mammographic views. Localised compression or paddle views are particularly helpful in deciding whether a lesion is real or just a summation shadow. Ultrasound of the area of mammographic concern can help to determine whether a lesion is truly present.

Microcalcifications

Microcalcifications are frequently encountered on routine screening mammograms. In many cases these microcalcifications turn out to be benign, but occasionally are an important feature of DCIS. Some calcifications have a characteristic benign appearance and require no further action. There is a considerable overlap between the appearance of benign and malignant microcalcifications, necessitating percutaneous biopsy in many cases.

Benign Microcalcifications

Many benign processes in the breast can cause microcalcifications, including fibrocystic change, duct ectasia, fat necrosis and fibroadenomatoid hyperplasia. Fibroadenomas and papillomas can also become calcified. Sometimes normal structures, such as the skin or small blood vessels, calcify. Calcifications can also develop in atrophic breast lobules or normal stroma.

Vascular calcifications have a characteristic 'tramline' appearance caused by calcification in both walls of the vessel (Fig. 2-20). Similarly, duct ectasia has a classical appearance that rarely causes diagnostic difficulty. In this condition, coarse rod and branching calcifications are recognised due to calcification of debris within dilated

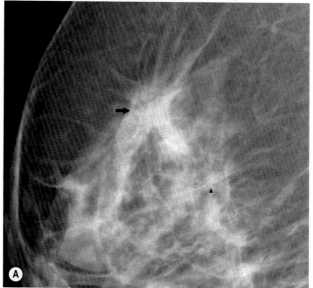
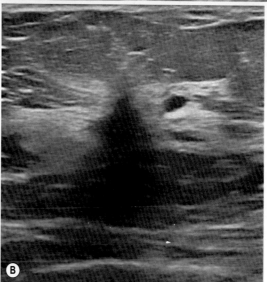

FIGURE 2-19 ■ **Radial scars.** Radial scars can mimic the appearance of malignancy on mammography and ultrasound. (A) A large spiculate mass (arrow) with an adjacent smaller lesion (arrowhead) is demonstrated on mammography. (B) Both were visible on ultrasound and were found to be radial scars on biopsy.

ducts. These calcifications have been described as having a 'broken needle' appearance and are usually bilateral (Fig. 2-21A). Sometimes the debris may extrude from the ducts into the adjacent parenchyma, leading to an inflammatory-type reaction. Fat necrosis may then occur and the calcifications take on a characteristic 'lead-pipe' appearance (Fig. 2-21B). In many cases the diagnosis is obvious, but sometimes biopsy may be required, particularly if the calcifications are unilateral or focal.

Fibrocystic change is a common cause of microcalcifications (Fig. 2-22). On a lateral magnification view, layering of calcific fluid contained within microcysts can be appreciated, producing a characteristic 'teacup' appearance. However, in many cases, percutaneous biopsy is required to exclude DCIS.

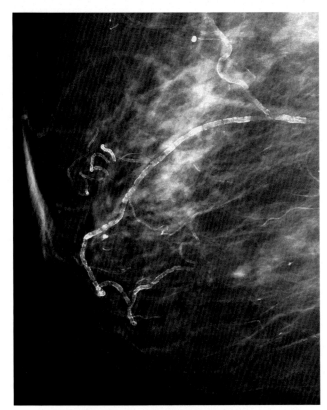

FIGURE 2-20 ■ Vascular calcifications.

Fat necrosis is a frequently encountered cause of benign calcifications, particularly when there is a history of trauma or previous surgery (Fig. 2-23). It may present as 'egg shell' calcifications within the wall of an oil cyst or as coarse dystrophic calcifications associated with areas of scarring (Fig. 2-18).

Fibroadenomas may become calcified, particularly after the menopause. Classically, the calcifications have a coarse, 'popcorn' appearance (Fig. 2-9). However, they can be small and punctate, necessitating a biopsy to establish the diagnosis. Fibroadenomatoid hyperplasia is an increasingly common cause of microcalcifications detected during screening. Histologically, there are features of a fibroadenoma and fibrocystic change. There is usually no associated mass lesion and in many cases biopsy is required to exclude DCIS (Fig. 2-24).

Skin calcifications are characteristically round, well defined, have a lucent centre and are very often bilateral and symmetrical. Talcum powder or deodorants on the skin, as well as tattoo pigments, can mimic microcalcifications.

Malignant Microcalcifications

Microcalcifications are found associated with invasive breast cancer and DCIS. Calcifications are more likely to be malignant if they are clustered rather than scattered throughout the breast, if they vary in size and shape (pleomorphic), and if they are found in a ductal or linear distribution. Malignant microcalcifications associated with high histological grade DCIS are classically rod

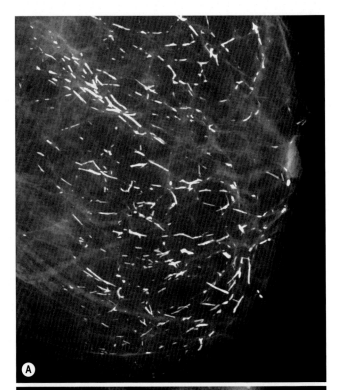

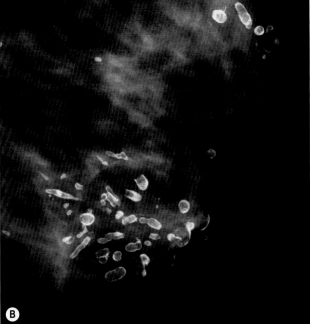

FIGURE 2-21 ■ Duct ectasia. (A) Broken needle appearance, typical of duct ectasia. (B) Sometimes thicker, more localised calcifications can be seen, giving a 'lead-pipe' appearance.

shaped and branched. These calcifications are known as casting or comedo microcalcifications and represent necrotic debris within the ducts; hence, their linear, branching structure (Fig. 2-25). Approximately one-third of malignant microcalcification clusters have an invasive focus within them at surgical excision.[32] The greater the number of flecks of microcalcification associated with an area of DCIS, the greater the risk of invasive disease.[32]

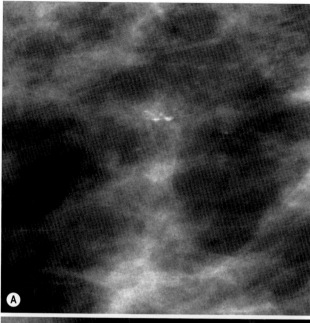

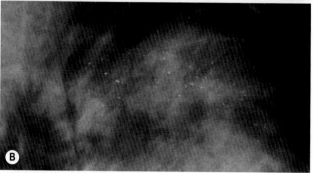

FIGURE 2-22 ■ **Fibrocystic change.** (A) 'Teacups' representing the layering out of calcific material in the dependent portion of microcysts on a lateral magnification view. (B) As calcifications associated with areas of fibrocystic change may not exhibit this characteristic appearance, stereotactic core biopsy is required.

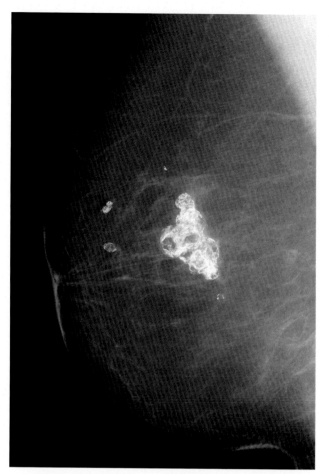

FIGURE 2-23 ■ **'Egg shell' calcifications of fat necrosis.**

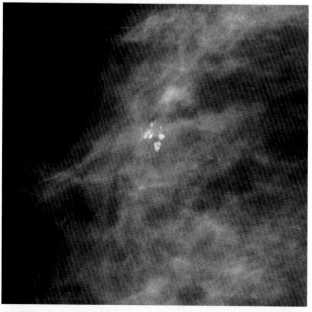

FIGURE 2-24 ■ **Small cluster of indeterminate microcalcifications.** Stereotactic biopsy revealed fibroadenomatoid change.

In the screening setting, it is often the presence of mammographically visible calcifications associated with high-grade DCIS that leads to the diagnosis of small, high-grade cancers.[33] Calcifications are much less frequently found in low-grade DCIS, as there is usually no intraductal necrosis. When they do occur, they are clustered, but otherwise have a non-specific appearance.

The sensitivity of ultrasound for detecting DCIS is significantly lower than that of mammography, which is one of the reasons why ultrasound is not a useful screening test for breast cancer. However, ultrasound may be able to identify areas of microcalcifications seen on a mammogram, aiding percutaneous biopsy.

ADDITIONAL IMAGING TECHNOLOGIES

Magnetic Resonance Imaging

Although mammography and ultrasound remain the most frequently used techniques for imaging the breast,

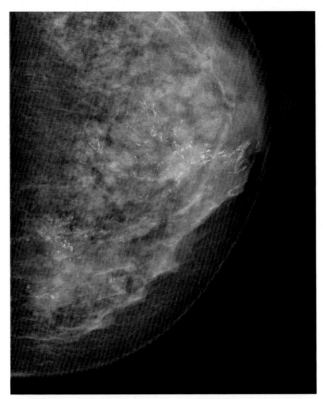

FIGURE 2-25 ■ **Ductal carcinoma in situ (DCIS).** Mammography shows the segmental distribution of pleomorphic microcalcifications. Granular, rod-shaped and branching calcifications can be identified. The appearances are typical of high-grade DCIS.

contrast-enhanced MRI is becoming increasingly important, largely because of its high sensitivity for detecting invasive breast cancer, which approaches 100% in many studies. MRI is the technique of choice for assessing the integrity of breast implants. It is more accurate than mammography, ultrasound or clinical examination in identifying implant failure.

Technique

Successful breast MR studies require at least a 1.5-tesla system and the use of a dedicated breast coil. Some breast coils have inbuilt compression devices to stabilise the breast and reduce the number of slices required to cover the whole of the breast. Patients are examined in the prone position, with the breast hanging down into the coil. The intravenous injection of gadolinium-based contrast agent is required; it is the presence of abnormal vasculature within the lesion that enables detection.

Some method of eliminating the signal from fat is needed as an enhancing lesion and fat display similar high signal on a T1-weighted image. Fat suppression may be active or passive: active fat suppression is typically achieved by the use of spectrally selective pulse sequences to suppress the signal from fat; passive fat suppression involves subtraction of the unenhanced images from the enhanced images. Subtraction allows faster imaging, with good spatial and temporal resolution, but it requires no patient movement between the two sets of images. Methods of active fat suppression, such as parallel

imaging, allow fat suppression to be achieved with shorter examination times while maintaining good spatial and temporal resolution.

Fast 3D gradient-echo pulse sequences provide the optimum method for imaging small lesions. Temporal resolution is important because the optimum contrast between malignancy and normal breast tissue is achieved in the first 2 min following the injection of gadolinium. Later, normal breast tissue may start to show non-specific enhancement, masking the presence of disease. Other signs of malignancy, such as a rapid uptake of contrast agent followed by a 'washout' phase, may only be apparent if images are acquired dynamically every minute over a period of 6–7 min after the gadolinium injection.

A higher temporal resolution allows rapid dynamic imaging but at the expense of spatial resolution or the volume of the breast imaged. Good spatial resolution can only be achieved at the expense of an increased examination time. With modern equipment it should be possible to achieve a slice thickness of <3 mm while maintaining a temporal resolution of 60–90 s, covering the whole of both breasts.

At 3 tesla there is an increase in the signal-to-noise ratio, leading to potential improvements in image quality. There are issues with field inhomogeneity at 3 tesla that can lead to problems, particularly with fat suppression.

Newer MRI techniques, such as diffusion-weighted imaging (DWI) and spectroscopy, are being investigated to try and improve the specificity of breast MRI. DWI is an unenhanced echoplanar sequence which measures the mobility of water molecules within the breast tissue. Cancers generally have a higher cellular density and extracellular water is less able to diffuse; thus values of apparent diffusion coefficient (ADC) are lower (typically $<1.5 \times 10^{-3}$ mm^2/s) compared to benign lesions or normal breast tissues (typically $>1.6 \times 10^{-3}$ mm^2/s). There is overlap between the ADC values of benign and malignant lesions, but the use of DWI has the potential to increase the specificity of breast MRI.[34,35]

Spectroscopy provides metabolic information about a tumour. Choline is an important substrate of phospholipid synthesis and so is a marker of membrane biosynthesis. Consequently, choline levels are elevated in rapidly proliferating breast cancer cells. The presence or absence of a choline peak on the MR spectra has been used as a way of differentiating malignant from benign lesions, although sometimes choline can be detected in benign or normal tissue. MRI spectroscopy can be performed as a single-voxel or multi-voxel technique enabling information to be gathered from a large volume of tissue. Multivoxel techniques, also referred to as spectroscopic or chemical shift imaging, have the ability to provide quantitative information of choline concentration.[36] MR spectroscopy is dependent on the signal-to-noise ratio of the examination and so the accuracy of spectroscopy is improved when imaging at field strengths of 3 tesla and above.

Lesion Characterisation

There are two main approaches to image interpretation: the first relates to lesion morphology and the second to assessment of enhancement kinetics. The architectural features that indicate benign and malignant disease are similar to those already described for mammography and ultrasound. Benign lesions tend to be well defined with smooth margins, whereas malignant lesions are poorly defined and may show spiculation or parenchymal deformity.

Malignant lesions tend to enhance rapidly following the injection of contrast agent and may show characteristic ring enhancement. Dynamic contrast-enhanced MRI enables more detailed enhancement curves to be calculated to aid characterisation. Malignant lesions usually show a rapid uptake of contrast agent in the initial phase of the examination, followed by a washout or plateau in the intermediate and late periods after injection, whereas benign lesions exhibit a steady increase in signal intensity throughout the time course of the examination.[37] There is some overlap in the enhancement characteristics of benign and malignant lesions. One of the strengths of breast MR imaging is that invasive cancer can be effectively excluded with a high degree of certainty if no enhancement is seen.

Investigators use a combination of architectural features and enhancement kinetics to differentiate benign from malignant lesions. The use of the breast imaging reporting and data system (BIRADS) lexicon aids reporting.[23] Using this system, lesions can be characterised into one of three morphological groups: (1) a focus (a lesion <5 mm, rarely worthy of further investigation); (2) a mass (>5 mm); and (3) non-mass enhancement (an area of enhancement without a morphological correlate). Further descriptors can then be used to describe the shape, margin and enhancement characteristics of mass lesions and the distribution and internal enhancement characteristics of non-mass lesions. Enhancement kinetics are helpful in the assessment of mass lesions, but are not useful in the assessment of non-mass enhancement where DCIS and lobular carcinoma are part of the differential diagnosis.

Normal breast tissue may enhance and this enhancement is in part dependent on the phase of the menstrual cycle. The optimum time for performing a breast MRI is during the second week of the menstrual cycle (between days 7 and 13) when background glandular enhancement should be least intense.[38] Timing the MRI examination with the second week of the menstrual cycle may not be possible for patients undergoing cancer staging, but should be undertaken for screening and follow-up studies.

Recent surgery or radiotherapy can interfere with image interpretation. Enhancement patterns return to normal between 3 and 6 months after radiotherapy.[39] Percutaneous breast biopsy (FNAC, core, or vacuum-assisted biopsy) rarely interferes with MRI interpretation.

Indications for Breast MRI

Contrast-enhanced breast MRI is used for local staging of primary breast cancer. MRI is the most accurate technique for sizing invasive breast carcinomas and will sometimes show unsuspected multifocal disease in the same breast or even additional tumour foci in the contralateral breast. MRI can be expected to show additional tumour foci in the affected breast away from the primary tumour site in around 16% of cases[40] and additional disease in the contralateral breast in around 4% of cases.[41] This may lead to a change in the therapeutic approach, potentially avoiding inappropriate breast-conserving surgery or unnecessary mastectomies. The routine use of MRI for the preoperative staging of primary breast cancer remains controversial and so careful patient selection is important. MRI is usually reserved for patients where estimating tumour size is proving difficult by conventional methods, including mammographically occult lesions, patients with mammographically dense breasts, and where there is significant discrepancy between size estimations at mammography, ultrasound and clinical examination.

Another group of patients who benefit from preoperative staging with MRI are those whose carcinomas have lobular features. Lobular carcinomas are more likely to be multifocal compared with ductal NST tumours. They are more difficult to detect and their size is more difficult to measure by conventional methods because of their infiltrating growth pattern. In approximately 50% of such patients MRI will show more extensive tumour (Fig. 2-26).[42]

Another important role of MRI is identifying an occult primary tumour in women presenting with malignant axillary lymphadenopathy with a normal mammogram and breast ultrasound. In this situation, MRI is highly sensitive for identifying an occult primary. MRI is also useful in the postsurgical breast, differentiating surgical scarring from tumour recurrence.

MRI can help to assess the response to treatment in women receiving neoadjuvant chemotherapy for locally advanced primary breast cancers. It can recognise responders to treatment earlier than other imaging methods by demonstrating a reduction in lesion size, or a change in the enhancement pattern, with the level of enhancement reducing or taking on a more benign appearance. Neoadjuvant chemotherapy can also be used to downstage large breast cancers to enable breast-conserving surgery to become a treatment option. MRI can be used to plan the extent of surgical resection in positive responders, with successful breast conservation possible in around 59% of women where mastectomy would have been necessary.[43]

MRI has become an important tool for screening younger women with a high familial risk of breast cancer. Some of these women (e.g. known gene mutation carriers) have a lifetime risk of developing breast cancer of around 85%. In these younger women the sensitivity of mammography for detecting malignancy is low, largely due to the presence of mammographically dense breast parenchyma. Screening with MRI is superior to mammography in detecting invasive breast cancer in such women, although mammography remains more sensitive for detecting DCIS.[44,45]

Managing MRI-Detected Lesions

Lesions detected at MRI require proper work-up, including histological diagnosis where appropriate. Findings should be correlated with mammography, but probably most useful is a targeted, second-look ultrasound of the

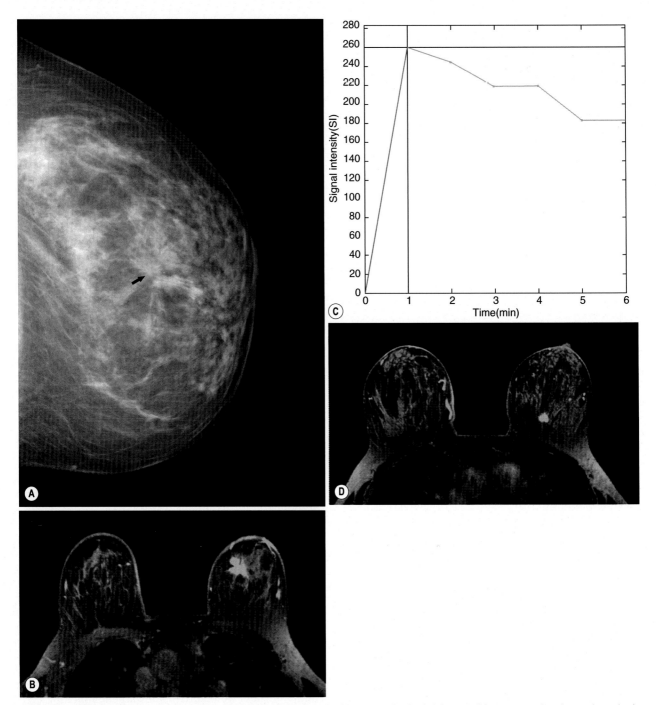

FIGURE 2-26 ■ **MRI for local tumour staging.** This patient presented with a mass in the left breast. Mammography showed a spiculate lesion (arrow) lying centrally within the breast, best appreciated on the CC view (A). Biopsy indicated a carcinoma with lobular features. MRI confirmed the presence of a malignant spiculate lesion (B) with a typically malignant enhancement curve (rapid uptake of contrast agent followed by a washout phase) (C). An additional tumour focus was identified away from the primary tumour site (D). This was confirmed at biopsy.

area. In many cases, ultrasound will identify any additional lesions and facilitate image-guided biopsy. Lack of an ultrasound correlate makes the chances of malignancy much less likely. In one study, carcinoma was found in 43% of MRI lesions that had an ultrasound correlate compared with 14% of MRI lesions that lacked an ultrasound correlate.[46] An ultrasound correlate is more likely for invasive carcinoma compared with DCIS.[46] However, where MRI lesions are suspicious or indeterminate, the absence of a corresponding ultrasound abnormality does not negate the need to pursue a histological diagnosis and MRI-guided biopsy should be considered. For lesions that are considered low risk, follow-up MRI after a suitable period of time, typically one year, is acceptable.

When MRI is used for staging breast cancer, problems arise when additional enhancing lesions are detected away from the primary tumour site. The same principles of mammographic review and second-look ultrasound apply. Surgical management should not be changed unless additional enhancing lesions are histologically proven to represent malignancy.

Controversies Surrounding the Use of Breast MRI

It would seem reasonable to assume that the identification of additional tumour foci in the breast at the time of diagnosis should improve surgical planning and long-time patient outcomes with a decrease in both tumour recurrence rates and the incidence of contralateral disease in the years following treatment. No robust evidence is yet available to support these assumptions. If the use of MRI for surgical planning is effective, a reduction in surgical re-excision rates would be expected in women who underwent preoperative MRI. A randomised controlled trial (COMICE, Comparative Effectiveness of MRI in Breast Cancer) found no significant difference in the re-excision rates between the group who underwent preoperative breast MRI and those that did not, with re-excision rates of 18.8 and 19.3%, respectively.[47] There is also very little evidence that MRI improves long-term outcomes for patients. In one study, local recurrence rates and the incidence of contralateral disease were assessed over an 8-year period in women who had undergone breast-conserving surgery: no significant difference was observed in women who underwent preoperative MRI compared with those who did not.[48] There is evidence that MRI does lead to changes in surgical treatment, typically from breast-conserving surgery to mastectomy. A recent meta-analysis has shown more extensive surgery than initially planned in 11.3% of women who underwent preoperative MRI.[40]

There are two factors to consider when explaining why routine preoperative staging MRI has not been shown to affect outcomes in breast cancer patients. The first relates to the specificity of MRI and the second to a form of overdiagnosis. Although MRI is very sensitive for detecting malignancy, reported specificities are lower, varying between 81 and 97%. Consequently, it is very important that any additional lesions identified at MRI are proven to be malignant before management changes are made, avoiding potential unnecessary mastectomies. Obtaining a tissue diagnosis can increase the number of percutaneous biopsies performed and the diagnostic uncertainty may precipitate some women choosing more radical surgery. The second, more important, factor is the clinical significance of any additional disease identified. There is no doubt that breast MRI does find additional disease, but some of this disease may not be clinically relevant in patients undergoing breast-conserving surgery followed by radiotherapy, chemotherapy and hormone treatments. It is well established that these adjuvant treatments are effective at reducing local recurrence rates by controlling foci of residual disease not excised at the time of breast-conserving surgery.

MRI for Imaging Breast Implants

MRI is the technique of choice for assessing the integrity of breast implants, with a sensitivity and specificity of over 90%. When imaging breast implants, no contrast agent is required unless malignancy is suspected. Imaging should be performed in the prone position using a dedicated breast coil. The main goal is to determine whether the implant has ruptured and, if so, to establish the location of the leaked filler (usually silicon).

When implants fail, the rupture may be either intracapsular or extracapsular: intracapsular rupture occurs when silicon has escaped from the plastic shell of the implant, but is contained within the fibrous implant capsule (Fig. 2-27); signs of intracapsular rupture include the 'wavy line', 'linguini', 'key-hole' and 'salad oil' signs.[49] False-positive interpretations can be made when normal implant folds are mistaken for signs of rupture.

Extracapsular rupture is diagnosed when silicon is demonstrated outside the fibrous capsule. In this situation, ultrasound can be diagnostic, demonstrating free silicon, silicon granulomas or silicon-containing axillary lymph nodes (Fig. 2-28).

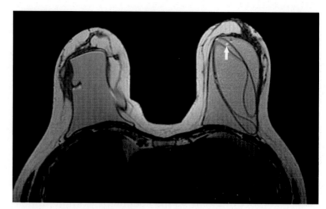

FIGURE 2-27 ■ **Intracapsular implant rupture.** On these T2-weighted fast spin-echo images, the plastic shell of the left breast implant can be seen floating within the silicon, producing a 'wavy line' or 'linguini' sign. Note the presence of a bright dot of water-like material (arrow), the 'salad oil' sign.

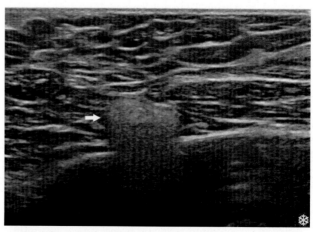

FIGURE 2-28 ■ **Extracapsular implant rupture.** A small silicon granuloma is visible, lying adjacent to a breast implant (arrow). The silicon granuloma has a characteristic 'snow storm' appearance.

Nuclear Medicine Techniques

Sestamibi imaging using ^{99m}Tc-MIBI and PET imaging techniques using ^{18}F-FDG have been developed following the observation that many breast cancers show uptake of these isotopes. Breast-specific gamma imaging (sometimes referred to as scintimammography) and FDG positron emission mammography (PEM) have significantly improved in recent years with the development of high-resolution mini-camera detectors designed specifically for imaging the breast. Indications for use overlap with those for MRI, including local staging, searching for a mammographically occult primary, particularly where there is dense mammographic background pattern, and detecting recurrence in the postsurgical breast. Research is continuing, but so far these techniques have failed to establish a place in routine practice.

BREAST CANCER SCREENING

Introduction

Breast cancer mortality in the UK is amongst the highest in the world. The causes of breast cancer are not well understood and, in the absence of any effective preventative measures, much effort and health care resources have been focused on the quest to reduce breast cancer mortality by early detection through screening. A number of randomised controlled trials (RCTs) and case control studies carried out since the mid-1960s have shown that screening by mammography can reduce breast cancer mortality.

The UK National Health Service Breast Screening Programme was set up following the publication of the Forrest Report in 1986.[50] This document, commissioned by the UK Department of Health under the chairmanship of Professor Sir Patrick Forrest, reviewed the scientific evidence for population breast cancer screening. It recommended the immediate introduction of screening by mammography in the UK.

Within a year of publication, population breast cancer screening, free at the point of delivery, was introduced into the UK National Health Service. This was the first population-based breast screening programme in the world. Currently in the UK, breast cancer screening by mammography is provided for all women over the age of 50. Women between the ages of 50 and 70 are invited every 3 years. Two-view mammography is used for all screens and the mammograms are double read. Women over 70 are not invited but are encouraged to attend by self-referral. There is an ongoing trial to assess the possible mortality benefits of extending the screening invitation from 47 to 73.

The Evidence for Screening

Data from RCTs provide the strongest evidence of the efficacy of screening in reducing breast cancer mortality. The design of RCTs enables the elimination of lead-time bias. Most of the RCTs of screening were carried out in Sweden. An overview of these trials was published in 2002 and included data from Malmo, Gothenburg, Stockholm and the Ostergotland arm of the Two Counties study.[51] Almost a quarter of a million women were included in these studies, with approximately half being invited for screening and the other half making up the control group. The median trial time was 6.5 years and the median follow-up 15.8 years. The overall results indicated a 21% reduction in breast cancer mortality. The mortality reduction was largest in women aged 60–69 (33%).

Due to continuing criticisms of RCTs of breast screening, which suggested that the overall mortality may be higher in those screened because of adverse effects of treatment, this study also looked at total cause mortality. This showed a relative risk of dying of any cause in the study arm of 0.98, which was of borderline statistical significance.[51] The precise mortality reduction attributable to screening is controversial, as RCTs may underestimate the benefit of screening due to non-attendance and contamination (mammography occurring within the control group). It has been suggested that regular attendance for mammographic screening may result in a 63% reduction in breast cancer deaths.[52]

Which Age Groups Should be Screened?

There is definite evidence from RCTs of a reduction in mortality in women aged 55–69; previous meta-analyses have supported the introduction of screening at age 50 but these data are based on 10-year age bands. Data analysis based on 5-year age bands of screening women aged 50–55 has never shown a mortality benefit in this age group. The reasons for this are unclear but it has been postulated that this may be due to the unusual behaviour of breast cancer in perimenopausal women.

There is no evidence from RCTs to support the screening of women over the age of 70. However, the number of women over the age of 70 in these studies is low. Although the mammograms of older women are easy to read and the incidence of cancer is high, there would be a significant risk of overdiagnosis and consequently overtreatment in this age group. Overdiagnosis is the detection and treatment of cancers that would not become clinically apparent or threaten life. Overdiagnosis probably occurs in about 10% of cancers detected when screening women aged 50–70, with significantly higher rates in women aged over 70 years. Pathological lesions that might be considered overdiagnosed and treated are low-grade DCIS and invasive tubular cancers. A number of studies are now addressing this issue by suggesting either less invasive treatment or a watch and wait policy for such lesions.

A recent meta-analysis of RCTs screening women aged 39–49 at random has shown a statistically significant mortality reduction of 17%.[53] The Malmo and Gothenburg studies have both shown statistically significant mortality reductions in this age group.[54,55] As breast cancer is only half as common in women in their 40s compared with women in their fifties, some authors have suggested that presenting data in terms of percentage reduction in population mortality may be misleading. On the other hand, preventing breast cancer deaths in younger women will result in a larger number of life years gained and it has been shown that breast cancers arising in women in their 40s account for 34% of life years lost to breast cancer.

The RCTs of screening were not designed to look at particular age groups and such subanalysis has been criticised. In particular, a proportion of the screening episodes occurring in women aged 40–49 at randomisation actually occurred when women were over the age of 50. In addition, women in the control groups of these studies were not always screened at 50. Therefore, it is possible that part of the mortality benefit demonstrated in these women may be due to screening episodes over the age of 50.

There are other issues to consider when screening women in their 40s. The lower cancer incidence results in the specificity of both recall and biopsy being lower than that in older women. The sensitivity of mammography for detecting malignancy is also lower for women in their 40s, although the introduction of digital mammography should substantially improve screening performance in this age group.[9]

The interval at which a screening mammogram needs to be repeated is determined by lead-time, which is age related. The lead-time of screening is that time between mammographic detection of breast cancer and clinical presentation. The lead-time of screening in women under the age of 50 in the Gothenburg screening trial was 2.2 years.[55] This suggests the ideal screening interval for women under the age of 50 is either every 18 or 12 months. The high frequency of screening required in younger women and the lower incidence of breast cancer have led to questions being raised regarding the cost-effectiveness of screening in this age group. These disadvantages may be partly negated by the large number of life years gained per life saved. On the other hand, the lead-time of screening for older women aged over 50 is 3–4 years, so the 3-year screening interval in the UK would seem appropriate. However, reducing the screening interval to 2 years for the over-fifites may be beneficial as a high rate of interval cancers are seen in the UK in the third year after screening.[56]

The Screening Process and Assessment

Screening mammograms are carried out by female radiographers, either at static sites or using mobile vans. In the UK, interpretation of screening mammograms is limited to practitioners who read a high volume of images (greater than 5000 examinations per year). Evidence suggests that high-volume readers have a significantly increased sensitivity for detection of breast cancer compared to medium- and low-volume readers.[57] In the UK, there has been a national shortage of breast screening radiologists. This has led to the introduction of radiographer film readers. Radiographers have been shown to have identical sensitivity and specificity when compared with screening radiologists once they have been trained.

Double reading is standard practice in the UK screening programme, with consensus or arbitration adopted to

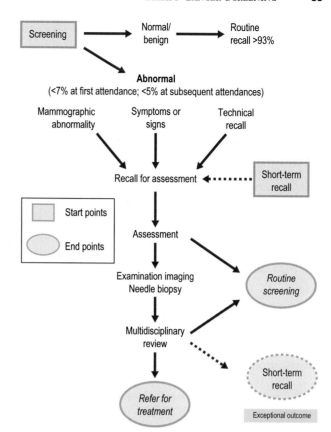

FIGURE 2-29 ■ **The screening assessment process.**

deal with discordant double-reading opinions. For consensus double reading, disparate opinions are discussed by the two film readers and a consensus achieved. Arbitration involves a third reader independently reviewing the mammograms and deciding whether recall is necessary. Data from the UK screening programme have shown that double reading with arbitration results in the best small invasive cancer detection rate with acceptable recall rates.[58]

Approximately 5% of women are called back for assessment. Figure 2-29 outlines the assessment process; typically it involves a combination of extra mammographic views, ultrasound and physical examination. Approximately one in seven of those recalled have breast cancer.

Interval Cancers

These are cancers that arise symptomatically in women who have had a normal screening mammogram before their next invitation to screening. Interval cancer analysis helps assess the effectiveness of a screening programme and enables radiologists to learn by reviewing the screening mammograms of women who later present with symptomatic cancers. Interval cancers have a prognosis similar to symptomatic cancers in the non-screening population, which is worse than that of cancers detected at screening.

Interval cancers in the NHSBSP are now divided into three subtypes:
- Type 1 interval cancers are cancers where the previous screening mammograms show no evidence of malignancy, even in retrospect.
- Type 2 interval cancers are cancers where the previous screening mammograms show uncertain features when viewed retrospectively.
- Type 3 interval cancers are cancers where there are malignant features on the previous screening mammograms.

The mammographic features most frequently missed or misinterpreted on screening mammograms are calcification and architectural distortion.[59]

How Does Mammographic Screening Reduce Breast Cancer Mortality?

Most of the benefit of mammographic screening is due to detection of small lymph node-negative invasive cancers. Finding high-grade invasive breast cancer less than 10 mm in size is particularly useful as the prognosis of such tumours is excellent, whereas grade 3 invasive breast cancers presenting symptomatically have a very poor prognosis.[60] However, some of the low-grade tubular cancers detected at screening are so indolent that a number of these lesions may never threaten life and mammographic screening in these instances may lead to overdiagnosis and overtreatment.[61]

Approximately 25% of cancers detected by mammographic screening are DCIS. High-grade DCIS is accepted by most authorities to be a precursor of high-grade invasive disease. Most DCIS diagnosed through screening is high-grade and so detection is beneficial. The merit of detecting low-grade DCIS is more controversial, with only approximately 40% of cases eventually developing low-grade invasive breast cancer.

Quality Assurance (QA)

In the UK, local performance is monitored by regional QA teams with the data collected centrally by the Department of Health. This is a statutory requirement and the teams are responsible for screening-unit performance monitoring and for individual performance appraisal. Some of the recent national performance figures are shown in Table 2-1. The standardised detection ratio is the actual number of cancers detected expressed as a ratio of the predicted number of cancers that need be detected to achieve a mortality reduction of 25%.

Interventional Breast Radiology

Breast radiology requires skills in interventional techniques, particularly ultrasound and X-ray stereotactic-guided needle sampling, percutaneous excision of benign lesions and localisation of abnormalities for surgical excision. Eighty per cent of abnormalities detected by screening mammography are impalpable and need to be biopsied and localised using image-guided techniques.

Needle biopsy is highly accurate in determining the nature of most breast lesions and is now used in place of

TABLE 2-1   UK National Health Service Breast Screening Programme Performance 2008–2010

	2008/2009	2009/2010
Number of women invited	2,702,876	2,754,885
Acceptance rate (% of invited)	73.7%	73.3%
Number of women screened (invited)	1,990,534	2,018,403
Number of women screened (self-referred)	87,661	84,467
Total number of women screened	2,078,195	2,102,870
Number of women recalled for assessment	91,395	89,164
Women recalled for assessment (%)	4.4%	4.2%
Number of benign open surgical biopsies	1746	1646
Number of cancers detected	16,535	16,476
Cancer detected per 1000 women screened	7.96	7.84
Number of in situ cancers detected	3438	3257
Number of invasive cancers less than 15 mm	6791	6939
Standardised detection ratio	**1.45**	**1.44**

Source: NHSBSP Annual Review 2011, NHSBSP Publications, Sheffield, UK.

open surgical biopsy. For patients with breast cancer, needle biopsy provides accurate information on the nature of malignant disease, such as histological type and grade, and allows assessment of tumour biology, cell markers and genetics.

The methods available for breast tissue diagnosis are:
- fine-needle aspiration for cytology (FNAC);
- needle core biopsy for histology;
- vacuum-assisted biopsy (VAB); and
- open surgical biopsy.

Fine-Needle Aspiration for Cytology and Needle Core Biopsy

FNAC involves the manual passage of a small-bore needle (usually 23 gauge) repeatedly through an abnormality to shear off clumps of cells into the needle lumen. This is usually performed while applying suction to the aspiration needle. The aspirate is then either smeared onto a microscope slide or washed into a buffer solution ready for cytological assessment. FNAC can be performed freehand on a palpable abnormality or carried out under image guidance. The procedure is quick to perform and associated with minimal morbidity. However, it is associated with significant false-positive and false-negative results, is operator dependent and relies greatly on the experience and skill of the cytopathologist.[62] It also does not provide reliable information about whether a cancer is in situ or invasive or the pathological type and grade.

Core biopsy of breast tissue is carried out using a 14G diameter needle with a 20-mm sample notch attached to an automated spring-loaded device. Smaller-gauge needles give less reliable results. The needle retrieves a core of tissue, approximately 15–20 mg in weight, which is suitable for histological assessment. This technique is less operator dependent than FNAC and breast tissue histological expertise is much more widely available. Core needle biopsy is associated with fewer false-positive and false-negative results than FNAC and is the technique of choice for routine use in breast diagnosis. FNAC is still favoured by some operators for sampling axillary lymph nodes, although most abnormal nodes lie low in the axilla, away from vascular structures, and are amenable to 14G core biopsy.[31]

The better overall performance of core biopsy compared with FNAC is illustrated in the performance of the NHS Breast Screening Programme in the UK. At the start of the programme, needle sampling by FNAC was almost universal but fewer than 10% of the 90 screening units were able to achieve the target of 90% preoperative diagnosis of breast cancer. After transferring to core biopsy, all of these units now routinely achieve greater than 90% preoperative diagnosis of breast cancer.

Vacuum-Assisted Biopsy

The predominant reasons for failure to achieve accurate diagnosis by needle biopsy are sampling error and failure to retrieve sufficient representative material. Vacuum-assisted biopsy (VAB) addresses these issues. Systems typically use 7 to 11G needles to obtain multiple cores, each weighing up to 300 mg.

VAB significantly improves the diagnostic accuracy for borderline breast lesions and lesions at sites in the breast difficult to biopsy using other techniques. The use of VAB to biopsy microcalcifications halves the risk of missing a coexisting invasive cancer in an area of DCIS compared with 14G core biopsy.[63] VAB is indicated for:

- very small mass lesions;
- architectural distortions;
- failed 'conventional' core biopsy;
- microcalcifications;
- papillary and mucocele-like lesions;
- diffuse non-specific abnormality;
- excision of benign lesions; and
- sentinel node sampling.

VAB can be used under ultrasound, stereotactic or MRI guidance. After needle placement in the breast, suction is applied pulling tissue into a sampling chamber. A rotating or cutting inner cannula automatically advances. In most systems, suction is then used to retrieve the specimen so that multiple cores can be obtained without the need to remove the needle from the breast. Contiguous core biopsies can be obtained by rotating the probe through 360°. Unlike core biopsy, the VAB probe does not have to pass directly through the area being sampled as the suction can be used to draw the abnormality into the sampling chamber, allowing a satisfactory sample to be obtained by placing the probe close to rather than through the abnormality. Ultrasound-guided hand-held vacuum-assisted devices can be used as an alternative to surgery to completely excise benign lesions, such as fibroadenomas, and to widely sample lesions that may be associated with an increased risk of malignancy, such as radial scars and papillary lesions.

Guidance Methods for Breast Needle Biopsy

Ultrasound guidance is the method of choice for biopsy of both palpable and impalpable breast lesions, as it provides real-time visualisation of the biopsy procedure and visual confirmation of adequate sampling. Between 80 and 90% of breast abnormalities that need to be biopsied are visible on ultrasound. For impalpable abnormalities not visible on ultrasound, stereotactic X-ray-guided biopsy is required. A few lesions are visible only on MRI and require MR-guided biopsy.

X-ray-guided stereotactic biopsy is used for impalpable lesions that are not visible on ultrasound. Most microcalcifications and mammographic architectural distortions need to be biopsied under X-ray guidance. There are two types of stereotactic equipment: add-on devices that attach to a conventional upright mammography machine and dedicated prone table devices (Fig. 2-30). Prone table devices are expensive and can only be used for breast biopsy; they require a room in the breast imaging department dedicated for this purpose. The main advantage of this type of device is that the patient cannot see the biopsy procedure while it is being done and vasovagal episodes are said to be less frequent.

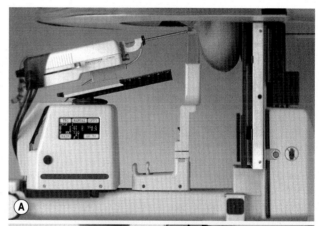

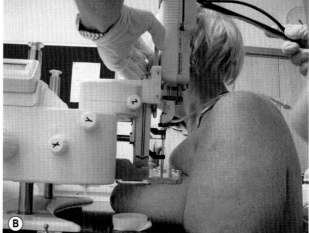

FIGURE 2-30 ■ Stereotactic breast biopsy. (A) A prone stereotactic X-ray breast biopsy table. (B) An upright add-on breast biopsy device showing vacuum-assisted biopsy being performed with vertical positioning of the biopsy needle.

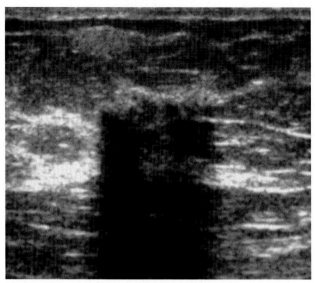

FIGURE 2-31 ■ **Ultrasound visible biopsy marker.** An ultrasound image of breast tissue containing gel pellets placed at the site of a stereotactic biopsy showing how the mass effect with distal shadowing allows the biopsy site to be easily identified on ultrasound.

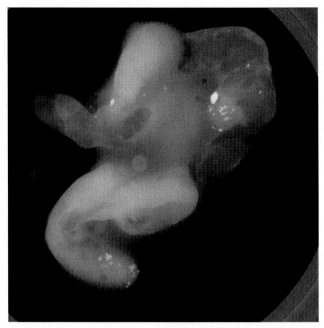

FIGURE 2-32 ■ **Core specimen radiography.** A specimen radiograph showing a good yield of microcalcifications in several vacuum-assisted biopsy samples.

Add-on devices can be attached to a mammography machine that is otherwise available for routine mammography. These are less expensive and do not require dedicated space. The two methods have equally high levels of accuracy (95% retrieval of representative material) and both are associated with low levels of morbidity and few complications. Vasovagal episodes can be minimised by giving the patient an anxiolytic agent such as sublingual Lorazepam 30 min before the procedure. Upright add-on systems can also be used with the patient lying in the lateral decubitus position.

Both the add-on and prone table stereotactic devices allow precise localisation of the lesion by acquiring two images, 15° on either side of the central axis of the X-ray gantry. The x, y and z coordinates of the lesion are calculated from the relative positions of the target lesion on the two stereotactic images compared with a fixed reference point. After injection of local anaesthetic, the biopsy needle is advanced into the breast via a small skin incision through a needle holder that guides it to the correct depth.

It is possible, particularly after VAB, that the whole of the mammographic abnormality may have been removed, so a marker should be placed at the biopsy site. A variety of metal clip and gel pellet markers are available for this purpose; combined gel and metal markers are ideal as these render the biopsy site ultrasound-visible, allowing subsequent localisation procedures to be carried out under ultrasound rather than stereotactic guidance (Fig. 2-31).

Number of Samples

Sufficient material must be obtained but it is unnecessary to take multiple cores as a matter of routine. For ultrasound-guided biopsy, a minimum of two core specimens is recommended. Stereotactic biopsy is typically used for abnormalities that are more difficult to define or sample, and so a minimum of five core specimens should be obtained. Core specimen radiography is performed when sampling microcalcifications to prove that representative material has been obtained (Fig. 2-32). The identification of microcalcifications in at least three separate cores and/or a total of five separate flecks of calcification in the biopsy specimen should allow an accurate diagnosis to be made.[64] When diagnostic uncertainty remains, larger-gauge VAB can be used to obtain greater tissue volumes (approximately 300 mg per core). The aim is to obtain at least 2 g of tissue.

MRI-Guided Biopsy

A few breast lesions are only visible with MRI and therefore have to be biopsied under MRI guidance. A number of different approaches have been developed for this procedure, but the most widely used system involves the patient lying prone within the breast coil with the breast immobilised between compression plates, one of which is in the form of a grid (Fig. 2-33A). Vacuum-assisted biopsy is the preferred method of tissue sampling under MRI guidance.

Compression is important to stabilise the breast and keep a lesion's location fixed once initially localised. It is important to avoid over-compression, as this can interfere with lesion conspicuity. A vitamin E capsule is placed over the expected lesion position and sagittal imaging performed following intravenous gadolinium injection. The position of the lesion within the breast relative to the skin can then be determined by reference to the skin marker and the gridlines; depth is calculated on the basis

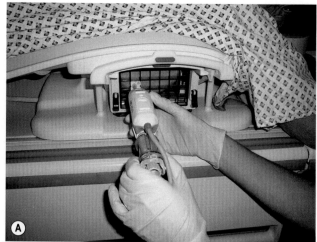

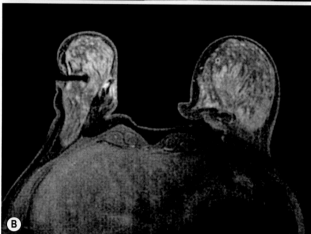

FIGURE 2-33 ■ MRI-guided breast biopsy. (A) The breast being biopsied is immmobilised by the grid compression plate and the vacuum biopsy device inserted via the introducing cannula. (B) The introducing cannula is visible on this axial MRI image, enabling the position to be checked before the biopsy.

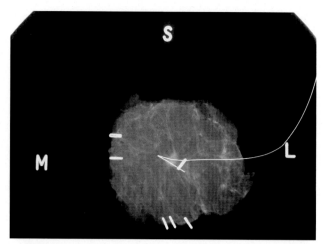

FIGURE 2-34 ■ Surgical specimen radiograph. A specimen radiograph of a marker localisation surgical biopsy showing the hook wire through the small mass lesion. The specimen is orientated by surgical clips showing the superior (S), lateral (L) and medial (M) margins. The radiograph shows clear margins of excision.

of the slice thickness and the number of slices between the skin and the lesion. Following the injection of local anaesthetic, an introducing cannula is inserted through a needle guide into the breast with the correct position confirmed by further imaging (Fig. 2-33B). The biopsy device is inserted through the introducing cannula and the biopsy samples obtained (Fig. 2-33A). The patient is re-imaged to ensure that the correct area has been sampled and a biopsy marker deployed.

MRI-guided biopsies are more challenging than other breast biopsies, due to lesion access and visibility. Most modern breast coils enable the breast to be accessed from both the medial and lateral directions, but problems can be encountered with posterior lesions that cannot be captured within the compression grid. Lesion visibility tends to decrease with time following the injection of gadolinium due to a combination of contrast washout from the lesion and increased background enhancement. Despite these limitations, vacuum-assisted MRI-guided biopsy offers a safe and accurate way of obtaining a tissue diagnosis from MRI-only-visible breast lesions.

Managing the Result of Needle Biopsy

It is important that the result of needle breast biopsy is correlated with the imaging and clinical findings. This is best achieved by reviewing each case at a multidisciplinary meeting at which the imaging, clinical and pathological findings are reviewed and management decisions and choices to be offered are discussed and agreed before the patient is seen with the results.

Preoperative Localisation of Impalpable Lesions

The purpose of preoperative localisation is to ensure that an impalpable lesion is accurately marked, facilitating complete surgical excision. For malignant lesions, the aim is to remove a minimum of 5 mm (and preferably 10 mm) of surrounding normal tissue at all margins. Without localisation, much larger volumes of tissue may be removed, with the potential to cause unnecessary deformity of the breast. Specimen radiography is used to confirm that the lesion has been removed and that adequate margins have been achieved (Fig. 2-34). The specimen is orientated using radio-opaque markers to identify the margins. If excision appears inadequate, further margin excision can be carried out at the same operation.

There are a number of methods available for preoperative localisation. These include simple skin marking over the lesion, insertion of a wire, or injection of carbon dye or radioisotope-labelled colloid. Ultrasound is the preferred method of image guidance.

The ideal wire is easy to deploy, maintains a stable position in the breast and is flexible enough to allow check mammography to take place following insertion. Several types of hook wire systems are available. All use an introducing needle through which the wire is advanced into the breast. For mass lesions and small clusters of microcalcification, the wire should be placed directly through the lesion or area, with the tip of the wire just beyond it. For a larger area of microcalcifications, several wires may be used to 'bracket' the area to be removed. Check mammograms should be performed to confirm that the correct area has been localised; these should be available to the surgeon.

Impalpable lesions can be localised using radio-labelled high-molecular-weight colloid. This technique is known as radio-opaque lesion localisation (ROLL). ^{99m}Tc-labelled colloid is injected under image guidance into the immediate vicinity of the tumour and the surgeon then localises the lesion using a fine-tipped gamma probe. The colloid must be large enough not to diffuse away from the injection site; the type of colloid used for lung scintigraphy is ideal.

CONCLUSION

Mammography and ultrasound continue to be the primary imaging tools for the assessment and diagnosis of breast disease. The development of digital mammography and high-resolution ultrasound has led to improvements in image quality and breast cancer detection. MRI is an important additional tool for local staging of breast cancer in carefully selected cases, aiding surgical planning.

The modern breast radiologist requires interventional radiology skills, with biopsies performed under ultrasound, X-ray and MRI guidance. Accurate preoperative diagnosis with image-guided percutaneous core biopsy is crucial in the management of breast disease, with surgery reserved for treatment rather than diagnosis. Increasingly sophisticated vacuum-assisted biopsy devices are available to improve the yield of representative tissue during biopsy, further improving preoperative diagnosis rates.

The past 20 years have seen a reduction in breast cancer mortality despite increasing incidence of the disease. Population-based breast cancer screening with mammography aims to reduce mortality by early detection. This remains a controversial area, but the benefits of screening in reducing mortality continue to outweigh the risks of overdiagnosis and overtreatment.

REFERENCES

1. Sickles EA. Practical solutions to common mammographic problems: tailoring the examination. Am J Roentgenol 1988;151: 31–9.
2. Feig SA. Importance of supplementary mammographic views to diagnostic accuracy. Am J Roentgenol 1988;151:40.
3. Eklund GW, Busby RC, Miller SH, et al. Improving imaging of the augmented breast. Am J Roentgenol 1988;151:469–73.
4. Review of Radiation Risk in Breast Screening 2003 Report by a joint working party of the NHSBSP National Coordinating Group for Physics, Quality Assurance and the National Radiological Protection Board. NHSBSP Publication No 54, Sheffield.
5. Davies HE, Wathen CG, Gleeson FV. Risks of exposure to radiological imaging and how to minimise them. BMJ 2011;342: 589–93.
6. Lewin JM, D'Orsi CJ, Hendrick RE, et al. Clinical comparison of full-field digital mammography and screen-film mammography for detection of breast cancer. Am J Roentgenol 2002;179:671–7.
7. Skaane P, Young K, Skjennald A. Population-based mammographic screening: comparison of screen-film and full-field digital mammography with soft-copy reading: Oslo I study. Radiology 2003; 229:877–84.
8. Skaane P, Skjennald A. Screen-film mammography versus full-field digital mammography with soft-copy reading: randomised trial in a population-based screening program: the Oslo II study. Radiology 2004;232:197–204.
9. Pisano ED, Gatsonis C, Hendrick E, et al. Diagnostic performance of digital versus film mammography for breast-cancer screening. N Engl J Med 2005;353:1846–7.
10. Castellino RA, Roehrig J, Zhang W. Improved computer-aided detection (CAD) algorithms for screening mammography. Radiology 2000;217:400.
11. Malich A, Marx C, Facius M, et al. Tumour detection rate of a new commercially available computer-aided detection system. Eur Radiol 2001;11:2454–9.
12. Freer TW, Ulissey MJ. Screening mammography with computer aided detection: prospective study of 12,860 patients in a community breast centre. Radiology 2001;220:781–6.
13. Fenton JJ, Abraham L, Taplin SH, et al. Effectiveness of computer-aided detection in community mammography practice. J Natl Cancer Inst 2011;103:1152–61.
14. Gur D, Sumkin JH, Rockette HE, et al. Changes in breast cancer detection and mammography recall rates after the introduction of a computer-aided detection system. J Natl Cancer Inst 2004;3: 185–90.
15. Gilbert FJ, Astley SM, Gillan MGC, et al. Single reading with computer-aided detection for screening mammography. N Engl J Med 2010;359:1675–84.
16. Guerriero C, Gillan MGC, Cairns J, et al. Is computer aided detection (CAD) cost effective in screening mammography? A model based on the CADET II study. BMC Health Services Research 2011;11:11.
17. Noroozian M, Hadjiiski L, Klein KA, et al. Digital breast tomosynthesis is comparable to mammographic spot views for mass characterization. Radiology 2012;262:61–8.
18. Wallis MG, Moa E, Zanca F, et al. Two-view and single-view tomosynthesis versus full-filed digital mammography: High-resolution X-ray imaging observer study. Radiology 2012;262: 788–96.
19. Berg WA, Cosgrove DO, Doré CJ, et al. Shear-wave elastography improves the specificity of breast US: The BE1 multinational study of 939 masses. Radiology 2012;262:435–49.
20. Stavros AT, Thickman D, Rapp CL, et al. Solid breast nodules: use of sonography to distinguish between benign and malignant lesions. Radiology 1995;196:123–34.
21. O'Malley FP, Pinder SE, Mulligan AM. Breast Pathology. 2nd ed. Philadelphia: Elsevier; 2011.
22. Wolfe JN. A study of breast parenchyma by mammography in the normal woman and those with benign and malignant disease. Radiology 1967;89:201–5.
23. American College of Radiology. Breast Imaging Reporting and Data Systems Atlas (BI-RADS Atlas). Reston, VA: American College of Radiology; 2003.
24. Yaghjyan L, Colditz GA, Collins LC, et al. Mammographic breast density and subsequent risk of breast cancer in postmenopausal women according to tumor characteristics. J Natl Cancer Inst 2011;103:1179–89.
25. Ellis IO, Galea M, Broughton N, et al. Pathological prognostic factors in breast cancer. II. Histological type. Relationship with survival in a large study with long-term follow-up. Histopathology 1992;20:479–89.
26. Lampejo OT, Barnes DM, Smith P, et al. Evaluation of infiltrating ductal carcinomas with a DCIS component: correlation of the histologic type of the in-situ component with the grade of the infiltrating component. Semin Diagn Pathol 1994;11:215–22.
27. Cornford EJ, Wilson ARM, Athanassiou E. Mammographic features of invasive lobular and invasive ductal carcinoma of the breast: a comparative analysis. Br J Radiol 1995;68:450–3.
28. Stutz JA, Pinder S, Ellis IO, et al. The radiological appearances of invasive cribriform carcinoma of the breast. Clin Radiol 1994; 49:693–5.
29. Chopra S, Evans AJ, Pinder SE, et al. Pure mucinous breast cancer—mammographic and ultrasound findings. Clin Radiol 1996;51:421–4.
30. McCulloch GL, Evans AJ, Yeoman LJ, et al. Radiological features of papillary carcinoma of the breast. Clin Radiol 1997;52:865–8.

31. Damera A, Evans AJ, Cornford EJ, et al. Diagnosis of axillary nodal metastases by ultrasound-guided core biopsy in primary operable breast cancer. Br J Cancer 2003;89:1310–13.

32. Bagnall MJC, Evans AJ, Wilson ARM, et al. Predicting invasion in mammographically detected microcalcification. Clin Radiol 2001;56:828–32.

33. Evans AJ, Pinder SE, Snead DRJ, et al. The detection of ductal carcinoma in situ at mammographic screening enables the diagnosis of small, grade 3 invasive tumours. Br J Cancer 1997;75:542–4.

34. Kul S, Cansu A, Alhan E, et al. Contribution of diffusion weighted imaging to dynamic contrast-enhanced MRI in the characterisation of breast tumours. Am J Roentgenol 2011;196:210–17.

35. Partridge SC, DeMartini WB, Kurland BF, et al. Quantitative diffusion-weighted imaging as an adjunct to conventional breast MRI for improved positive predictive value. Am J Roentgenol 2009;193:1716–22.

36. Dorrius MD, Pijnappel RM, Jansen-van der Weide MC, et al. Determination of choline concentration in breast lesions: quantative multivoxel proton MR spectroscopy as a promising noninvasive assessment tool to exclude benign lesions. Radiology 2011;259:695–703.

37. Kuhl CK, Mielcareck P, Klaschik S, et al. Dynamic breast MR imaging: are signal intensity time course data useful for differential diagnosis of an enhancing lesion? Radiology 1999;211:101–10.

38. Kuhl CK, Bieling HB, Gieske J, et al. Healthy premenopausal breast parenchyma in dynamic contrast enhanced MR imaging of the breast: normal contrast medium enhancement and cyclical phase dependency. Radiology 1997;203:137–44.

39. Morakkabati N, Leutner CC, Schmiedel A, et al. Breast MR imaging during or seen after radiation therapy. Radiology 2003;229:893–901.

40. Houssami N, Ciatto S, Macaskill P, et al. Accuracy and surgical impact of magnetic resonance imaging in breast cancer staging: systematic review and meta-analysis in detection of multifocal and multicentric cancer. J Clin Oncol 2008;26:3248–58.

41. Brennan M, Houssami N, Lord SJ, et al. MRI screening of the contralateral breast in women with newly diagnosed breast cancer: Systematic review and meta-analysis of incremental cancer detection and impact on surgical management. J Clin Oncol 2009;27:5640–9.

42. Weinstein SP, Orel SG, Heller R, et al. MR imaging of the breast in patients with invasive lobular carcinoma. Am J Roentgenol 2001;176:399–406.

43. Bhattacharyya M, Ryan D, Carpenter R, et al. Using MRI to plan breast-conserving surgery following neoadjuvant chemotherapy for early breast cancer. Br J Cancer 2008;98:289–93.

44. MARIBS Study Group. Screening with magnetic resonance imaging and mammography of a UK population at high familial risk of breast cancer: a prospective multicentre cohort study (MARIBS). Lancet 2005;365:1769–78.

45. Kriege M, Brekelmans CTM, Boetes C, et al. Efficacy of MRI and mammography for breast-cancer screening in women with a familial or genetic predisposition. N Engl J Med 2004;351:427–37.

46. La Trenta LR, Menell JH, Morris EA, et al. Breast lesions detected with MRI imaging: utility and histopathologic importance of identification with US. Radiology 2003;227:856–61.

47. Turnbull LW, Brown SR, Harvey I, et al. Comparative effectiveness of MRI in breast cancer (COMICE) trail: a randomized control trial. Lancet 2010;375:563–71.

48. Solin LJ, Orel SG, Wei-Ting H, et al. Relationship of breast magnetic resonance imaging after breast-conservation treatment with radiation for women with early-stage invasive breast carcinoma of ductal carcinoma in situ. J Clin Oncol 2008;26:386–91.

49. Middleton MS. Magnetic resonance evaluation of breast implants and soft-tissue silicon. Top Magn Reson Imaging 1998;9:92–137.

50. Forrest APM (Chairman): Working Group on Breast Cancer Screening. Report to the Health Ministers of England, Wales, Scotland and Northern Ireland. London: HMSO; 1986.

51. Nystrom L, Andersson I, Bjurstam N, et al. Long-term effects of mammographic screening: update overview of the Swedish randomised trials. Lancet 2002;359:909–19.

52. Tabar L, Vitak B, Tony HH, et al. Beyond randomised controlled trials: organised mammographic screening substantially reduces breast carcinoma mortality. Cancer 2001;91:1724–31.

53. Magnus MC, Ping M, Shen MM, et al. Effectiveness of mammography screening in reducing breast cancer mortality in women 39-49 years: a meta-analysis. J Womens Health 2011;20:845–52.

54. Andersson I, Janzon L. Reduced breast cancer mortality in women under age 50: updated results from the Malmo mammographic screening program. J Natl Cancer Inst Monogr 1997;22:63–8.

55. Bjurstam N, Bjorneld L, Duffy SW, et al. The Gothenburg Breast Screening Trial. First results on mortality, incidence and mode of detection for women ages 39–49 years at randomisation. Cancer 1997;80:2091–9.

56. Day N, McCann J, Camilleri-Ferrante C, et al. Monitoring interval cancers in breast screening programmes: the East Anglian experience. J Med Screen 1995;2:180–5.

57. Moss SM, Blanks RG, Bennett RL. Is radiologists' volume of mammography reading related to accuracy? A critical review of the literature. Clin Radiol 2005;60:623–6.

58. Blanks RG, Wallis MG, Moss SM. A comparison of cancer detection rates achieved by breast cancer screening programmes by number of readers, for one and two view mammography: results from the National Health Service breast screening programme. J Med Screen 1998;5:195–201.

59. Burrell H, Sibbering D, Wilson A, et al. The mammographic features of interval cancers and prognosis compared with screen detected symptomatic breast cancers. Radiology 1996;199:811–17.

60. Tabar L, Duffy SW, Vitak B, et al. The natural history of breast cancer: what have we learned from screening? Cancer 1999;86:449–62.

61. Evans AJ, Pinder SE, Burrell HC, et al. Detecting which invasive cancers at mammographic screening saves lives? J Med Screen 2001;8:86–90.

62. Britton PD. Fine needle aspiration or core biopsy. The Breast 1999;8:1–4.

63. Brennan ME, Turner RM, Ciatto S, et al. Ductal carcinoma in situ at core-needle biopsy: meta-analysis of underestimation and predictors of invasive cancer. Radiology 2011;260:119–28.

64. Bagnall MJC, Evans AJ, Wilson ARM, et al. When have mammographic calcifications been adequately sampled at needle core biopsy? Clin Radiol 2000;55:548–53.

CHAPTER 3

Reticuloendothelial Disorders: Lymphoma

Sarah J. Vinnicombe • Norbert Avril • Rodney H. Reznek

CHAPTER OUTLINE

EPIDEMIOLOGY

HISTOPATHOLOGICAL CLASSIFICATION

STAGING, INVESTIGATION AND MANAGEMENT

LYMPH NODE DISEASE IN LYMPHOMA

EXTRANODAL DISEASE IN LYMPHOMA

MUCOSA-ASSOCIATED LYMPHOID TISSUE LYMPHOMAS

BURKITT'S LYMPHOMA

LYMPHOMA IN THE IMMUNOCOMPROMISED

MONITORING RESPONSE TO THERAPY

SURVEILLANCE AND DETECTION OF RELAPSE

CONCLUSION

The lymphomas are complex, but may be divided into two broad groups: Hodgkin's lymphoma (HL) and non-Hodgkin's lymphoma (NHL). The overall incidence of NHL has increased steadily since 1960, with age-adjusted incidence rates being highest in more developed countries. It is estimated that there will be 70,000 new cases in 2012, an age-adjusted incidence of 19 per 100,000 persons per year, representing a 73% increase since the early 1970s.[1] This is due in part to secondary lymphoma arising in the setting of acquired immune deficiency syndrome (AIDS), though the incidence had started to increase before the AIDS epidemic. In the corresponding period, the incidence of HL has remained relatively steady at around 3 per 100,000.

EPIDEMIOLOGY

Age

HL has a peak incidence in the 20–30-year age group, with a second peak in the elderly population. The incidence of NHL increases exponentially with age after 20 years. The subtypes of lymphoma encountered differ in frequency between adult and paediatric groups, with a strong bias towards precursor B- and T-lymphoblastic lymphoma and Burkitt's lymphoma (BL) in childhood. Lymphomas with less typical age distribution include mediastinal large B-cell lymphoma, which has a peak incidence between 25 and 35 years, and mantle cell lymphoma, which is more common in those over 60 years.

Infectious Agents

Oncogenic lymphotrophic viruses have been implicated in many types of NHL. The single most important agent in this regard is Epstein–Barr virus (EBV). The EBV genome was first detected in cultured African Burkitt's lymphoma cells and is present in over 90% of such cases. EBV is important as a trigger for lymphoproliferations/lymphomas occurring in congenital immunodeficiencies, immunosuppressed organ transplant recipients, patients receiving maintenance chemotherapy and patients receiving combined immunosuppressive therapy for collagen disorders. EBV is also found in HL (mostly the mixed cellularity type); patients who have had infectious mononucleosis are at increased risk of HL. The retrovirus human lymphotropic virus type 1 (HTLV–1) is implicated in the causation of adult T-cell lymphoma, which is endemic in certain areas of East Africa, the Caribbean, southwest Japan and New Guinea. Human herpesvirus 8 (HHV–8) has been implicated as a cause of primary effusion lymphoma, a rare type of large cell lymphoma confined to serous-lined body cavities, which occurs with highest frequency in the HIV-positive population. Bacterial overgrowth can also promote lymphomagenesis. In gastric lymphoma of mucosa-associated lymphoid tissue (MALT) type, *Helicobacter pylori* infection has been shown to be necessary for the development and early proliferation of the lymphoma.

Immunosuppression

A variety of NHL is associated with pre-existing immunosuppression. The degree of immunosuppression is important in determining the lymphoma type that may emerge. In organ-specific autoimmune diseases, such as Hashimoto's thyroiditis and Sjögren's syndrome, extranodal marginal zone lymphomas of MALT type can arise within the affected organ. In severe immunodeficiency states, such as the congenital immunodeficiencies, AIDS and after organ transplantation, the lymphomas are very often EBV-driven large B-cell lymphomas. Infection with human immunodeficiency virus (HIV) explains much of the massive increase in the incidence of NHL in the past two decades. In the setting of systemic collagen diseases, there is an increase in haematological malignancy and patients receiving immunosuppressive therapy for these conditions are at still greater risk. The types of haematological malignancy that arise are quite varied, but there is a slight excess of myeloma and small B-lymphocytic lymphoma.

Genetic Factors

It is known that the risk of developing haematological malignancy is increased in patients with a family history of disease. This increased risk does not extend to the histological type or lineage of the tumours in question, such that one family member may have HL whereas a relative may have NHL or myeloid leukaemia.

Gender and Race

There is a slight predominance of NHL and HL in men (1.1–1.4 to 1). The incidence of NHL and HL varies by race, with higher frequencies in whites than blacks or Asians. Certain NHL types cluster according to race: for example, the natural killer (NK) T-cell lymphomas are most frequently encountered in oriental populations.

HISTOPATHOLOGICAL CLASSIFICATION

Hodgkin's Lymphoma

Biological studies have shown that HL is a true lymphoma. The defining malignant cell of HL is the Reed–Sternberg cell, a large, binucleated blast cell. Mononuclear counterparts are called Hodgkin's cells. The Reed–Sternberg cells and their variants form a minority population within any involved lymph node. The balance is made up of reactive non-neoplastic T cells, histiocytes, plasma cells, eosinophils and fibroblasts, varying in proportion according to the histological subtype. Since the 1960s, so-called classical HL has been subclassified into four histological types, indicated below along with their relative frequencies in Western populations:
- Lymphocyte-rich—5%
- Mixed cellularity (MC)—20–25%
- Nodular sclerosing (NS)—70%
- Lymphocyte-depleted (LD)—<5%.

In the nodular sclerosing type, substantial fibroblastic activity results in segmentation of involved nodes into cellular nodules separated by thick bands of collagen. It typically presents as a bulky mediastinal mass. In mixed cellularity HL, classical Reed–Sternberg cells are mixed with sheets of inflammatory elements. It is commoner in developing countries and in patients with HIV infection, as is the rare lymphocyte-depleted HL. Both have an aggressive clinical course. All four classical subtypes share the same immunophenotype and together constitute 95% of all cases of HL. A second distinct entity is nodular lymphocyte predominant HL, which was probably misdiagnosed as lymphocyte-rich classical HL in the past. It has a different morphology, immunophenotype and clinical course from classical HL; latent EBV infection is not a feature.

Non-Hodgkin's Lymphoma

Many of the difficulties that beset early taxonomists in the classification of NHL have been overcome with improved immunological and molecular methods of diagnosis. The Revised European–American Lymphoma (REAL) classification in 1994 depended on a triad of morphology, immunophenotype and molecular methods as well as clinical features for defining disease entities,[2] differentiating it from earlier morphologically based classifications. The scheme forms the backbone of the World Health Organisation (WHO) classification of tumours of haematopoietic and lymphoid tissues.[3] A summary of the WHO classification (4th edition) is given in Table 3-1. The WHO classification stratifies neoplasms by lineage into clinically distinct disease entities and is a real advance in the ability to identify disease accurately and consistently. Further, it can be refined so as to improve patient management.[4] For example, it has recently been shown that gene expression profiling in diffuse large B-cell lymphoma (DLBCL) enables recognition of discrete subsets (germinal centre B-cell type and activated B-cell type) which have independent prognostic significance, and this has been included in the 4th edition of the classification.[3] Other additions include paediatric follicular lymphoma, primary DLBCL of the central nervous system (PCNSL), and two so-called 'grey zone' lymphomas: B-cell lymphoma with features intermediate between DLBCL and classical HL, and B-cell lymphoma with features intermediate between DLBCL and BL.

STAGING, INVESTIGATION AND MANAGEMENT

Hodgkin's Lymphoma

Clinical Features and Staging

Most patients present with lymph node enlargement, most often in the cervical chains. Up to 40% have B symptoms (fever, drenching night sweats and weight loss of more than 10% of the person's bodyweight). Other constitutional symptoms can occur, such as pruritus, fatigue, anorexia and rarely alcohol-induced pain at the site of enlarged lymph nodes. Clinical examination usually reveals lymphadenopathy, most commonly in the neck. Axillary nodal enlargement occurs in up to 20% and inguinal disease in up to 15%, although exclusive infradiaphragmatic nodal disease is seen in up to 10% of patients at presentation. Splenomegaly may be evident on clinical examination in up to 30%.

Tissue biopsy is essential to make the diagnosis. Though a diagnosis of lymphoma may be made from a cutting needle biopsy, surgical excision biopsy of an entire node is preferable, so that the architecture of the node can be evaluated. Investigations will comprise a

TABLE 3-1   **WHO Classification of Lymphoid Neoplasms**

Neoplasm	Percentage of NHL*
B-CELL NEOPLASMS	85.0
Precursor B-cell neoplasms	
Precursor B-lymphoblastic leukaemia/ lymphoma	
Mature B-cell neoplasms	
CLL/small lymphocytic lymphoma	6.7
B-cell prolymphocytic leukaemia	
Lymphoplasmacytic (lymphoplasmacytoid) lymphoma	1.2
Splenic marginal zone lymphoma	<1.0
Hairy cell leukaemia	
Plasma cell myeloma	
Solitary plasmacytoma of bone	
Extraosseous plasmacytoma	
Extranodal marginal zone B-cell lymphoma of mucosa-associated lymphoid tissue (MALT)	7.6
Nodal marginal zone lymphoma	1.8
Follicular lymphoma	22.0
Mantle cell lymphoma	6.0
Diffuse large B-cell lymphoma (BCL)	32.0
Mediastinal (thymic)	2.4
Intravascular	
Primary effusion lymphoma	
Burkitt's lymphoma/leukaemia	1.0
B-CELL PROLIFERATIONS OF UNCERTAIN MALIGNANT POTENTIAL	
Lymphomatoid granulomatosis	
Post-transplant lymphoproliferative disorder, polymorphic	
T-CELL AND NK-CELL NEOPLASMS	14.0
Precursor T-cell neoplasms	
Precursor T-lymphoblastic lymphoma/ leukaemia	1.7
Blastic NK-cell lymphoma	
Mature T-cell and NK-cell neoplasms	
T-cell prolymphocytic leukaemia	
T-cell large granular lymphocytic leukaemia	
Aggressive NK-cell leukaemia	
Adult T-cell leukaemia/lymphoma	2.4
Extranodal NK-/T-cell lymphoma, nasal type	<1.0
Enteropathy-type T-cell lymphoma	
Hepatosplenic T-cell lymphoma	<0.001
Subcutaneous panniculitis-like	1.0
T-cell lymphoma	
Mycosis fungoides	
Sézary syndrome	1.2
Primary cutaneous anaplastic large cell lymphoma	
Peripheral T-cell lymphoma, unspecified	
Angioimmunoblastic T-cell lymphoma	7.0
Anaplastic large cell lymphoma	
T-CELL PROLIFERATIONS OF UNCERTAIN MALIGNANT POTENTIAL	
Lymphoid papulosis	
HODGKIN'S LYMPHOMA	
Nodular lymphocyte-predominant HL	
Classical HL	
Nodular sclerosis classical HL	
Lymphocyte-rich classical HL	
Mixed cellularity classical HL	
Lymphocyte-depleted classical HL	

*Approximate frequency—refers to lymph node biopsies in adults, with 1% accounting for the very rare entities.

TABLE 3-2   **Cotswold's Modification of the Ann Arbor Staging Classification of Hodgkin's Disease**

Stage	Classification
I	Involvement of a single lymph node region (I) or a single extralymphatic organ or site (IE)
II	Involvement of two or more lymph node regions on the same side of the diaphragm (II) or one or more lymph node regions plus an extralymphatic site (IIE)
III	Involvement of lymph node regions on both sides of the diaphragm (III) (the spleen is included in stage III) subdivided into: III(1): involvement of spleen and/or splenic hilar, coeliac and portal nodes III(2): with para-aortic, iliac, or mesenteric nodes
IV	Involvement of one or more extralymphatic organs, e.g. lung, liver, bone, bone marrow, with or without lymph node involvement
Additional qualifiers denote the following:	A: asymptomatic B: fever, night sweats and weight loss of >10% body weight X: bulky disease (defined as a lymph node mass >10 cm in diameter or, if involving the mediastinum, a mass greater than one-third of the intrathoracic diameter at the level of T5 E: involvement of a single extranodal site, contiguous with a known nodal site

blood count and erythrocyte sedimentation rate (ESR), together with liver biochemistry, renal function and serum urate. A staging computed tomography (CT) or a diagnostic positron emission tomography (PET)/CT imaging with 2-[F-18]fluoro-2-deoxy-D-glucose (FDG) is mandatory and may show involvement of intrathoracic, abdominal or pelvic lymph nodes. The so-called Cotswold's modification[5] of the original Ann Arbor staging classification (Table 3-2) was designed to take into account prognostic factors such as the volume of lymph node masses as identified with CT. A bone marrow aspirate and trephine biopsy should be performed in all patients except those with stage I disease, in whom the likelihood of bone marrow infiltration is negligible.

Prognosis and Treatment

For HL a poorer prognosis is noted with:
- Older patients
- Tumour subtype
- Raised ESR
- Mutiple sites of disease
- Bulky mediastinal disease
- B symptoms.

Treatment is almost invariably given with curative intent. The choice of treatment will depend predominantly on stage, and the presence/absence of adverse prognostic factors. HL is highly radiosensitive, and until recently many patients were treated with 'mantle' radiotherapy, which encompassed the cervical nodal chains, the axillae and the mediastinum down to the level of T10. However, there has been a steady trend towards the avoidance of radiotherapy in young patients because of the significant increase in secondary cancers, notably of the thyroid and breast (areas included in the radiotherapy field), and death through coronary artery disease.

Localised Disease (Stages IA and IIA). The majority of patients with early-stage favourable disease (non-bulky) are treated with combination chemotherapy. The use of interim FDG/PET imaging may allow escalation or de-escalation of therapy, with the goal of avoiding radiotherapy in patients who have a good response to combination chemotherapy and who are therefore in a very good prognostic group.

Advanced Disease (Stages IIB, IIIA/B and IVA/B). Patients presenting with a large mediastinal mass (i.e. a mass greater than 10 cm in diameter at CT) are generally treated with more intense chemotherapy initially, so as to shrink the mass. Consolidative radiotherapy may then be given. For advanced-stage disease, treatment comprises extensive combination chemotherapy, with or without subsequent consolidatory radiotherapy to sites of 'bulky' disease.

Failure to achieve an initial complete or almost complete response to first-line treatment and recurrence in the first year are both associated with a poor prognosis. Patients who develop recurrent HL more than once will generally ultimately die of the disease. By comparison, patients who develop recurrent HL some years after receiving treatment for localised disease can be given further combination chemotherapy and still be cured.

Non-Hodgkin's Lymphoma

Accurate diagnosis requires adequate tissue biopsy and an experienced histopathologist. Some lesions, for example, retroperitoneal, mediastinal and mesenteric masses, may be amenable to ultrasound or CT-guided core-needle biopsy, which may safely yield adequate tissue for histological diagnosis and immunophenotyping[6] but, as with HL, an entire lymph node is preferable for diagnosis.

Clinical Features and Staging

Most patients present with painless lymph node enlargement, but B symptoms are less frequent compared to HL, occurring in approximately 20%. In contradistinction to HL, the histological subtype of NHL is the major determinant of treatment rather than the stage. Nonetheless the stage of the disease has strong prognostic significance, a more advanced stage being associated with a significantly worse prognosis.[7] As with HL, the modified Ann Arbor staging system is generally used. Around 80% of patients will have advanced disease (stage III or IV) at presentation, so all newly diagnosed patients should undergo detailed physical examination, including examination of the fauces and testes. As with HL, CT or FDG-PET/CT of the neck, chest, abdomen and pelvis is mandatory, together with a bone marrow aspirate and trephine biopsy, owing to the propensity of most NHL

to infiltrate the bone marrow at presentation. Depending on the pattern of symptoms, other radiological investigations such as MRI may be indicated, especially for central nervous system lymphoma.

Prognosis and Treatment

The prognosis of NHL varies tremendously, depending upon the histological subtype. In order to evaluate therapies better and to choose the most appropriate treatment for a given patient, the International Prognostic Index (IPI) was developed.[7] The IPI is strictly speaking only applicable to aggressive lymphomas such as diffuse large B-cell lymphoma (DLBCL). Five factors were statistically associated with significantly inferior overall survival:

- Age >60 years
- Elevated serum lactate dehydrogenase (LDH)
- Performance status >1 (i.e. non-ambulatory)
- Advanced stage (III or IV)
- Presence of >1 extranodal site of disease.

A similar prognostic index (FLIPI) has been developed for more indolent follicular lymphoma (FL), where the important factors are considered to be:

- Age >60 years
- Elevated serum LDH
- Haemoglobin <12 g/dL
- Advanced stage (III or IV)
- More than four nodal sites of disease.

A recent modification (FLIPI 2) includes elevated serum β_2-microglobulin and longest diameter of the largest involved lymph node over 6 cm.[8]

The histological subtype determines not only the type of treatment but also when treatment should start. For asymptomatic patients with FL, surveillance alone may be appropriate until symptoms develop or transformation to a more aggressive DLBCL occurs. On the other hand, patients with relatively localised DLBCL require treatment with multi-agent anthracycline-containing chemotherapy immediately. Standard treatment for DLBCL and higher-grade FL comprises cyclophosphamide, doxorubicin, vincristine and prednisone (CHOP) combined with rituximab, a chimeric monoclonal antibody against the CD20 receptor, expressed by over 95% of B-cell NHL (CHOP-R). Radiotherapy alone is considered for the small proportion of patients with stage I disease and no adverse factors, in whom surgical excision alone is considered inappropriate.

LYMPH NODE DISEASE IN LYMPHOMA

In HL, lymph node involvement is usually the only manifestation of disease, whereas in NHL nodal disease is frequently associated with extranodal involvement. There are differences in the patterns of lymph node involvement in HL and NHL at presentation. Lymph nodes tend to be larger in NHL than HL; indeed, in nodular sclerosing and lymphocyte-depleted HL, nodal enlargement may be minimal. Typically, involved nodes tend to displace adjacent structures rather than invade them, except in the case of primary mediastinal large B-cell lymphoma (PMBL), which is characterised by local invasion of adjacent structures.

Imaging Nodal Disease

At present, size is the only criterion by which lymph nodes demonstrated on CT or MRI are considered to be involved, though clustering of multiple small lymph nodes, for example within the anterior mediastinum or the mesentery, is suggestive. A maximum short-axis diameter of 10 mm is taken to be the upper limit of normal, depending upon the exact site within the neck, thorax, abdomen, or pelvis. There are exceptions: normal neck jugulodigastric node can measure up to 13 mm short-axis diameter; nodes in the gastrohepatic ligament and porta hepatis are considered abnormal if they measure more than 8 mm in diameter; retrocrural nodes greater than 6 mm are taken as enlarged;[9] and in the pelvis the upper limit of normal is 8 mm.[10] Lymph nodes at some sites, such as the splenic hilum, presacral and perirectal areas, are not usually visualised on cross-sectional imaging and, whenever demonstrated, are likely to be abnormal.

Enlarged lymph nodes in both HL and NHL are usually homogeneous, of soft-tissue density on CT. Mild or moderate uniform enhancement occurs after intravenous injection of contrast medium. Calcification is uncommon but may be seen on post-treatment images. Necrosis is rarely seen in large nodal masses in both HL (particularly nodular sclerosing HL) and aggressive NHL, more frequently after treatment. On MRI, involved lymph nodes have low-to-intermediate signal intensity on T1-weighted images, and they may have very high signal intensity on fat-suppressed T2-weighted and short tau inversion recovery (STIR) sequences. Though the signal intensity of involved nodes and the presence of necrosis do not appear to have much prognostic significance, there is some evidence that within large lymphomatous masses, heterogeneous T2 signal at magnetic resonance imaging (MRI), or heterogeneous enhancement at CT, is associated with a worse outcome.

Choice of Imaging Technique

CT has been the technique of choice for the staging and follow-up of lymphoma for some time, and enables localisation of the most appropriate lesion for consideration of percutaneous image-guided biopsy. Ultrasound has no value in whole-body staging. Ultrasonographic appearances of lymphomatous nodal disease are non-specific, though the pattern of vascular perfusion as demonstrated by power Doppler interrogation may suggest the diagnosis, lymphomatous nodes having rich central and peripheral perfusion. The main value of ultrasound in lymphoma lies in confirming the nature of a palpable mass and assessing the major viscera. The accuracy of MRI in detecting lymph node involvement is equal to that of CT (and is better in some areas such as the supraclavicular fossa and within the pelvis), but it has no particular advantage over CT in this respect and its role is essentially adjunctive, to solve problems or monitor response to treatment. Recent advances in MRI technology (high

field strength magnets and parallel imaging) have enabled MRI to be used for whole-body staging: the role of whole-body diffusion-weighted imaging in staging and response assessment is a field of active research.[11] Major advantages in patients with HL in particular (who are often young) include the lack of ionising radiation.

Detection of disease in normal-sized nodes is not possible with cross-sectional imaging, nor is it possible to differentiate between nodal enlargement secondary to lymphoma or reactive hyperplasia. Functional imaging is often able to make this distinction. The superior diagnostic accuracy and more favourable imaging characteristics of PET with FDG and, latterly, PET/CT, has resulted in a dramatic decline in the use of gallium-67 scintigraphy, which no longer has a role as an isolated tool in the staging of lymphoma.

Numerous studies have shown that FDG-PET is at least as accurate as CT in the depiction of nodal and extranodal disease[12,13] and more sensitive than Ga-67 scintigraphy. It results in clinically significant upstaging in up to 10–20% of patients compared to CT, which may result in changes in therapy, particularly in HL.[14] Most NHLs are FDG-avid, though false-negative studies can occur with low-grade lymphomas such as small lymphocytic lymphoma, cutaneous lymphoma, some peripheral T-cell lymphomas and MALT types. For these subtypes, contrast-enhanced CT remains the standard of care. The development of PET/CT with accurate co-registration means that both morphological and functional abnormalities can be assessed simultaneously with improved diagnostic performance of FDG-PET as a result.[15] It is important to recognise that lymphomatous involvement of certain organs can be very difficult to recognise with FDG-PET/CT, because of physiological uptake—for example, in the stomach and central nervous system.[16] Debate continues as to whether it is necessary to carry out a full diagnostic CT imaging as part of the PET/CT study and often a low-dose CT, for the purposes of attenuation correction and anatomical correlation, is sufficient.[17,18]

Neck

Between 60 and 80% of patients with HL present with cervical lymphadenopathy. The spread of the disease is most frequently to contiguous nodal groups, with involvement of the internal jugular chain and spread to other deep lymphatic chains in the neck. Patients with supraclavicular or bilateral neck adenopathy are at increased risk of infradiaphragmatic disease.

Cervical adenopathy is less common in NHL, but commonly occurs in association with extranodal disease in Waldeyer's ring. Approximately 40–60% of patients who present with head and neck involvement will have disseminated NHL. Involved nodal groups tend to be non-contiguous. Central necrosis within a lymph node is rarely seen. Imaging with contrast-enhanced CT or MRI has a useful role in evaluating the neck in patients with lymphoma, as it may identify enlarged nodes which are impalpable. It is helpful in response assessment, particularly in patients treated with radiotherapy, where post-treatment fibrosis renders clinical assessment difficult.

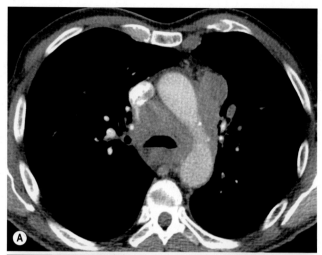

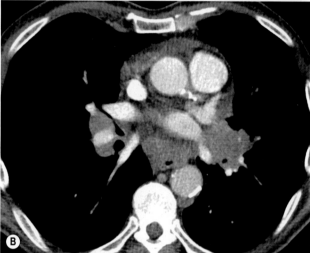

FIGURE 3-1 ■ **Anterior and middle mediastinal nodal disease.** (A) Contrast-enhanced CT showing marked confluent enlargement of the middle mediastinal nodes, extending laterally into the aortopulmonary window and extending into the prevascular left para-aortic region. (B) Subcarinal, bilateral hilar and paraaortic nodal involvement in the same patient.

Thorax

Intrathoracic nodes are involved at presentation in 60–85% of patients with HL and 25–40% of patients with NHL.[19] Nodes larger than 1 cm short-axis diameter are considered enlarged. Any intrathoracic group of nodes may be affected, but all the mediastinal sites other than paracardiac and posterior mediastinal nodes are more frequently involved in HL than NHL. Nearly all patients with nodular sclerosing HL have disease in the anterior mediastinum. The frequency of nodal involvement in HL is as follows:[19] prevascular and paratracheal—84% (Fig. 3-1); hilar—28% (Fig. 3-1); subcarinal—22% (Fig. 3-1); others—5% (aortopulmonary, anterior diaphragmatic, internal mammary (Fig. 3-2)). In NHL involvement of the hilar and subcarinal groups is rarer, occurring in 9 and 13%, respectively, whereas superior mediastinal nodes are involved in 35%.[20]

The great majority of cases of HL show enlargement of two or more nodal groups, whereas only one nodal

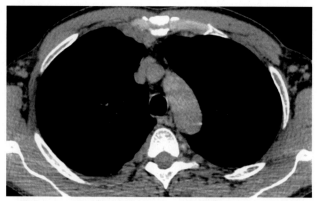

FIGURE 3-2 ■ **Internal mammary lymphadenopathy.** Axial CT showing marked enlargement of the right internal mammary lymph nodes. Note the minimal bilateral axillary lymph node enlargement and paravertebral extrapleural disease bilaterally.

group is involved in up to half of the cases of NHL. Hilar nodal enlargement is rare without associated mediastinal involvement, particularly in HL. Although paracardiac and internal mammary nodes are rarely involved at presentation in HL, they may be involved in recurrent disease, as they are not included in the classical 'mantle' radiation field. In HL and NHL, large anterior mediastinal masses usually represent thymic infiltration as well as a nodal mass (Fig. 3-3). A large anterior mediastinal mass in HL is recognised as an adverse prognostic feature and, as such, defines the need for more aggressive initial therapy. CT will demonstrate unsuspected mediastinal nodal enlargement despite a normal chest radiograph in 10% of patients with HL, and these patients have a poorer prognosis. CT of the chest has been shown to alter management in up to 25% of patients with HL. The therapeutic impact is less in patients with NHL, who are likely to receive chemotherapy regardless of stage. Impalpable axillary nodal enlargement is also frequently detected on CT in HL and NHL.

Abdomen and Pelvis

At presentation the retroperitoneal nodes are involved in 25–35% of patients with HL but up to 55% of patients with NHL.[21] Mesenteric lymph nodes are involved in more than half the patients with NHL and less than 5% of patients with HL.[21] Other sites such as the porta hepatis and splenic hilum are also less frequently involved in HL than NHL (Fig. 3-4). In HL, nodal spread is predictably from one lymph node group to another through directly connected lymphatic pathways. Nodes are frequently of normal size or only minimally enlarged. Spread from the mediastinum occurs through the lymphatic vessels to the retrocrural nodes, coeliac axis and so on. Around the coeliac axis, multiple normal-sized nodes may be seen, which can be difficult to evaluate because involved, normal-sized nodes are frequent in HL[22] (Fig. 3-4). The coeliac axis, splenic hilar and porta hepatis nodes are involved in about 30% of patients and splenic hilar nodal involvement is almost always associated with diffuse splenic infiltration (Fig. 3-4). The node of the foramen of Winslow (porta caval node), lying between

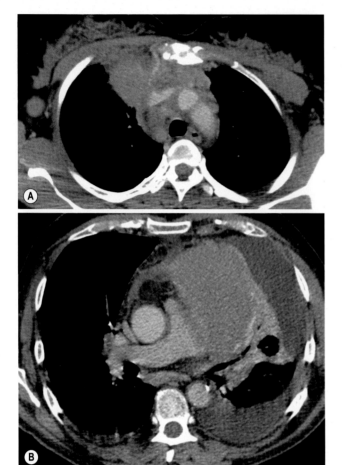

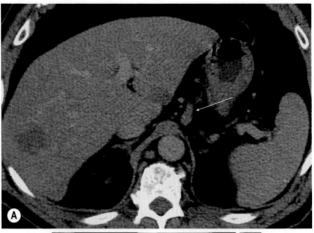

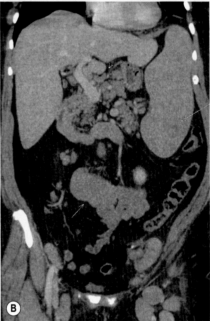

FIGURE 3-3 ■ **Mediastinal masses in lymphoma.** (A) Contrast-enhanced CT showing a large anterior mass involving the chest wall in a young patient with Hodgkin's lymphoma. Note the right axillary nodal disease. (B) Contrast-enhanced CT in a patient with primary mediastinal large B-cell lymphoma (PMBL) in the anterior and middle mediastinum. Note the pericardial involvement, compressive atelectasis of the left upper lobe and large left pleural effusion.

FIGURE 3-4 ■ **Upper abdominal lymph node enlargement.** (A) Contrast-enhanced CT showing an enlarged lymph node in the gastrohepatic ligament (arrow). Minimal lymph node enlargement (exceeding 6 mm) is also seen in the right retro-crural region Two liver deposits are present in this patient with HL. (B) Coronal reformatted contrast-enhanced CT showing lymph node enlargement around the coeliac axis and porta hepatis (arrowhead), the splenic hilum, the mesentery (short arrow), the left external iliac chain and both inguinal regions. There is splenomegaly and a focal splenic lesion (long arrow).

the portal vein and the inferior vena cava, is important, as it is often overlooked and may be the only site of disease relapse. It has a triangular shape; its normal long-axis diameter is up to 3 cm and in the anteroposterior plane is approximately 1 cm.

In NHL, nodal involvement is frequently non-contiguous and bulky and is more frequently associated with extranodal disease. Discrete mesenteric nodal enlargement or masses may be seen with or without retroperitoneal nodal enlargement. Large-volume nodal disease in both mesentery and retroperitoneum may give rise to the so-called 'hamburger' sign, in which a loop of bowel is compressed between two large nodal masses (Fig. 3-5). Multiple normal-sized mesenteric nodes should be regarded with suspicion for the diagnosis of lymphoma and lymphoma is a recognised cause of the 'misty mesentery'. In NHL, regional nodal involvement is frequently seen in patients with primary extranodal lymphoma involving an abdominal viscus. Involved nodes tend to enhance uniformly and the presence of multilocular enhancement should suggest an alternative diagnosis such as tuberculosis or atypical infection.

In the pelvis, any nodal group may be involved in both HL and NHL. Presentation with enlarged inguinal or femoral lymphadenopathy is seen in less than 20% of HL, and its presence should prompt close scrutiny of the pelvic nodal groups. In patients with massive pelvic disease, MRI is helpful for delineating the full extent of tumour and the effect on the adjacent organs.

EXTRANODAL DISEASE IN LYMPHOMA

Involvement of extranodal sites by lymphoma usually occurs in the presence of widespread advanced disease elsewhere. Such secondary involvement is a recognised

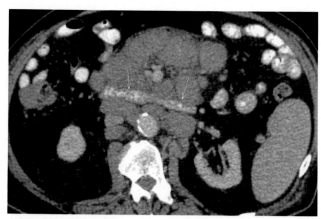

FIGURE 3-5 ■ **Extensive mesenteric nodal disease.** Nodal enlargement in the mesentery and the retroperitoneum in a patient with NHL, compressing the third part of the duodenum (arrows) resulting in the hamburger sign.

adverse prognostic feature in HL and NHL but is much commoner in the latter. However, in approximately 35% of cases of NHL, primary involvement of an extranodal site occurs, with lymph node involvement limited to the regional lymph nodes: stages I–IIE. Primary extranodal HL is extremely rare and rigorous exclusion of disease elsewhere is essential before this diagnosis can be made. The incidence of extranodal involvement in NHL depends on factors such as the age of the patient, the presence of pre-existing immunodeficiency and the pathological subtype of lymphoma. Extranodal disease is commoner in children, (particularly in the gastrointestinal tract, the major abdominal viscera and extranodal locations in the head and neck)[23] and in the immunocompromised host. The high incidence of extranodal involvement in these patient groups is a reflection of the fact that such lymphomas are usually aggressive histological subtypes.

The incidence of extranodal NHL is rising faster than that of nodal NHL. For example, primary lymphomas of the CNS were increasing in frequency at a rate of 10% per annum until the introduction of highly active antiretroviral therapies.[24] Of the various pathological subtypes of NHL, mantle cell (a diffuse B-cell lymphoma), lymphoblastic lymphomas (80% of which are T-cell), BL (small cell non-cleaved) and MALT lymphomas demonstrate a propensity to arise in extranodal sites.

CT generally performs well in the depiction of extranodal disease, though there are certain instances where other techniques are preferable. FDG-PET is more sensitive than CT chiefly because of its ability to identify splenic and bone marrow infiltration[13] (Fig. 3-6). PET or PET/CT can upstage as many as 40% of cases, though the CT component remains essential: for example, in low-grade lymphoma and in the lungs, where small nodules may be below the resolution of PET technology.

Thorax

Pulmonary Parenchymal Involvement

Several categories of lung involvement can be identified including:

- lymphomatous involvement associated with existing or previously treated intrathoracic nodal disease;
- lymphomatous involvement associated with widespread extrathoracic disease;
- primary pulmonary HL; and
- primary pulmonary NHL.

Some authors also separate out AIDS-related lymphoma (ARL) and the post-transplant lymphoproliferative disorder (PTLD),[25] both of which commonly affect the lungs.

Lung involvement at presentation occurs in just under 4% of patients with NHL, but in approximately 12% of patients with HL. It is usually secondary to direct extension of nodal disease into the adjacent parenchyma, hence its paramediastinal or perihilar location. In this circumstance there is no effect on stage; the 'E' lesion. Patients with HL presenting with an intrapulmonary lesion in the absence of demonstrable mediastinal disease are unlikely to have lymphomatous disease of the lung unless there has been previous mediastinal or hilar irradiation, when recurrence may be confined to the lungs. Conversely, in NHL, nodal disease is absent in 50% of those patients with pulmonary or pleural involvement. As nodal disease progresses or relapses, lung involvement becomes commoner in HL and NHL, such that 30–40% of patients with HL have pulmonary involvement at some stage during the course of the disease.

The radiographic appearances are extremely variable, but the commonest pattern is of one or more discrete nodules, with or without cavitation, which tend to be less well defined than those of primary or metastatic carcinoma, which they otherwise resemble (Figs. 3-7 and 3-8).[26] The disease often spreads along lymphatic channels and involves lymphoid follicles around bronchovascular divisions, resulting in peribronchial nodulation spreading out from the hila, which can result in streaky shadowing visible on chest radiographs and at CT (Fig. 3-7).

Less commonly, lymphomatous cells fill the pulmonary acini, producing rounded or segmental areas of consolidation with air bronchograms (Fig. 3-8). Nodulation along the bronchial wall may enable differentiation from infective consolidation. A rare pattern of disease is widespread interstitial reticulonodular shadowing, producing a lymphangitic picture. Another rare manifestation is atelectasis, which usually results from endobronchial lymphoma rather than extrinsic compression by nodal disease.

The differential diagnosis of pulmonary involvement in lymphoma is extensive, and includes drug-induced changes, the effect of radiotherapy, and opportunistic infection during or following chemotherapy, particularly in patients with antecedent immunosuppression. Precise clinical correlation is essential in determining the most likely diagnosis.

Primary Pulmonary Lymphoma

Primary pulmonary lymphoma accounts for less than 1% of all lymphomas and is usually low-grade B-cell NHL, arising from MALT or bronchus-associated lymphoid tissue (BALT). BALT lymphomas tend to occur in the fifth to sixth decades, have an indolent course with 5-year survivals of over 60% and tend to remain extranodal, although lymph node involvement can occur with advanced disease.[27] Many patients will have a prior history of inflammatory or autoimmune disease, such as Sjögren's syndrome, collagen vascular disease and dysgammaglobulinaemia.[28] The imaging findings are non-specific with the single commonest manifestation being a solitary nodule. Multiple nodules, or one or more rounded or segmental areas of consolidation,[29] are also seen. These can persist unchanged for long periods. Pleural effusions are seen in up to 20% of cases.[28]

In the remaining 15–20% of patients, primary lung lymphoma is due to high-grade NHL. The most common finding on a chest radiograph is of a solitary or multiple pulmonary nodules, which characteristically grow rapidly. Chest wall and nodal involvement occurs more frequently than with pulmonary MALT-type lymphomas.[27] Primary pulmonary HL is extremely rare. The most frequently described finding is single or multiple nodules with upper zone predominance and a relatively high incidence of cavitation.

Pleural Disease

Pleural effusions are usually accompanied by mediastinal lymphadenopathy (Fig. 3-9) and may be detected on CT in 50% of patients with mediastinal nodal disease. They are usually exudates secondary to central lymphatic or

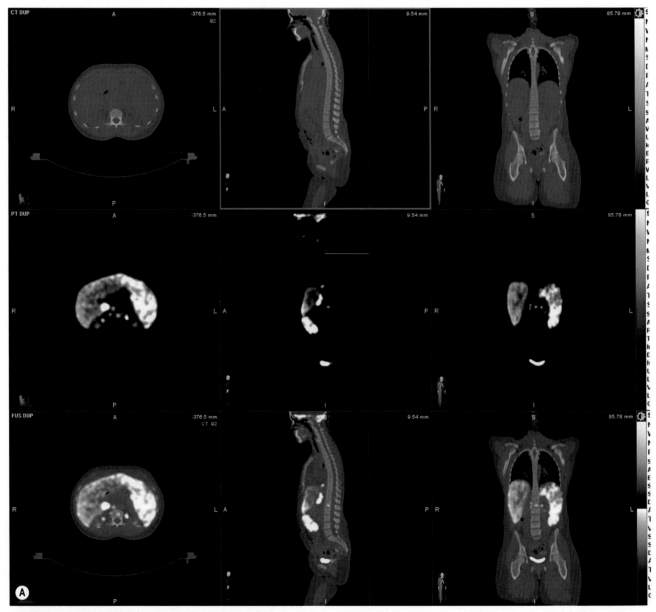

FIGURE 3-6 ■ **PET/CT image resulting in upstaging.** There is metabolically active disease in lymph nodes above and below the diaphragm with splenomegaly, but the PET/CT also demonstrates disease in the liver and the body of L1, making this stage IV disease.

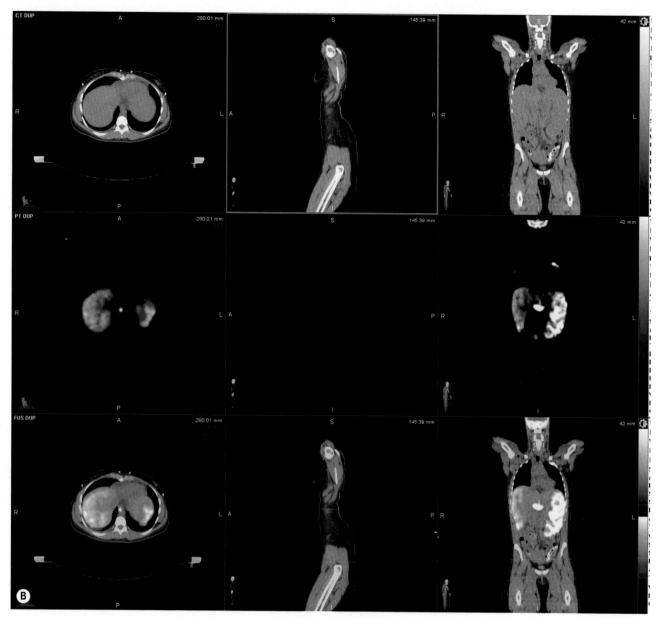

FIGURE 3-6, Continued ■

venous obstruction and therefore clear promptly with treatment of the mediastinal disease. Pulmonary involvement need not be present. Focal pleural masses do occur at presentation but are more commonly seen in recurrent disease, when they are generally accompanied by an effusion.

Pericardium and Heart

Direct pericardial and cardiac involvement can occur with high-grade peripheral T-cell and large B-cell lymphomas. It is rare at presentation, except in patients with AIDS-related lymphoma (ARL) and PTLD who may present with acute onset of heart block, tamponade, or congestive cardiac failure. Pericardial effusions occur in 6% of patients with HL at the time of presentation and are associated with large masses adjacent to the heart.

They are also common in primary mediastinal large B-cell lymphoma (PMBL) (Fig. 3-3B). Effusions are regarded as evidence of pericardial involvement, although this does not alter disease stage. Small pericardial effusions of uncertain aetiology are often seen at CT during treatment. They usually resolve with time, although some pericardial thickening may persist.

Thymus

Thymic involvement by HL in association with mediastinal nodal disease occurs in around 30% of patients at presentation. PMBL characteristically involves the thymus, occurring typically in young women between the ages of 25 and 40 years (Fig. 3-3B). Rapidly growing bulky disease is usual and up to 40% have superior vena caval obstruction, which is rare with other lymphomas.

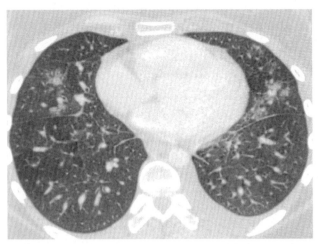

FIGURE 3-7 ■ **Pulmonary involvement in a patient with Hodgkin's lymphoma.** CT performed at the time of presentation, showing widespread ill-defined intrapulmonary nodular shadowing scattered throughout both lungs with a bronchocentric distribution. Note also the abnormal thickened interlobular septae and patchy ground-glass opacity.

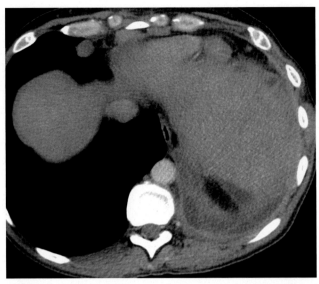

FIGURE 3-9 ■ **Pleural disease in lymphoma.** CT showing a typical appearance of pleural involvement in a patient with NHL. There is uniform pleural thickening with an accompanying pleural effusion. Note also the right and left paracardiac lymph node enlargement.

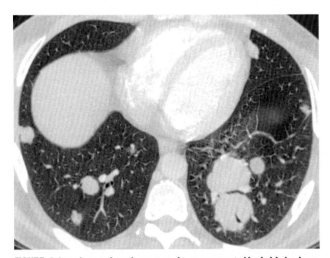

FIGURE 3-8 ■ **Lung involvement in recurrent Hodgkin's lymphoma.** CT showing multiple rounded nodules: the left lower lobe nodule is beginning to cavitate.

On CT, differentiation of enlarged mediastinal lymph nodes from thymic involvement is often difficult as the thymus involved by lymphoma usually has a homogeneous soft-tissue density or a heterogeneous nodular appearance. On MRI as well, the gland is often of mixed signal intensity similar to that of involved nodes. Nodal masses tend to be more lobulated, whereas thymic involvement is generally diffuse. Cystic change can be recognised at CT and MRI with PMBL and HL. These cysts can persist or even increase in size following regression of the rest of the involved gland with successful treatment. Calcification may be present at the outset or may develop during treatment.[30] Benign thymic rebound hyperplasia can develop after completion of chemotherapy, and can be difficult to differentiate from recurrent disease. Unfortunately, functional imaging with

FDG-PET may not always differentiate between the two and clinical correlation combined with follow-up studies may be necessary.

Chest Wall

In HL, spread into the chest wall usually occurs by direct infiltration from an anterior mediastinal mass, especially from the internal mammary chain. However, chest wall masses can arise de novo, especially in NHL. Bony destruction is rare and should suggest an alternative diagnosis. Thoracic wall disease is better shown by MRI than CT, particularly on T2-weighted or STIR sequences, where there is excellent contrast between the mass and normal low signal intensity muscle. PET/CT can also demonstrate chest wall involvement and these techniques may facilitates more accurate planning of radiotherapy portals.[31]

Breast

Lymphoma of the breast is usually associated with widespread disease elsewhere. There may be multiple nodules, with associated large-volume adenopathy. Primary NHL of the breast is rare, accounting for approximately 2% of all lymphomas and under 1% of all breast malignancies. The age distribution is bimodal, with the first peak occurring during pregnancy and lactation, often high-grade or Burkitt's lymphoma (BL) and affecting both breasts diffusely with an inflammatory picture at ultrasound and mammography.[32] There is a second peak at around 50 years when patients present with discrete masses which are usually solitary, but multiple masses occur and disease is bilateral in over 10%. The masses are usually fairly well defined, with little accompanying architectural distortion. Calcification has not been described.

Hepatobiliary System and Spleen

Liver

Liver involvement is present in up to 15% of adult patients with NHL at presentation. This figure is higher in the paediatric population and in recurrent disease. In HL, liver involvement occurs in about 5% of patients at presentation, almost invariably in association with splenic HL. Pathologically, diffuse microscopic infiltration around the portal tracts is the most common form of involvement. CT and MRI are therefore insensitive in the detection of liver involvement. However, hepatomegaly strongly suggests the presence of diffuse infiltration (in contradistinction to the significance of splenomegaly). Larger focal areas of infiltration are present in only 5–10% of patients with hepatic lymphoma. Cross-sectional imaging may demonstrate miliary nodules or larger solitary or multiple masses, resembling metastases (Fig. 3-10) and with entirely non-specific features on all forms of cross-sectional imaging. At MRI, as with metastases, deposits have moderate T2 hyperintensity. Superparamagnetic iron oxide particles and hepatocyte-specific contrast agents can increase the conspicuity of focal deposits. Occasionally, especially in children, periportal infiltration is manifest as periportal low-attenuation tissue at CT (Fig. 3-11).

True primary hepatic lymphoma, indistinguishable radiologically from hepatocellular carcinoma, is rare but the incidence is rising, up to 25% of affected patients being hepatitis B or C positive. Non-Hodgkin's lymphoma of the bile ducts and gallbladder is rare but occurs with relatively high frequency in patients with ARL.

Spleen

The spleen is involved in 30–40% of patients with HL at the time of presentation, usually in the presence of nodal disease above and below the diaphragm (stage III), but in a small proportion it is the sole focus of intra-abdominal disease (designated stage IIIS). In the majority of patients, the involvement is microscopic and diffuse and thus particularly difficult to identify on cross-sectional imaging. Splenomegaly is an unreliable sign of involvement; 33% of patients have splenomegaly without infiltration and, conversely, 33% of normal-sized spleens are found to contain tumour following splenectomy. Measurements of splenic volume and splenic indices are not generally utilised.

Focal splenic deposits occur in only 10–25% of cases and may be demonstrated by any form of cross-sectional imaging when they are more than 1 cm in diameter (Fig. 3-4B). Up to 40% of patients with NHL have splenic involvement at some stage. Imaging findings include a

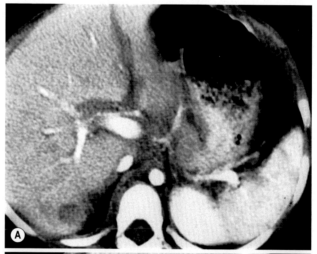
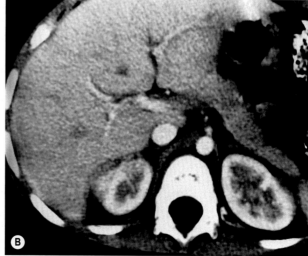

FIGURE 3-11 ■ **Periportal lymphoma.** (A) Contrast-enhanced CT in a child with NHL, showing infiltration of low-density lymphomatous tissue from the porta hepatis, encasing the main portal vein, extending alongside the right portal vein. A solitary focal abnormality is seen posteriorly within the liver. (B) Follow-up after chemotherapy shows complete resolution of the disease.

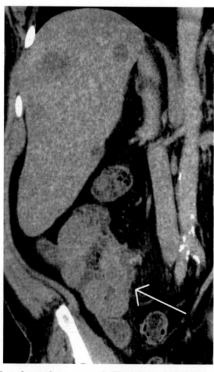

FIGURE 3-10 ■ **Lymphomatous infiltration of the liver.** There are multiple poorly defined low-density lesions in the liver in this patient with T-cell NHL of the small bowel (arrowed).

solitary mass, miliary nodules or multiple masses, all of which have a non-specific appearance. The differential diagnosis of multiple masses includes opportunistic infection and granulomatous disease.

In early studies, the sensitivity of ultrasound and CT for the detection of splenic involvement was extremely low (about 35%). Detection of small nodules has improved with the advent of contrast-enhanced multidetector CT (MDCT) with optimisation of splenic parenchymal opacification. MRI with superparamagnetic iron oxide may improve diagnostic accuracy but is seldom undertaken outside the research arena. However, FDG-PET can detect splenic disease more accurately than either CT or gallium scintigraphy.[33] In the past, the poor sensitivity of imaging for the detection of splenic involvement in HL necessitated staging laparotomy with splenectomy, but the development of effective combination chemotherapy with good salvage regimens has led to this practice being abandoned.

Primary splenic NHL is rare, accounting for 1% of all patients with NHL. Patients present with splenomegaly, often marked and focal masses are usual. Splenic involvement is also a particular feature of certain other pathological subtypes of NHL, such as mantle cell lymphoma and splenic marginal zone lymphoma. Infarction is a well-recognised complication.

Gastrointestinal Tract

The gastrointestinal (GI) tract is the commonest site of primary extranodal NHL, accounting for 30–45% of all extranodal presentations and constituting about 1% of all GI tumours. It is the initial site of lymphomatous involvement in up to 10% of all adult patients and up to 30% of children.[23] As elsewhere, primary HL of the gastrointestinal tract is most unusual. Secondary involvement of the gastrointestinal tract via direct extension from involved mesenteric or retroperitoneal lymph nodes is extremely common, and consequently multiple sites of involvement occur.

Primary lymphomas arise from lymphoid tissue of the lamina propria and the submucosa of the bowel wall and occur most frequently below the age of 10 years (usually BL) and in the sixth decade (MALT type and enteropathy-associated T-cell type). Primary gastrointestinal lymphoma is usually unifocal.

Accepted criteria for the diagnosis of primary disease include:
- No superficial or intrathoracic lymph node enlargement
- No involvement of the liver or spleen
- A normal white cell count
- No more than local regional lymph node enlargement.

In both primary and secondary cases, the stomach is most frequently involved (50%), followed by the small bowel (35%) and large bowel (15%).

Stomach

Primary lymphoma accounts for about 2–5% of all gastric tumours.[34] It originates in the submucosa, affecting the

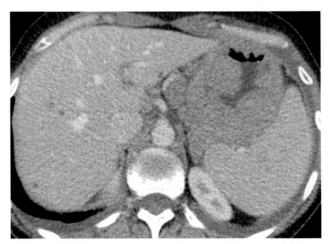

FIGURE 3-12 ■ **Gastric lymphoma.** Axial contrast-enhanced CT showing gross gastric mural and rugal thickening with adjacent enlarged gastrohepatic lymph node.

antrum more commonly than the body or cardia. Radiologically the appearances reflect the gross pathological findings; common appearances are multiple nodules, some with central ulceration, or a large fungating lesion with or without ulceration. About a third of patients have diffuse infiltration, with marked thickening of the wall and narrowing of the lumen, sometimes with extension into the duodenum, indistinguishable from linitis plastica. Only about 10% are characterised by diffuse enlargement of the gastric folds, similar to the pattern seen in hypertrophic gastritis (Fig. 3-12).

As the disease originates in the submucosa, the signs described above are best demonstrated on barium studies or endoscopically, but CT better reflects the true extent of gastric wall thickening and accompanying nodal involvement. Typically, infiltration of adjacent organs is unusual but it may occur in DLBCL. In gastric MALT lymphomas, mural thickening may be minimal; CT is of limited value even with dedicated studies, and endoscopic ultrasound with biopsy is more useful in staging, prognostication and assessment of response (Fig. 3-13). Low-grade MALT lymphoma is more likely to cause shallow ulceration and nodulation, whereas high-grade lymphoma can produce more massive gastric infiltration and polypoid masses (Fig. 3-11).

Small Bowel

Lymphoma accounts for up to 50% of all primary tumours of the small bowel, occurring most frequently in the terminal ileum, and becoming progressively less frequent proximally; duodenal lymphomas are rare (Fig. 3-14). In children, the disease is almost exclusively ileocaecal. Most bowel lymphomas are of B-cell lineage. The disease is multifocal in up to 50% of cases; mural thickening with constriction of bowel segments is typical. Patients commonly present with obstructive symptoms. Bowel wall thickening is well demonstrated on CT (Figs. 3-10 and 3-15). With progressive tumour spread through the submucosa and muscularis mucosa, aneurysmal dilatation of long segments of bowel can develop, presumably due to

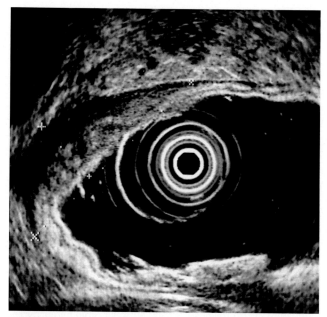

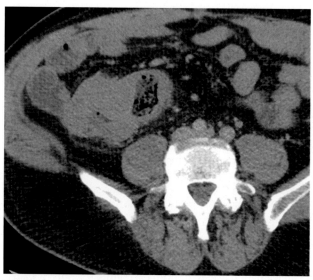

FIGURE 3-15 ■ **Involvement of large bowel in non-Hodgkin's lymphoma.** CT showing marked and extensive diffuse thickening of the wall of the caecum and ascending colon.

FIGURE 3-13 ■ **MALT lymphoma.** Endoscopic ultrasound showing a narrow sheet of low echogenic tissue in the submucosa (arrowed). (Image courtesy of Dr A. McLean, Department of Diagnostic Imaging, St Bartholomew's Hospital, London.)

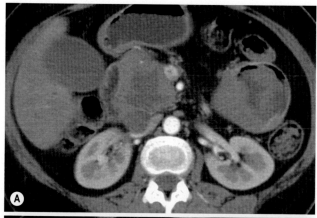

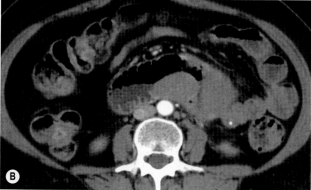

FIGURE 3-14 ■ **Burkitt's lymphoma involving the duodenum.** (A, B) There is a large mass in the head of the pancreas and the wall of the second part of the duodenum, causing obstruction of the common bile duct posteriorly, with involvement of the fourth part of the duodenum. (B) Disease involving the third part of the duodenum.

infiltration of the autonomic plexus. Alternating areas of dilatation and constriction are a common manifestation of infiltration and are well demonstrated by CT.

If lymphomatous infiltration is predominantly submucosal, multiple nodules or polyps of varying size result, mostly in the terminal ileum. It is this form of lymphoma that typically causes intussusception, usually in the ileocaecal region. Lymphoma is the commonest cause of intussusception in children older than 6 years.

Enteropathy-associated T-cell lymphoma and immunoproliferative small intestinal disease (alpha-chain disease) commonly present with clinical and imaging features of malabsorption, but acute presentations with perforation are common. Often the whole small intestine is affected, especially the duodenum and jejunum. In the small bowel (and colon), MALT lymphoma is manifest as mucosal nodularity, which can be appreciated in barium studies. Secondary invasion of the small bowel is commonly seen when large mesenteric lymph node masses cause displacement, encasement or compression of the bowel. Peritoneal disease identical to that seen with ovarian carcinoma generally occurs late in advanced disease, although it may be seen at presentation in BL.

Colon and Rectum

Primary colonic lymphomas are usually of Burkitt's or MALT subtypes, but account for under 0.1% of all colonic neoplasms, most arising in the caecum and rectum (Fig. 3-15). The most common pattern of disease is a diffuse or segmental distribution of small nodules 0.2–2.0 cm in diameter, typically with intact mucosa. A less common form of the disease is a solitary polypoid mass, often in the caecum, indistinguishable from carcinoma on imaging unless there is concomitant involvement of the terminal ileum.

In advanced disease, there may be marked thickening of the colonic or rectal folds, resulting in focal strictures, fissures or ulcerative masses with fistulation. Lymphomatous strictures are generally longer than carcinomatous strictures and irregular excavation of the mass strongly suggests lymphoma. Involvement of the anorectum is a feature of ARL. Patients usually present with obstruction and rectal bleeding.

Oesophagus

Involvement of the oesophagus is extremely unusual and begins as a submucosal lesion, usually in the distal third of the oesophagus. Ulceration is a later phenomonem. Secondary involvement by contiguous spread from adjacent nodal disease is more common but rarely results in dysphagia.

Pancreas

Primary pancreatic lymphoma accounts for only 1.3% of all pancreatic malignancies and 2% of patients with NHL. It usually presents with a solitary mass, often in the head of the pancreas, indistinguishable from primary adenocarcinoma on US, CT, or MRI.[35] Biliary or pancreatic ductal obstruction can occur (Fig. 3-14). Calcification and necrosis are rare. Less commonly, diffuse uniform enlargement of the pancreas is seen. Involvement is far more common in NHL than in HL. Secondary pancreatic involvement usually results from direct infiltration from adjacent nodal masses, either focal or massive.

Genitourinary Tract

The genitourinary tract is not commonly involved at the time of presentation (<5%); however, >50% of patients will have involvement of some part of the genitourinary tract at autopsy. The testicle is the most commonly involved organ, followed by the kidney and the perirenal space; only rarely are the bladder, prostate, uterus, vagina or ovaries involved. True primary genitourinary lymphoma is rare, as there is normally very little lymphoid tissue within the genitourinary tract.

Kidneys

CT is sensitive in the diagnosis of lymphomatous renal masses, but since renal involvement is generally a late phenomenon, renal involvement is identified in only around 3% of patients undergoing staging CT. Close to 90% of cases are associated with high-grade NHL and detection of renal involvement rarely alters the disease stage. In over 40% of patients the disease occurs at the time of recurrence only and renal function is usually normal.[36]

The commonest pattern of disease, seen in 60%, is multiple masses (Fig. 3-16). On CT, the masses may show a typical 'density reversal pattern' before and after administration of contrast medium, lesions being more dense than the surrounding parenchyma before contrast medium administration and less dense after. A solitary renal mass is seen in only 5–15% of cases and may be indistinguishable from renal cell carcinoma (Fig. 3-17).[36]

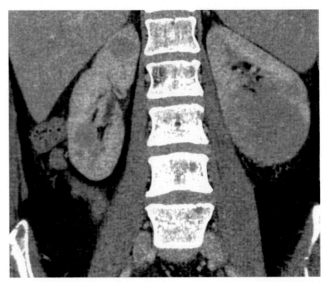

FIGURE 3-16 ■ Multiple lymphomatous renal masses. Coronal reformatted CT showing multiple masses, hypodense compared with the normally enhancing adjacent renal parenchyma. There are also multiple lytic bone lesions in this patient with NHL.

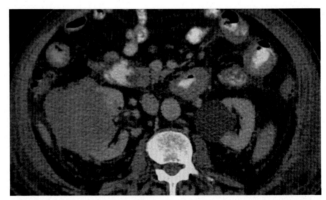

FIGURE 3-17 ■ Renal lymphomatous mass. A large right renal mass extends into the perinephric space on contrast-enhanced CT in a patient with NHL. There is also a lymphomatous mass in the left perinephric space; multiple peritoneal and retroperitoneal nodules; mesenteric nodal disease and extensive small bowel involvement.

Importantly, in over 50% of lymphomatous renal masses, there is no accompanying retroperitoneal lymph node enlargement on CT.

Direct infiltration of the kidney by contiguous retroperitoneal nodal masses is the second most common type of renal involvement, occurring in 25% of cases. Associated encasement of the renal vessels and extension into the renal hilum and sinus is common and radiologically this pattern can closely resemble transitional cell carcinoma of the renal pelvis. In a further 10%, soft-tissue mass(es) are seen in the perirenal space, occasionally encasing the kidney without any evidence of invasion of the parenchyma (Fig. 3-17).

Diffuse intrinsic infiltration of the kidney resulting in global enlargement is the least common manifestation of renal lymphomatous involvement. This pattern can occur with high-grade and paediatric lymphomas such as BL.

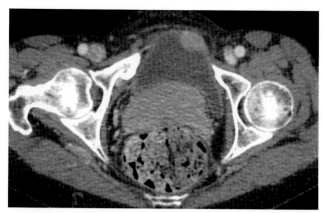

FIGURE 3-18 ■ **Bladder lymphoma.** Contrast-enhanced CT of the pelvis in a female patient showing a polypoid soft-tissue mass arising from the wall of the bladder. There is involvement of the vagina.

On ultrasound, the kidneys are diffusely enlarged and uniformly hypoechoic. On CT, the appearance following intravenous injection of contrast medium is variable, but usually the normal parenchymal enhancement is replaced by homogeneous non-enhancing tissue.

Bladder

The urinary bladder is a rare site of primary extranodal involvement, accounting for less than 1% of all bladder tumours.[37] Small cell and MALT types are seen, the latter often in middle-aged women with a history of recurrent cystitis. Large multilobular submucosal masses with minimal or no mucosal ulceration are typical (Fig. 3-18). Transmural spread into adjacent pelvic organs can occur and is well demonstrated on cross-sectional imaging. The prognosis is generally good. Secondary lymphoma of the bladder is found in 10–15% of patients with lymphoma at autopsy, resulting from contiguous spread from adjacent involved pelvic lymph nodes. Microscopic involvement is far more common than gross infiltration, but both can be associated with haematuria. On CT the appearances are usually non-specific and indistinguishable from transitional cell carcinoma, producing either diffuse widespread thickening of the bladder wall or a large nodular mass.

Prostate

Primary prostatic lymphoma is also extremely rare, but in contradistinction to primary bladder NHL it carries a very poor prognosis. It is generally intermediate-to-high grade and histological examination usually shows diffuse infiltration with spread into the periprostatic tissues. More frequently, prostatic involvement is secondary to spread from the adjacent nodes in the setting of advanced disease.

Testis

Testicular lymphoma accounts for about 5% of primary testicular tumours overall and is the commonest primary

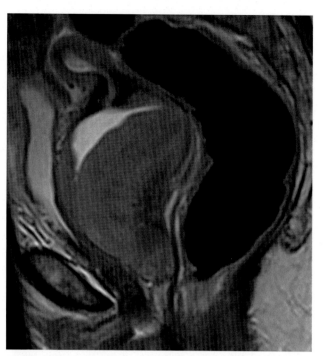

FIGURE 3-19 ■ **Lymphoma involving the vagina.** Sagittal T2-weighted MRI of the patient described in the legend to Fig. 3-18 demonstrates a large intermediate-to-high signal intensity mass, substantially larger than seen usually in a squamous carcinoma of the cervix. Biopsy showed an aggressive B-cell lymphoma.

tumour in patients over the age of 60 years. It is vanishingly rare in HL but is seen at presentation in approximately 1% of all patients of NHL, usually with DLBCL or BL. There is an association with lymphoma of Waldeyer's ring, the skin and central nervous system. Patients usually present with a painless testicular swelling and in up to 25% of cases the involvement is bilateral. Relapse can occur in the contralateral testis. Ultrasonically, the lesions usually have a non-specific appearance, with focal areas of decreased echogenicity, or a more diffuse decrease in reflectivity of the testicle without any focal abnormality. Because of the association with disease elsewhere, staging must always include ultrasonic evaluation of the contralateral testis and whole-body cross-sectional imaging. Cranial CT or MRI, and CSF examination should also be considered.

Female Genital Tract

Isolated lymphomatous involvement of the female genital organs is rare, accounting for approximately 1% of extranodal NHL. Nearly 75% of women affected are postmenopausal and present with vaginal bleeding. The cervix is affected more frequently than the uterus and vagina. Involvement of the gynaecological tract is best demonstrated by MRI, where primary lymphoma of the cervix and/or vagina is characterised by a large soft-tissue mass with homogeneous intermediate-to-high T2 signal intensity (Fig. 3-19).[38] Involvement of the uterine body usually produces diffuse enlargement, often with a lobular contour similar to a fibroid. Characteristically,

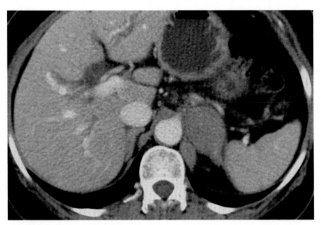

FIGURE 3-20 ■ Adrenal lymphoma. Contrast-enhanced CT showing a large homogeneous left adrenal mass. Note biliary obstruction which was secondary to a mass in the duodenum and head of the pancreas (same patient as that described in the legend to Fig. 3-14).

the mucosa and underlying junctional zone are intact. Primary uterine lymphoma has a good prognosis and MRI can demonstrate complete resolution after treatment. Primary ovarian lymphoma, by contrast, has a very poor prognosis as it often presents late and disease is frequently bilateral. It is less common than uterine lymphoma. The usual pathological subtypes are DLBCL or BL. Imaging appearances are identical to those of ovarian carcinoma, although haemorrhage, necrosis and calcification are relatively rare.

Adrenal Glands

Primary adrenal lymphoma is extremely rare, usually occurring in men over the age of 60. Secondary involvement of the adrenals is detected in about 6% of patients undergoing routine abdominal staging CT, usually in the presence of widespread retroperitoneal disease. Adrenal insufficiency is unusual, even with bilateral disease. The appearance on cross-sectional imaging is indistinguishable from that of metastases (Fig. 3-20). Bilateral adrenal hyperplasia in the absence of metastatic involvement is also recognised.[39]

Musculoskeletal System

Involvement of the bone, bone marrow and skeletal muscles can occur in both HL and NHL. Bone and bone marrow are particularly important sites of disease relapse and any skeletal symptoms following previous treatment for lymphoma should always raise the suspicion of bone disease. Involvement of osseous bone does not necessarily imply bone marrow involvement and the two have different prognostic implications. Neither skeletal radiography nor isotope bone imaging have any predictive value in determining marrow involvement.

Bone Marrow

Since the bone marrow is an integral part of the reticuloendothelial system, lymphoma may arise within the marrow as true primary disease, which is then categorised as stage IE disease. More often, however, the marrow is involved as part of a disseminated process, when it is categorised as stage IV disease. In NHL, marrow involvement is present in 20–40% of patients at presentation and is associated with a poorer prognosis than liver or lung involvement. Bone marrow biopsy is therefore included in the staging of NHL and will increase the stage in up to 30% of cases, usually from stage III to stage IV.[40] In FL infiltration is often paratrabecular rather than diffuse, whereas in high-grade NHL the marrow is more likely to be affected focally; hence the increased incidence of marrow positivity with bilateral iliac crest biopsies. In HL, marrow involvement at presentation is rare but will develop during the course of the disease in 5–15% of patients. Bone marrow biopsy, therefore, is not considered necessary as part of the initial staging of patients with clinical early-stage HL.

Magnetic resonance imaging is extremely sensitive in detecting bone marrow involvement, involved areas having low signal intensity on T1-weighted images and high signal on STIR sequences; T1-weighted sequences are the most sensitive.[41] It can upstage as many as 30% of patients with negative iliac crest biopsies and a positive MRI study appears to confer a poorer prognosis regardless of bone marrow biopsy status. Whole-body diffusion-weighted imaging with background suppression (DWIBS) can be used to stage and monitor treatment,[11] though limited availability has precluded widespread adoption of this technique in the UK.

FDG-PET is moderately sensitive for bone marrow involvement at presentation,[42] upstaging a similar proportion of patients as MRI when compared to bone marrow biopsy. However, as with MRI, false-negative studies occur especially with microscopic infiltration (under 5%) and low-grade lymphoma which is FDG-PET negative elsewhere.[43] On the other hand, diffuse or heterogeneously increased uptake in a pretreatment image may indicate reactive marrow hyperplasia rather than infiltration. FDG-PET/CT can also be used to assess treatment response, though reactive marrow hyperplasia can limit specificity, especially where granulocyte colony stimulating factors have been administered. Neither MRI nor FDG-PET can replace histological examination of the bone marrow, firstly because of their relatively low negative predictive value (NPV) and secondly because composite lymphomas are not infrequent.

Bone

True primary lymphoma of bone is nearly all NHL and accounts for almost 1% of all NHL and 5% of extranodal lymphoma. The criteria for the diagnosis of primary lymphoma of bone require that:
- only a single bone is involved;
- there is unequivocal histological evidence of lymphoma;
- other disease is limited to regional areas at the time of presentation; and
- the primary tumour precedes metastases by at least 6 months.

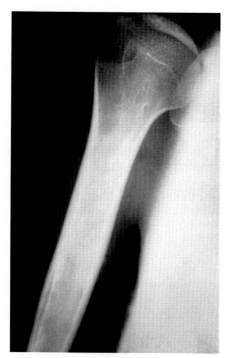

FIGURE 3-21 ■ **Primary non-Hodgkin's lymphoma of bone.** Plain radiograph of the humerus of a 14-year-old child showing a poorly defined sclerotic lesion in the proximal humerus. Further investigation revealed no other sites of lymphomatous disease.

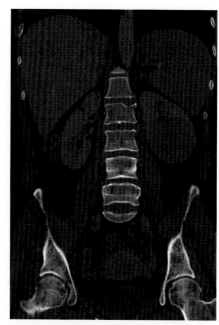

FIGURE 3-22 ■ **Non-Hodgkin's lymphoma of bone.** Coronal CT on bone settings (same patient as that described in the legend to Fig. 3-16) showing multiple lytic lesions throughout the visualised skeleton with pathological fractures in a right rib, L2 and the right iliac blade.

The diagnosis of true primary bone lymphoma is made less often than in the past, probably because better imaging has allowed detection of synchronous disease elsewhere, indicating that the apparent 'primary' osseous involvement is in fact secondary. This is particularly the case in children. The median age at presentation is 40–50 years with a slight male predominance and usually occurs in the pelvis or appendicular skeleton, involving the femur, tibia and humerus in descending order of frequency.[44]

Infiltration of bone can also occur secondarily by direct invasion from adjacent soft-tissue masses. Radiographic evidence of secondary bone involvement is present during the course of the disease in 20% of patients with HL, appearing in 4% at initial presentation. Secondary involvement of bone is present in 5–6% of patients with NHL, although it is more frequent in children with NHL.[23] The axial skeleton is much more commonly affected than the appendicular skeleton.

Whether primary or secondary, bone lesions in NHL are permeative and osteolytic in just under 80% of cases, sclerotic in only 4% and mixed in 16% (Fig. 3-21).[45] By comparison, HL typically gives sclerotic or mixed sclerotic and lytic lesions (86%) and is far less frequently lytic (14% of cases). In HL, most lesions are found in the skull, the spine and the femora. The classic finding is the sclerotic 'ivory' vertebra. Nevertheless, radiographically, primary and secondary NHL, HL and other bone tumours (such as Ewing's sarcoma and other small round cell tumours) may be indistinguishable. Soft-tissue disease typically may involve adjacent bones; anterior mediastinal and paravertebral masses not infrequently involve the

sternum and vertebrae, respectively, resulting in scalloping or destruction.

CT will often demonstrate bony disease if there is a prominent lytic or sclerotic process (Fig. 3-22). Screening for bone involvement is reserved for patients with specific complaints. Radionuclide radiology has a sensitivity of close to 95% in the detection of bone involvement, but is of limited value compared with FDG-PET or PET/CT. MRI depicts primary bone lymphoma in exquisite anatomical detail (Fig. 3-23), and is the method of choice in local staging of primary bone lymphoma,[46] often demonstrating a greater extent of associated extraosseous involvement and degree of marrow infiltration. It is also of value in the assessment of response to treatment, but there is some evidence that FDG-PET can demonstrate response to treatment earlier and more accurately than conventional techniques including MRI.[47]

Central Nervous System

Primary

Primary CNS lymphoma (PCNSL) is restricted to the cranio-spinal axis, with no evidence of systemic disease and is nearly always intracranial. It increased dramatically in incidence in the 1990s, and accounts for over 3% of all primary brain tumours and up to nearly 30% of cases of NHL in some series. The increase in younger adults can be explained by the association with AIDS and iatrogenic immunosuppression and until the advent of highly active antiretroviral therapy up to 6% of patients with AIDS could be expected to develop PCNSL during the course of the disease. However, the incidence is also rising steadily in the over 60 year olds, for reasons

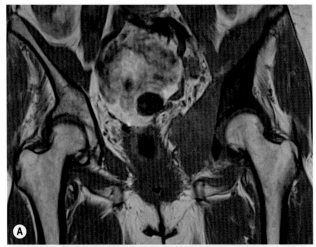

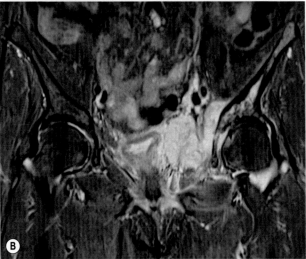

FIGURE 3-23 ■ **Non-Hodgkin's lymphoma of bone.** Coronal T1-weighted (A) and STIR (B) images of a patient with NHL of the left hemipelvis involving the adjacent obturator internus muscle and bladder. There is extensive involvement of the left hemipelvis manifest as low T1 and high T2 signal. Note exquisite depiction of the extent of bony and soft-tissue involvement with this combination of sequences.

masses are typically isointense on T1- and T2-weighted sequences. As at CT, there is homogeneous enhancement after the administration of gadolinium-DTPA (Fig. 3-23), though atypical forms with rim enhancement can occur with AIDS-related PCNSL.[51]

Secondary

Secondary CNS involvement is exceptionally rare in HL but occurs during the course of the disease in 10–15% of patients with NHL. Certain groups are known to be at risk: those with stage IV disease, testicular or ovarian presentation; those with high-grade histology (lymphoblastic and immunoblastic histologies) and also BL. Although intra-axial masses do occur, appearing identical to primary forms, secondary involvement much more commonly involves the extracerebral spaces (epidural, subdural and subarachnoid) as well as the spinal epidural and subarachnoid spaces. Presentation with cranial nerve palsies is common. MRI with intravenous injection of gadolinium-based contrast medium is superior to CT in the detection of such subdural and leptomeningeal disease, which is seen as enhancing plaques over the cerebral convexities and around the basal meninges.[52]

Contrast-enhanced MRI can also demonstrate spinal leptomeningeal disease, but there is a significant false-negative rate, higher than that for leptomeningeal carcinomatosis.[53] Disease in the spinal epidural space can cause spinal cord compression and cauda equina syndromes. This is a late manifestation of HL, but can be the presenting feature of NHL (Fig. 3-25). Epidural extension of tumour into the spinal canal from a paravertebral mass is the commonest cause, resulting in a so-called 'dumb-bell' tumour. The dura itself usually acts as an effective barrier to the intrathecal spread of tumour, and disease may be limited to the neural foramen. Less commonly, vertebral involvement results in epidural spread and extrinsic compression of the theca. Though all these patterns of epidural spread can occasionally be depicted at CT, subtle disease is readily missed unless actively sought and is much better demonstrated by MRI.

Orbit

Primary orbital lymphomas are nearly all NHL, which constitutes the most common primary orbital malignancy in adults, accounting for 10–15% of orbital masses and 4% of all primary extranodal NHL. They occur most commonly in patients between 40 and 70 years of age and typically present as a slow-growing, diffusely infiltrative tumour for which the main differential diagnosis is from the non-malignant condition, orbital pseudotumour. Secondary orbital involvement occurs in approximately 3.5–5.0% of both HL and NHL. Any component of the orbit can be involved and in both the primary and secondary forms, the clinical manifestations will depend on the site of involvement. Retrobulbar lymphoma infiltrates around and through the extraocular muscles, causing proptosis and ophthalmoplegia, but rarely disturbing visual acuity. Lacrimal gland involvement displaces the globe downwards and is bilateral in 20% of cases. Bilaterality does not appear to alter prognosis, which is generally good in

unknown. Peak incidence is in the fifth and sixth decades. Presentation is that of an intracranial space-occupying lesion or personality changes, as the lesions are often frontal.[48] Fits are rare, but are reported.

More than 50% of tumours occur within the cerebral white matter, close to or within the corpus callosum[49] and often abutting the ependyma. A butterfly distribution with spread across the corpus callosum is a typical finding. The deep grey matter of the thalamus and basal ganglia is affected in about 15% (Fig. 3-24). Only approximately 10% arise in the posterior fossa, usually near the midline. In about 15% of cases the disease is multifocal, though the incidence of multifocality is much higher in AIDS-related PCNSL.

Up to 70% of tumour masses are typically isodense or hyperdense on unenhanced CT and in 90% of cases, enhance homogeneously[49] (Fig. 3-24). Calcification virtually never occurs and there is relatively little surrounding vasogenic oedema or mass effect.[50] On MRI, the

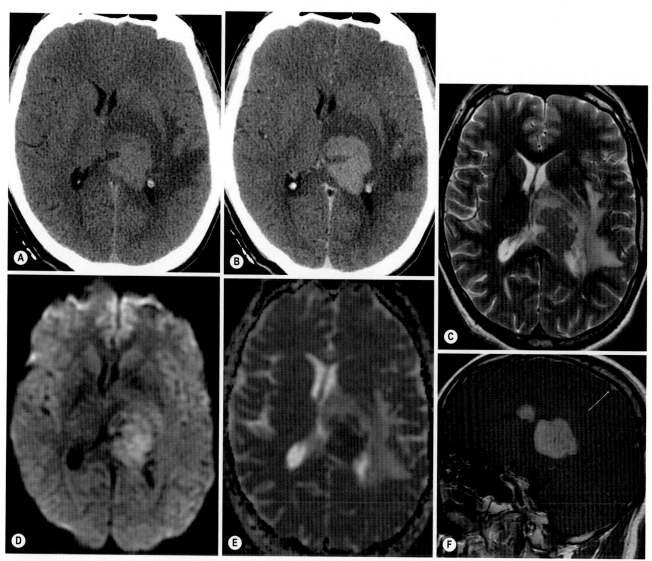

FIGURE 3-24 ■ **Cerebral non-Hodgkin's lymphoma.** (A) Unenhanced axial CT showing a hyperdense mass in the left thalamus extending into the splenium of the corpus callosum. (B) Post-contrast image demonstrating uniform enhancement of the mass. (C) Axial T2-weighted MRI image demonstrating the typical location of the lymphomatous mass and moderate surrounding vasogenic oedema. (D, E) Diffusion-weighted image (b800) and ADC map showing restriction of diffusion within the mass. (F) Sagittal T1-weighted MRI image post-intravenous gadolinium demonstrates a second intraventricular mass and dural involvement (arrow).

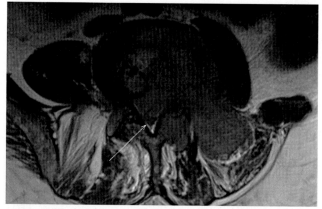

FIGURE 3-25 ■ **Epidural lymphoma.** T2-weighted axial MRI showing a mass of intermediate-to-high signal intensity in the paravertebral soft tissues, extending into the vertebral body and into the spinal canal as well as the paraspinal musculature. The mass is displacing and compressing the theca (arrowed).

all the primary forms. MALT lymphomas of the lacrimal glands can present as a mass or periorbital swelling. CT and MRI depict uni- or bilateral enhancing masses with a non-specific appearance. In patients with an orbital lymphomatous mass, about half will be found to have an extracentral nervous system primary site of origin. MRI best depicts the extent of disease and the presence, if any, of intracranial extension.

Head and Neck Lymphoma

Although HL typically involves the cervical lymph nodes as the presenting feature, true extranodal involvement of sites in the head and neck region with HL is rare. In contrast, 10% of patients with NHL present with extranodal head and neck involvement. About half of these will prove to have disseminated lymphoma. Extranodal NHL accounts for approximately 5% of head and neck cancers.

Waldeyer's Ring

Waldeyer's ring comprises lymphoid tissue in the nasopharynx, oropharynx, the faucial and palatine tonsil and the lingual tonsil. It is the commonest site of head and neck lymphoma and there is a close link with involvement of the gastrointestinal tract, either synchronous or metachronous, possibly reflecting the fact that up to 20% of these NHL are the MALT type. Accordingly some centres include endoscopy as well as whole-body cross-sectional imaging as part of staging, since up to 30% of patients will have advanced disease at presentation. The tonsils are most commonly affected, the commonest pattern being asymmetrical thickening of the pharyngeal mucosa, which is well shown by CT and MRI. A diagnosis of NHL is suggested by circumferential involvement or multifocality. Secondary invasion from adjacent nodal masses is also common.

NHL comprises 8% of tumours of the paranasal sinuses. In the West, the disease affects middle-aged men and the maxillary sinus is most commonly involved, commonly by DLBCL, whereas the aggressive diffuse T-cell type (that forms part of the 'lethal midline granuloma' syndrome) typically affects younger Asians and is linked to EBV. Paranasal sinus involvement often presents with acute facial swelling and pain, and disease often spreads from one sinus to the other in a contiguous fashion, though bony destruction is considerably less marked than in squamous cell carcinomas. These tumours are locally aggressive; spread through the skull base into the cranium is seen in up to 40%. Thus prophylactic intrathecal chemotherapy is often administered. MRI is the preferred imaging technique for evaluating head and neck lymphoma. Multiplanar fat-suppressed T1-weighted images pre-and post-intravenous gadolinium-based contrast medium are the most helpful in defining the full extent of disease and depicting tumour spread into the cranial cavity from the infratemporal fossa and skull base foramina.

Salivary Glands

All the salivary glands may be involved in lymphoma but the parotid gland is most frequently affected, usually by MALT lymphoma. Single or multiple well-defined masses are seen, which are of higher density than the surrounding gland on CT, hypoechoic on ultrasound and of intermediate signal intensity on T1- and T2-weighted MRI sequences. Many of the patients are middle-aged women and a history of Sjögren's disease is common.

Thyroid

NHL accounts for 2–5% of malignant tumours of the thyroid. MALT-type lymphomas arise in women in association with Hashimoto's disease. Presentation is with diffuse enlargement or large discrete nodules. However, DLBCL and anaplastic forms also occur, such patients presenting with a rapidly growing mass and obstructive symptoms. Direct spread of tumour beyond the gland and involvement of adjacent lymph nodes is common. At ultrasound these masses are relatively hypoechoic. At CT they usually have a lower attenuation than the normal gland and may show peripheral enhancement following injection of intravenous contrast medium.

MUCOSA-ASSOCIATED LYMPHOID TISSUE LYMPHOMAS

The MALT lymphomas arise from mucosal sites that normally have no organised lymphoid tissue, but within which acquired lymphoid tissue has arisen as a result of chronic inflammation or autoimmunity. Examples include Hashimoto's thyroiditis, Sjögren's syndrome and *Helicobacter*-induced chronic follicular gastritis. Patients with Sjögren's syndrome (lymphoepithelial sialadenitis) are at a 44-fold increased risk of developing lymphoma, of which over 80% are MALT type, and patients with Hashimoto's thyroiditis have a 3-fold increased risk of thyroid lymphoma. The histological hallmark of MALT lymphoma is the presence of lymphomatous cells in a marginal zone around reactive follicles, which can spread into the epithelium of glandular tissues to produce the characteristic lymphoepithelial lesion. In up to 30%, transformation to large cell lymphoma occurs.

Adults with a median age of 60 are most often affected, with a female preponderance. Most patients present with stage IE or IIE disease, which tends to be indolent. Bone marrow involvement is unusual (occurring in around 10%) but the frequency varies depending on the primary site. Multiple extranodal sites are involved in up to 25%, but this does not appear to have the same poor prognostic import as in other forms of NHL. Nonetheless, extensive staging investigations may be necessary.[54]

The commonest site of involvement is the gastrointestinal (GI) tract (50%) and within the GI tract, the stomach is most often affected (around 85% of cases) (Fig. 3-13). The small bowel and colon are involved in immunoproliferative small intestinal disease (IPSID), previously known as alpha-chain disease. Other sites commonly affected include the lung, head, neck, ocular adnexae, skin, thyroid and breast.

BURKITT'S LYMPHOMA

Burkitt's lymphoma (BL) is a highly aggressive B-cell variant of NHL, associated with EBV in a variable proportion of cases. Three clinical variants are recognised:
- Endemic (African) type
- Sporadic (non-endemic)
- Immunodeficiency associated.

Though these tumours are extremely aggressive and rapidly growing, they are potentially curable with intensive combination chemotherapy. They account for only 2–3% of NHL in immunocompetent adults, but 30–50% of all childhood lymphoma is BL. Immunodeficiency-associated BL is seen chiefly in association with HIV infection and may be the initial manifestation of AIDS. EBV is identified in up to 40% of cases. Extranodal disease is common and all three variants are at risk for CNS disease.

In the endemic form, the jaws and orbit are involved in 50% of cases, producing the 'floating tooth sign' on plain radiography. The ovaries, kidneys and breast may be involved. The sporadic forms have a predilection for the ileocaecal region and patients can present with acute abdominal emergencies such as intussusception (Fig. 3-14). Again, ovaries, kidneys and breasts are commonly involved. Retroperitoneal and paraspinal disease can cause paraplegia, the presenting feature in up to 15%. Disease is confined to the abdomen in approximately 50% of patients[55] and thoracic disease is relatively rare. Leptomeningeal disease can be seen at presentation, and as a site of relapse.

LYMPHOMA IN THE IMMUNOCOMPROMISED

The WHO classification recognises four broad groupings associated with an increased incidence of lymphoma and lymphoproliferative disorders:[3]
- lymphoproliferative diseases associated with primary immune disorders;
- lymphomas associated with HIV infection;
- post-transplant lymphoproliferative disorders; and
- other iatrogenic immunodeficiency-associated lymphoproliferative disorders.

The development of lymphoma in these settings is multifactorial, but mostly related to defective immune surveillance, with or without chronic antigenic stimulation.

Lymphomas Associated with HIV

The incidence of all subtypes of NHL is increased 60- to 200-fold in patients with HIV. However, the risk has declined markedly since the introduction of highly active antiretroviral therapy (HAART). Despite the lower risk with HAART, lymphoma is more often the first AIDS-defining illness. Prior to the advent of HAART, the incidence of PCNSL and BL was increased 1000-fold compared with the general population. Most are aggressive B-cell lymphomas and various types are seen, including those seen in immunocompetent patients, such as BL and DLBCL. Others occur much more frequently in the HIV population (e.g. primary effusion lymphoma and plasmablastic lymphoma of the oral cavity). The incidence of HL is also increased up to eightfold and has increased further since HAART was introduced. DLBCL tends to occur later, when CD4 counts are under $100 \times 10^{6-}$ L[1], whereas BL occurs in less immunodeficient patients. EBV positivity occurs in a variable proportion; PCNSL is associated with EBV in over 90% of cases and EBV positivity is seen in nearly all cases of HL associated with HIV.

Most tumours are aggressive, with advanced stage, bulky disease and a high serum LDH at presentation. Most have a marked propensity to involve extranodal sites, especially the GI tract, CNS (less frequent with the advent of highly active antiretroviral therapy), liver and bone marrow. Multiple sites of extranodal involvement are seen in over 75% of cases.[56] Peripheral lymph node enlargement is relatively uncommon.

In the chest, NHL is usually extranodal; pleural effusions and lung disease are common, with nodules, acinar and interstitial opacity being described. Hilar and mediastinal nodal enlargement is generally mild. There is a wide differential diagnosis and in one study the presence of cavitation, small nodules under 1 cm in diameter and nodal necrosis predicted for mycobacterial infection rather than lymphoma. Within the abdomen, the GI tract, liver, kidneys, adrenal glands and lower genitourinary tract are commonly involved. Mesenteric and retroperitoneal nodal enlargement is less common than in immunocompetent patients, but there are no real differences in the CT features of patients with or without AIDS.

Regarding PCNSL, certain features such as rim enhancement and multifocality are seen more often than in the immunocompetent population. This can cause confusion with cerebral toxoplasmosis, though the location of PCNSL in the deep white matter is suggestive. Quantitative FDG-PET uptake can help in the differentiation of PCNSL, toxoplasmosis and progressive multifocal leucoencephalopathy.

Post-transplant Lymphoproliferative Disorders

These occur in 2–4% of solid organ transplant recipients depending on the type of transplant, the lowest frequency being seen in renal transplant recipients (1%) and the highest in heart–lung or liver–bowel allografts (5%). Marrow allograft recipients are at low risk (1%). Most appear to represent EBV-induced monoclonal or, more rarely, polyclonal B- or T-cell proliferation as a consequence of immune suppression and reduced T-cell immune surveillance.[3] The clinical features are variable, correlating with the type of allograft and type of immunosuppression. PTLD develops earlier in patients receiving ciclosporin rather than azathioprine (mean interval 48 months). EBV-positive cases occur earlier than EBV-negative cases, the latter occurring 4–5 years after transplantation. In all cases, extranodal disease is disproportionately commoner, though CNS disease is rare. Involvement of the allograft itself is commoner in early-onset EBV-driven PTLD. In patients who have received ciclosporin, the GI tract is frequently affected. The bone marrow, liver and lung are often involved, with multiple intrapulmonary masses, pleural effusions, involvement of multiple segments of bowel and the transplanted organ all being reported.[57]

MONITORING RESPONSE TO THERAPY

Achievement of complete response after treatment is the most important factor for predicting prolonged survival in both HL and NHL. A complete response is designated when there is no clinical or radiological evidence of disease after treatment. Imaging plays a critical role in monitoring response and the advent of FDG-PET and FDG-PET/CT has resulted in a paradigm shift in response assessment in lymphoma. For large-volume intrathoracic disease, the chest radiograph remains useful

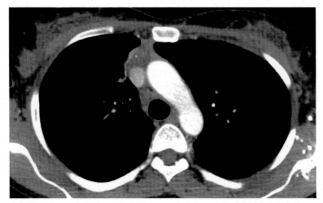

FIGURE 3-26 ■ **Thoracic residual mass in Hodgkin's lymphoma.** This is the same patient as that described in the legend to Fig. 3-3A. After treatment, follow-up CT at 6 months shows a residual anterior mediastinal mass; the right axillary lymph node has completely resolved. The mass has been stable for 2 years.

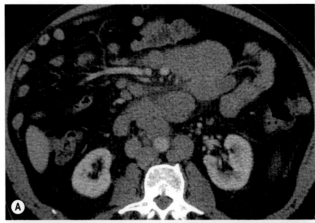

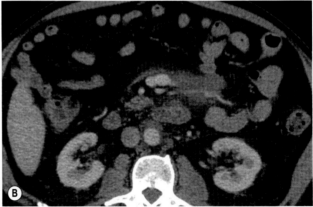

FIGURE 3-27 ■ **Mesenteric residual mass.** (A) Contrast-enhanced CT in a patient with NHL presenting with a large mesenteric nodal mass and bilateral para-aortic nodal disease. (B) Follow-up CT performed 1 year after treatment shows a persistent low-density soft-tissue mass within the mesentery encasing the mesenteric vessels, whilst the retroperitoneal nodal enlargement has resolved.

in assessing early response. However, changes due to radiotherapy, rebound thymic hyperplasia or thymic cyst formation make the mediastinum difficult to assess on a chest radiograph, particularly in children. Therefore, cross-sectional imaging is essential in final assessment of response in the chest, as well as the abdomen and pelvis (Figs. 3-26 and 3-27). Assessment of response requires the measurement of a number of marker lesions before, during and after therapy, for which the reproducibility and reliability of contrast medium-enhanced CT is a great advantage. Since there is significant interobserver variation in the measurement of masses, wherever possible well-defined regular masses above and below the diaphragm should be assessed.[58] Many centres favour an interim CT or FDG-PET/CT study after two cycles of chemotherapy for certain lymphomas, especially HL, and this is mandatory in many clinical trials. The optimal timing of final response assessment depends on the technique chosen and the availability of resources. Most centres assess patients with CT one month after completion of therapy, but if FDG-PET/CT is used, a longer interval is required (6–8 weeks for chemotherapy alone and 12 weeks if radiotherapy has been given).

Prognostication

Numerous studies have shown that an interim FDG-PET imaging yields much more prognostic information than CT alone, since FDG-PET can detect and quantify changes in functional/metabolic activity long before structural changes have taken place (Fig. 3-28). Interim FDG-PET also has a role to direct further treatment (escalation or de-escalation of treatment) and to avoid potential toxicity from an ineffective therapy. FDG-PET performed after one to three cycles of chemotherapy appears to predict progression-free and overall survival in 'aggressive' NHL more accurately than PET at the end of treatment and more accurately than conventional imaging.[59,60] The same is true of HL,[61,62] even after only one cycle of chemotherapy.[63] A large body of evidence shows that the NPV of the test exceeds 80% in patients

with aggressive NHL and 90% in patients with HL. In one multicentre study of patients with HL, the 2-year progression-free survival for interim PET-negative and -positive patients was 95% and 12%, respectively.[62] This suggests that early FDG-PET imaging could allow response-adapted modification of treatment, but it is as yet unknown whether this will translate into overall survival benefits. There are currently five ongoing trials evaluating de-escalation of therapy in early responders with limited-stage HL (for example, the RAPID trial, a quality-assured multicentre trial designed to establish whether interim PET can identify early responders, who may not require radiotherapy).[64] For NHL, the data are more heterogeneous, and therefore interim imaging is only recommended in the context of clinical trials.

It is recommended that the time from chemotherapy to imaging should be as close as possible to the next cycle to reduce the risk of false-negative results due to the 'tumour stunning'. Various response criteria have been proposed for interim PET images, including a category of 'minimal residual uptake' (MRU) lower or equal to that in the liver, but a semi-quantitative standardised uptake value approach may be more useful.[65]

Response Criteria

Standardised response criteria are essential for clinical research and comparison of different therapies. In 1999, a report set out standardised international criteria for assessment of response in NHL, similar to those already in use for HL.[66] The International Working Group (IWG) radiological criteria are essentially morphological and are as follows.

Complete Remission (CR)

- Complete disappearance of all radiological evidence of disease.

- All nodal masses to have decreased to normal: (A) < 1.5 cm in greatest transverse diameter for nodes that were > 1.5 cm pretherapy; (B) nodes initially between 1 and 1.5 cm must have decreased to 1 cm or less.
- The spleen, if previously enlarged on CT, must be normal in size and any focal deposits should have resolved.

Complete Remission, Unconfirmed (CR$_u$)

- A residual mass > 1.5 cm short-axis diameter (SAD) which has regressed by more than 75% of the sum of the products of the greatest diameters (SPD) of the original mass.

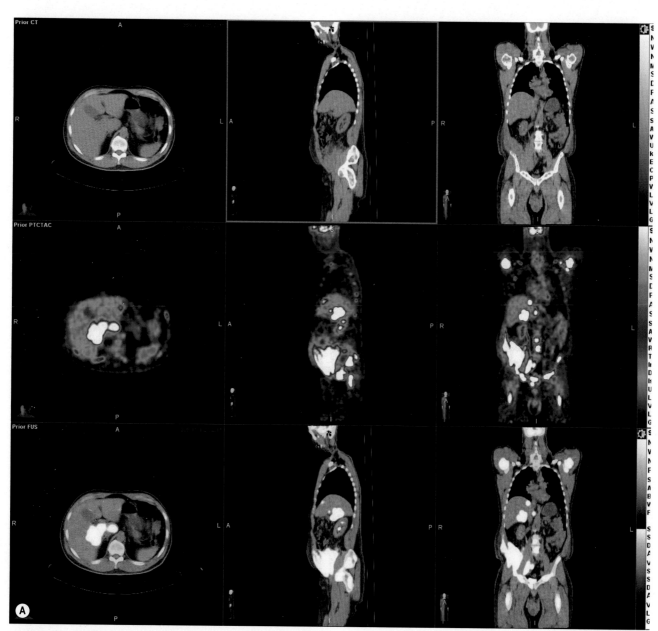

FIGURE 3-28 ■ **PET/CT in interim response assessment.** (A) Initial staging PET/CT in a patient with stage IVB DLBCL. Unenhanced CT, PET and fused images demonstrate extensive bony disease, a large confluent nodal mass in the right hemipelvis and hepatic involvement.

Continued on following page

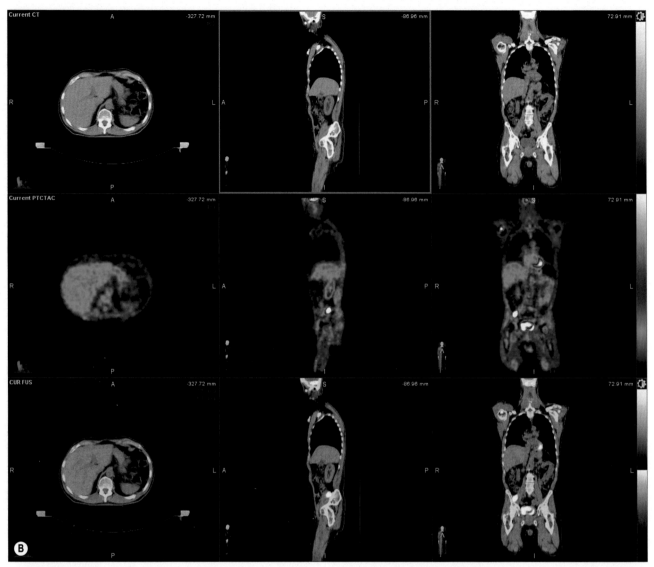

FIGURE 3-28, Continued ■ (B) After two cycles of CHOP-R, there has been a marked response to treatment with resolution of the disease in the liver and the right hemipelvis. Some osseous disease persists, especially in the right humerus (SUV reduced from 16.8 pretreatment to 10.5).

Partial Response (PR)

- > 50% decrease in the SPD of largest nodes/masses.
- No increase in size of spleen, liver or lymph nodes.
- Splenic or hepatic nodules decreased by 50%.

Stable Disease (SD)

- No evidence of progressive disease.
- Decrease in SPD less than 50%.

Progressive Disease (PD)

- ≥50% increase from nadir in the SPD of an established node/mass.
- Appearance of a new lesion during or at the end of therapy.

Residual Masses

Successfully treated, enlarged nodes often return to normal size in both HL and NHL. However, a residual mass of fibrous tissue can persist in up to 80% of patients treated for HL (usually within the mediastinum) and 20–60% of patients with NHL[30,67] who are in clinical CR (Figs. 3-26, 3-27 and 3-29). Residual masses occur more frequently in patients with bulky disease but how often such masses lead to relapse is uncertain. Until the advent of FDG-PET, determination of the nature of a residual mass was a major challenge in oncological radiology.

Computed Tomography

CT cannot distinguish between fibrotic tissue and residual active disease on the basis of density or size; hence the consistently low specificity and positive predictive

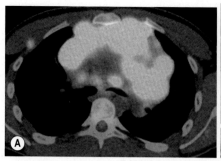 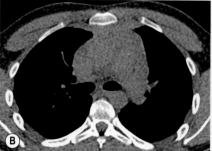 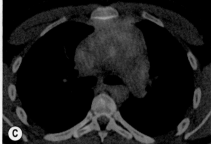

FIGURE 3-29 ■ **PET in assessment of the residual mass.** (A) Fused PET/CT image demonstrating a large metabolically active anterior/middle mediastinal mass and metabolically active but normal-sized right subpectoral lymph node. (B) Post-treatment CT shows a residual anterior mediastinal mass. (C) The mass has normal levels of FDG uptake, identical to that of the remainder of the mediastinum (a metabolic CR by the IHP criteria).

value (PPV) of CT after treatment in determining the likelihood of relapse in the presence of a residual mass. Until recently, serial CT every 2–3 months was used and masses that remained stable for 1 year were considered inactive.

MRI

MRI may help to differentiate active tumour from a fibrotic mass. Most tumours have high T2-signal intensity, which diminishes in response to treatment. Persistent heterogeneous or recurrent high T2 signal suggests residual or recurrent disease, respectively. However, small foci of tumour can persist undetected within a residual mass; hence the fairly low sensitivity of MRI. In addition, false-positive studies are common, especially soon after treatment because of non-specific inflammation and necrosis. Evidence for the value of diffusion-weighted imaging and measurement of the apparent diffusion coefficient (ADC) is not compelling at present.

Functional Imaging

Although gallium–67 scintigraphy is a far better predictor of disease relapse in patients with a residual mass than CT alone, it has many drawbacks. Thus it has been superseded by FDG-PET. At the end of treatment, FDG-PET has a very high PPV for early relapse, with or without a residual mass at CT.[68–70] However, false-negative and false-positive images occur. Recent evidence suggests that the PPV of FDG-PET may be lower in patients treated with rituximab.[71] Therefore, clinical correlation is essential when interpreting FDG-PET results.[72]

FDG-PET in Response Assessment

FDG-PET is more accurate than CT in response assessment, with a PPV at least double that of CT. In one follow-up study, all PET-positive/CT-negative patients relapsed, whereas only 5% of PET-negative/CT-positive patients relapsed[73] (Fig. 3-29). The few studies directly comparing FDG-PET and gallium–67 suggest that FDG-PET is more sensitive and has a greater overall accuracy.[74] However, it should be recognised that FDG-PET predicts for early relapse and that false-negative studies do occur with late relapse.

The profound impact of PET on the IWG criteria was first evaluated by Juweid et al. in a retrospective analysis of 54 patients with aggressive NHL who underwent PET and CT after completion of treatment.[75] Patients with a PR by standard IWC who were PET-negative did as well as those who were in CR by IWC and IWC + PET, indicating superior discriminative ability with FDG-PET. As a result of such studies, an International Harmonisation Project was convened to revise the IWC criteria.[76] These guidelines support the use of FDG-PET for end-of-therapy response assessment in DLBCL and HL, but not for other NHL, unless the CR rate is a primary endpoint of a clinical trial. In the revised criteria, patients with any residual mass can be assigned to the CR category provided that it is FDG-PET negative at the end of treatment and was (or can reasonably be expected to have been) PET positive before treatment. The CR$_u$ category is eliminated. A PR exists when there is residual FDG-PET positivity in at least one previously involved site.

The group has also issued guidance on timing, performance and interpretation of FDG-PET images.[77] Specifically, simple visual assessment of tracer uptake is deemed sufficient and it is not necessary to measure the standardised uptake value (SUV) or utilise cut-off values. Mediastinal blood pool activity is recommended as the reference background activity to define PET positivity for a residual mass ≥ 2 cm in greatest transverse diameter, regardless of its location. A smaller residual mass or a normal-sized lymph node should be considered positive if its activity is above that of the surrounding background.[77] Imaging should be performed at least 3 weeks and preferably at 6 to 8 weeks after completion of chemotherapy or chemoimmunotherapy, and 8 to 12 weeks after radiation or chemoradiotherapy. FDG-PET is also extremely useful in prognostication for patients about to undergo high-dose treatment and autologous stem cell transplantation.[78] Patients commencing high-dose therapy with a positive pre-treatment PET image have a much poorer prognosis.

SURVEILLANCE AND DETECTION OF RELAPSE

Relapse after satisfactory response to initial treatment occurs in 10–40% of patients with HL and approximately

50% of patients with NHL. In HL, relapse usually occurs within the first 2 years after treatment and patients are followed up closely during this period, although CT is not required unless clinical features suggest the possibility of recurrence.

For patients who attain a CR, there is very little evidence for routine surveillance with imaging. A number of studies have shown that relapse is rarely identified by conventional imaging before patients become symptomatic.[79–82] Functional imaging is able to identify early relapse before CT and, indeed, before the development of clinical signs. However, there is as yet little evidence for the efficacy of FDG-PET in this role. In one series of a cohort of patients treated for HL, relapses were identified by FDG-PET before there was any other evidence of relapse[83] but the false-positive rate was high. In another study it was concluded that there was no benefit from surveillance studies for HL or aggressive NHL beyond 18 months.[84] In these and other studies, true positive images in the absence of clinical suspicion of relapse were rare. On the other hand, in suspected relapse, the development of a positive PET image is highly suggestive and in this situation PET-CT is likely to have a significant therapeutic impact, allowing image-guided biopsies which can target the most metabolically active lesion and thereby direct therapy by establishing relapse or transformation.[6]

CONCLUSION

Management of patients with lymphoma depends heavily on the imaging findings, which are vital in initial staging of the disease, prognostication and monitoring response to treatment. The radiologist needs to understand the fundamental aspects of tumour behaviour and must appreciate the factors that will influence therapy. The radiological report should document the number of sites of nodal disease; the presence and sites of bulky disease; the presence of any extranodal disease; and factors which may influence delivery of therapy, such as central venous thrombosis or hydronephrosis. FDG-PET/CT has revolutionised the imaging of lymphoma, providing unprecedented insight into the functional behaviour of this diverse group of tumours, but further research is needed to establish the precise roles of PET and PET/CT and their place in the investigative algorithm. For all of these reasons, the radiologist has become a pivotal member of the multidisciplinary team managing patients with lymphoma.

REFERENCES

1. Cancer incidence—UK statistics. Cancer Research UK. Available at <http://info.cancerresearchuk.org/cancerstats/incidence/>. Accessed March 2012.
2. Harris NL, Jaffe ES, Stein H, et al. A revised European–American classification of lymphoid neoplasms: a proposal from the International Lymphoma Study Group. Blood 1994;84:1361–92.
3. Swerdlow SH, Campo E, Harris NL, et al, editors. World Health Organization Classification of Tumours of Haematopoietic and Lymphoid Tissues. 4th ed. Lyon: IARC Press; 2008.
4. Jaffe ES. The 2008 WHO classification of lymphomas: implications for clinical practice and translational research. Hematology Am Soc Hematol Educ Program 2009;523–31.
5. Lister TA, Crowther D, Sutcliffe SB, et al. Report of a committee convened to discuss the evaluation and staging of patients with Hodgkin's disease. J Clin Oncol 1989;7:1630–6.
6. Pappa VI, Hussain HK, Reznek RH, et al. The role of image-guided core needle biopsy in the management of patients with lymphoma. J Clin Oncol 1996;14:2427–30.
7. Shipp M, Harrington D, Anderson J, et al. Development of a predictive model for aggressive lymphoma: the international NHL prognostic factors project. N Engl J Med 1993;329:987–94.
8. Federico M, Bellei M, Marcheselli L, et al. Follicular lymphoma international prognostic index 2: a new prognostic index for follicular lymphoma developed by the international follicular lymphoma prognostic factor project. J Clin Oncol 2009;27:4555–62.
9. Callen PW, Korobkin M, Isherwood I. Computed tomography evaluation of the retrocrural prevertebral space. Am J Roentgenol 1997;129:907–10.
10. Vinnicombe S, Norman A, Nicolson V, Husband JE. Normal pelvic lymph nodes: documentation by CT scanning after bipedal lymphangiography. Radiology 1995;194:349–55.
11. Lin C, Luciani A, Itti E, et al. Whole-body diffusion magnetic resonance imaging in the assessment of lymphoma. Cancer Imaging 2012;12:403–8.
12. Moog F, Bangerter M, Diederichs CG, et al. Lymphoma: role of whole-body 2-deoxy-2-[F-18]fluoro-D-glucose (FDG) PET in nodal staging. Radiology 1997;203:795–800.
13. Moog F, Bangerter M, Diederichs CG, et al. Extranodal malignant lymphoma: detection with FDG-PET versus CT. Radiology 1998;206:475–81.
14. Bangerter M, Moog F, Buchmann I, et al. Whole-body 2-[^{18}F]-fluoro-2-deoxy-D-glucose positron emission tomography (FDG-PET) for accurate staging of Hodgkin's disease. Ann Oncol 1998;9:1117–22.
15. Kwee TC, Kwee RM, Nievelstein RA. Imaging in staging of malignant lymphoma: a systematic review. Blood 2008;111:504–16.
16. Chua SC, Rozalli FI, O'Connor SR. Imaging features of primary extranodal lymphomas. Clin Radiol 2009;64(6):574–88.
17. Rodríguez-Vigil B, Gómez-León N, Pinílla I, et al. PET/CT in lymphoma: prospective study of enhanced full-dose PET/CT versus unenhanced low-dose PET/CT. J Nucl Med 2006;47: 1643–8.
18. Elstrom R, Leonard J, Coleman M, et al. Combined PET and low dose, noncontrast CT scanning obviates the need for additional diagnostic contrast-enhanced CT scans in patients undergoing staging or restaging for lymphoma. Ann Oncol 2008;19:1770–3.
19. Castellino R, Blank N, Hoppe R, et al. Hodgkin's disease: contribution of chest CT in the initial staging evaluation. Radiology 1986;160:603–5.
20. Castellino R, Hilton S, O'Brien J, et al. Non-Hodgkin's lymphoma: contribution of chest CT in the initial staging evaluation. Radiology 1996;199:129–31.
21. Castellino RA, Marglin S, Blank N. Hodgkin's disease, the non-Hodgkin's lymphomas and the leukaemias in the retroperitoneum. Semin Roentgenol 1980;15:288–301.
22. Stomper PC, Cholewinski SP, Park J, et al. Abdominal staging of thoracic Hodgkin disease: CT-lymphangiography-Ga-67 scanning correlation. Radiology 1993;187:381–6.
23. Ng YY, Healy JC, Vincent JM, et al. The radiology of non-Hodgkin's lymphoma in childhood: a review of 80 cases. Clin Radiol 1994;49:594–600.
24. International Collaboration on HIV and Cancer. Highly active antiretroviral therapy and the incidence of cancer in human immunodeficiency virus-infected adults. J Natl Cancer Inst 2000; 92(22):1823–30.
25. Lee KS, Kim Y, Primack SL. Imaging of pulmonary lymphomas. Am J Roentgenol 1997;168:339–45.
26. Lewis ER, Caskey CI, Fishman EK. Lymphoma of the lung: CT findings in 31 patients. Am J Roentgenol 1991;156:711–14.
27. Shenkier T Connors J. Primary extranodal non-Hodgkin's lymphomas. In: Canellos G, Lister TA, Young B, editors. The Lymphomas. Philadelphia: Saunders Elsevier; 2006. pp. 339–41.
28. O'Donnell PG, Jackson SA, Tung KT, et al. Radiological appearances of lymphoma arising from mucosa associated lymphoid tissue (MALT) in the lung. Clin Radiol 1998;53:258–63.
29. Murray KA, Chor PJ, Turner JF. Intrathoracic lymphoproliferative disorders and lymphoma. Curr Probl Diagn Radiol 1996;25: 77–108.

30. Spiers AS, Husband JE, MacVicar AD. Treated thymic lymphoma: comparison of MR imaging with CT. Radiology 1997;203: 369–76.

31. Carlsen SE, Bergin CJ, Hoppe RT. MR imaging to detect chest wall and pleural involvement in patients with lymphoma: effect on radiation therapy planning. Am J Roentgenol 1993;160:1191–5.

32. Liberman L, Giess CS, Dershaw DD, et al. Non-Hodgkin lymphoma of the breast: imaging characteristics and correlation with histopathologic findings. Radiology 1994;192:157–60.

33. Rini JN, Manalili EY, Hoffman MA, et al. F-18 FDG versus Ga-67 for detecting splenic involvement in Hodgkin's disease. Clin Nucl Med 2002;27:572–7.

34. Brady LW, Asbell SO. Malignant lymphoma of the gastrointestinal tract. Radiology 1980;137:291–8.

35. Shirkhoda A, Ros PR, Farah J, et al. Lymphoma of the solid abdominal viscera. Radiol Clin North Am 1990;28:785–99.

36. Reznek RH, Mootoosamy I, Webb JA, et al. CT in renal and perirenal lymphoma: a further look. Clin Radiol 1990;42:233–8.

37. Aigen AB, Phillips M. Primary malignant lymphoma of the urinary bladder. Urology 1986;28:235–7.

38. Kim YS, Koh BH, Cho OK, et al. MR imaging of primary uterine lymphoma. Abdom Imaging 1997;22:441–4.

39. Vincent JM, Morrison ID, Armstrong P, et al. Non-metastatic enlargement of the adrenal glands in patients with malignant disease. Clin Radiol 1994;49:456–60.

40. Pond GD, Castellino RA, Horning S, et al. Non-Hodgkin's lymphoma: influence of lymphography, CT and bone marrow biopsy on staging and management. Radiology 1989;170: 159–64.

41. Yasumoto M, Nonomura Y, Yoshimura R, et al. MR detection of iliac bone marrow involvement by malignant lymphoma with various MR sequences including diffusion-weighted echo-planar imaging. Skeletal Radiol 2002;31:263–9.

42. Pakos EE, Fotopoulos AD, Ioannidis JP. 18F-FDG PET for evaluation of bone marrow infiltration in staging of lymphoma: a meta-analysis. J Nucl Med 2005;46(6):958–96.

43. Elstrom R, Guan L, Baker G, et al. Utility of FDG-PET scanning in lymphoma by WHO classification. Blood 2003;101(10): 3875–6.

44. Kim SY, Shin DY, Lee SS, et al. Clinical characteristics and outcomes of primary bone lymphoma in Korea. Korean J Haematol 2012;47:213–18.

45. Ngan H, Preston BJ. Non-Hodgkin's lymphoma presenting with osseous lesions. Clin Radiol 1975;26:351–6.

46. Stroszczynski C, Oellinger J, Hosten N, et al. Staging and monitoring of malignant lymphoma of the bone: comparison of ^{67}Ga scintigraphy and MRI. J Nucl Med 1999;40:387–93.

47. Park YH, Kim S, Choi SJ, et al. Clinical impact of whole-body FDG-PET for evaluation of response and therapeutic decision-making of primary lymphoma of bone. Ann Oncol 2005;16(8): 1401–2.

48. Bataille B, Delwail V, Menet E. Primary intracerebral malignant lymphoma: report of 248 cases. J Neurosurg 2001;92:261–6.

49. Erdag N, Bhorade R, Alberico R, et al. Primary lymphoma of the central nervous system. Am J Roentgenol 2001;176:1319–26.

50. Jenkins CN, Colquhoun IR. Characterization of primary intracranial lymphoma by computed tomography: an analysis of 36 cases and a review of the literature with particular reference to calcification haemorrhage and cyst formation. Clin Radiol 1998;53: 428–34.

51. Tang Y, Booth T, Bhogal P, et al. Imaging of primary central nervous system lymphoma. Clin Radiol 2011;66:768–77.

52. Chamberlain MC, Sandy AD, Press GA. Leptomeningeal metastasis: a comparison of gadolinium-enhanced MR and contrast-enhanced CT of the brain. Neurology 1990;40:435–8.

53. Yousem DM, Patrone PM, Grossman RI. Leptomeningeal metastases: MR evaluation. J Comput Assist Tomogr 1990;14: 255–61.

54. Raderer M, Vorbeck F, Formanek M, et al. Importance of extensive staging in patients with mucosa-associated lymphoid tissue (MALT)-type lymphoma. Br J Cancer 2000;83:454–7.

55. Johnson KA, Tung K, Mead G, et al. The imaging of Burkitt's and Burkitt-like lymphoma. Clin Radiol 1998;53:835–41.

56. Radin DR, Esplin JA, Levine AM, et al. AIDS-related non-Hodgkin's lymphoma: abdominal CT findings in 112 patients. Am J Roentgenol 1993;160:1133–9.

57. Pickhardt PJ, Siegel MJ. Abdominal manifestations of posttransplantation lymphoproliferative disorder. Am J Roentgenol 1998; 171:1007–13.

58. Hopper KD, Kasales CJ, Van Slyke MA, et al. Analysis of interobserver and intraobserver variability in CT tumor measurements. Am J Roentgenol 1996;167:851–4.

59. Spaepen K, Stroobants S, Dupont P, et al. Early restaging positron emission tomography with (18)F-fluorodeoxyglucose predicts outcome in patients with aggressive non-Hodgkin's lymphoma. Ann Oncol 2002;13:1356–63.

60. Haioun C, Itti E, Rahmouni A, et al. [18F]fluoro-2-deoxy-D-glucose positron emission tomography (FDG-PET) in aggressive lymphoma: an early prognostic tool for predicting patient outcome. Blood 2005;106(4):1376–81.

61. Hutchings M, Loft A, Hansen M, et al. FDG-PET after two cycles of chemotherapy predicts treatment failure and progression-free survival in Hodgkin lymphoma. Blood 2006;107(1):52–9.

62. Gallamini A, Hutchings M, Rigacci L, et al. Early interim 2-[18F] fluoro-2-deoxy-D-glucose positron emission tomography is prognostically superior to international prognostic score in advanced-stage Hodgkin's lymphoma: a report from a joint Italian-Danish study. J Clin Oncol 2007;25(24):3746–52.

63. Kostakoglu L, Goldsmith SJ, Leonard JP, et al. FDG-PET after 1 cycle of therapy predicts outcome in diffuse large cell lymphoma and classic Hodgkin disease. Cancer 2006;107(11):2678–87.

64. Barrington SF, Mackewn JE, Schleyer P, et al. Establishment of a UK-wide network to facilitate the acquisition of quality assured FDG-PET data for clinical trials in lymphoma. Ann Oncol 2011;22:739–45.

65. Lin C, Itti E, Haioun C, et al. Early 18F-FDG PET for prediction of prognosis in patients with diffuse large B-cell lymphoma: SUV-based assessment versus visual analysis. J Nucl Med 2007;48: 1626–32.

66. Cheson BD, Horning SJ, Coiffier B, et al. Report of an international workshop to standardize response criteria in non-Hodgkin's lymphoma. J Clin Oncol 1999;17:1244–53.

67. Surbone A, Longo DL, de Vitra VT, et al. Residual abdominal masses in aggressive non-Hodgkin's lymphoma after combination chemotherapy: significance and management. J Clin Oncol 1988; 6:1832–7.

68. Jerusalem G, Beguin Y, Fassotte MF, et al. Whole-body positron emission tomography using ^{18}F-fluorodeoxyglucose for post-treatment evaluation in Hodgkin's disease and non-Hodgkin's lymphoma has higher diagnostic and prognostic value than classical computed tomography scan imaging. Blood 1999;94:429–33.

69. Naumann R, Vaic A, Beuthien-Baumann B, et al. Prognostic value of positron emission tomography in the evaluation of post-treatment residual mass in patients with Hodgkin's disease and non-Hodgkin's lymphoma. Br J Haematol 2001;115:793–800.

70. Weihrauch MR, Re D, Scheidhauer K, et al. Thoracic positron emission tomography using ^{18}F-fluorodeoxyglucose for the evaluation of residual mediastinal Hodgkin disease. Blood 2001;98: 2930–4.

71. Han HS, Escalon MP, Hsiao B, et al. High incidence of false positive PET scans in patients with aggressive non-Hodgkin's lymphoma treated with rituximab-containing regimens. Ann Oncol 2009;20:309–18.

72. Bakheet SM, Powe J. Benign causes of 18-FDG uptake on whole body imaging. Semin Nucl Med 1998;28:352–8.

73. Zinzani PL, Chierichetti F, Zompatori M, et al. Advantages of positron emission tomography (PET) with respect to computed tomography in the follow-up of lymphoma patients with abdominal presentation. Leuk Lymphoma 2002;43:1239–43.

74. Van Den Bosche B, Lambert B, De Winter F, et al. ^{18}FDG-PET versus high-dose ^{67}Ga scintigraphy for restaging and treatment follow-up of lymphoma patients. Nucl Med Commun 2002;23: 1079–83.

75. Juweid M, Wiseman GA, Vose J, et al. Response assessment of aggressive non-Hodgkin's lymphoma by integrated International Workshop Criteria and fluorine-18-fluorodeoxyglucose positron emission tomography. J Clin Oncol 2005;23:4652–61.

76. Cheson BD, Pfistner B, Juweid ME, et al. Revised response criteria for malignant lymphoma. J Clin Oncol 2007;25:579–86.

77. Juweid ME, Stroobants S, Hoekstra OS, et al. Use of positron emission tomography for response assessment of lymphoma:

consensus of the Imaging Subcommittee of International Harmonization Project in Lymphoma. J Clin Oncol 2007;25:571–8.

78. Becherer A, Mitterbauer M, Jaeger U, et al. Positron emission tomography with [^{18}F]2-fluoro-D-2-deoxyglucose (FDG-PET) predicts relapse of malignant lymphoma after high-dose therapy with stem cell transplantation. Leukemia 2002;16:260–7.

79. Weeks JC, Yeap BY, Canellos GP, et al. Value of follow-up procedures in patients with large-cell lymphoma who achieve a complete remission. J Clin Oncol 1991;9:1196–203.

80. Guadagnolo BA, Punglia RS, Kuntz KM, et al. Cost-effectiveness analysis of computerized tomography in the routine follow-up of patients after primary treatment for Hodgkin's disease. J Clin Oncol 2006;24:4116–22.

81. Radford JA, Eardley A, Woodman C, et al. Follow up policy after treatment for Hodgkin's disease: too many clinic visits and routine tests? A review of hospital records. Br Med J 1997;314: 343–6.

82. Elis A, Blickstein D, Klein O, et al. Detection of relapse in non-Hodgkin's lymphoma: role of routine follow-up studies. Am J Hematol 2002;69:41–4.

83. Jerusalem G, Beguin Y, Fassotte M, et al. Early detection of relapse by whole-body positron emission tomography in the follow-up of patients with Hodgkin's disease. Ann Oncol 2003;14:123–30.

84. Zinzani PL, Stefoni V, Ambrosini V, et al. FDG-PET in the serial assessment of patients with lymphoma in complete remission. Blood 2007;110:71 (abstr 216).

CHAPTER 4

BONE MARROW DISORDERS: HAEMATOLOGICAL NEOPLASMS

Asif Saifuddin

CHAPTER OUTLINE

Primary Myelofibrosis
Systemic Mastocytosis
Leukaemia
LYMPHOMA
Primary Lymphoma of Bone
Hodgkin's Lymphoma

Non-Hodgkin's Lymphoma
Burkitt's Lymphoma
PLASMA CELL DISORDERS
Plasmacytoma
Multiple Myeloma

Chapters 4 and 5 deal with a variety of blood-related disorders that have a major influence on imaging of the skeletal system. The 2008 World Health Organisation (WHO) classification of myeloproliferative neoplasms is complex and includes a variety of conditions of differing malignant potential.[1] Only those that have significant radiological manifestations in the skeletal system will be discussed.

PRIMARY MYELOFIBROSIS[2]

Primary myelofibrosis (PMF) is a myeloproliferative neoplasm characterised by stem cell-derived clonal myeloproliferation resulting in bone marrow fibrosis, anaemia, splenomegaly and extramedullary erythropoiesis. The diagnosis is based on bone marrow morphology, showing evidence of fibrosis, and is supported by a variety of genetic abnormalities.

Clinical Features

It affects men and women equally, with an age range of 20–80 years (median age 60 years). The disorder presents insidiously with weakness, dyspnoea and weight loss due to progressive obliteration of the marrow by fibrosis or bony sclerosis, which leads to a moderate normochromic normocytic anaemia. Extramedullary erythropoiesis takes place in the liver and spleen, which become enlarged in 72 and 94% of cases, respectively, but is also reported in lymph nodes, lung, choroid plexus, kidney, etc. The natural history is one of slow deterioration, with death typically occurring 2–3 years after diagnosis. Progression to leukaemia is also a feature.

Radiological Features[3]

Bone sclerosis is the major radiological finding, being evident in approximately 30–70% of cases. Typically, this is diffuse (Fig. 4-1) but occasionally patchy, occurring most often in the axial skeleton and metaphyses of the femur, humerus and tibia. Sclerosis is due to trabecular and endosteal new bone formation, resulting in reduced marrow diameter. In established disease, lucent areas are due to fibrous tissue reaction. Periosteal reaction occurs in one-third of cases, most often in the medial aspects of the distal femur and proximal tibia. The skull may show a mixed sclerotic and lytic pattern.

MRI appearances vary depending upon the tissue contained in the marrow. Typically, the hyperintensity of marrow fat is replaced on both T1- and T2-weighted (T1W, T2W) sequences by hypointensity, which may be diffuse or heterogeneous (Fig. 4-2). Additional features include arthropathy due to haemarthrosis and secondary gout, occurring in 5–20% of cases. Also, infiltration of the synovium by bone marrow elements may result in polyarthralgia and polyarthritis. Leukaemic conversion may manifest radiologically by the development of an extraosseous soft-tissue mass (Fig. 4-3).

Radiological differentiation between other causes of increased bone density may be difficult, but the presence of anaemia and splenomegaly should suggest the diagnosis in this age group. Radiological differential diagnosis includes osteopetrosis, fluorosis, mastocytosis, carcinomatosis and adult sickle cell disease (SCD).

SYSTEMIC MASTOCYTOSIS[4]

Systemic mastocytosis represents a clonal disorder of mast cells, which is classified according to the WHO 2008 system into indolent mastocytosis, systemic mastocytosis with an associated haematological non-mast cell disorder, aggressive systemic mastocytosis and mast cell leukaemia. The majority of cases are associated with a pathological increase in the number of mast cells in both skin and extracutaneous tissues, although bone marrow involvement can occur without skin disease.

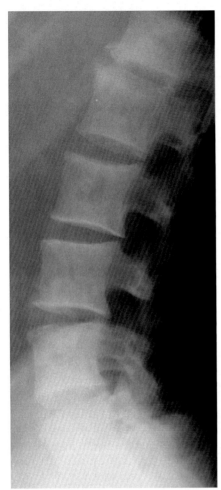

FIGURE 4-1 ■ **Myelofibrosis.** Lateral radiograph of the lumbar spine showing heterogeneous marrow sclerosis throughout the vertebral bodies.

Clinical Features

The condition presents in the fifth to eighth decades with equal frequency in men and women. Bone marrow involvement is present in approximately 90% of cases and is often asymptomatic, but may produce thoracic and lumbar spinal pain and arthralgia. The condition may be associated with myelodysplastic syndromes, myeloproliferative neoplasia, leukaemia and lymphoma. The prognosis is variable.

Radiological Features

Imaging, including radiography, scintigraphy, bone densitometry, CT and MRI, plays a role in the diagnosis, staging and monitoring of the disease. Skeletal changes are due to both the direct effect of mast cells and the indirect effect of secreted mediators such as histamine, heparin and prostaglandins. They include both osteolytic and osteosclerotic lesions, which may be either diffuse or focal. Small (4–5 mm) lytic lesions may be surrounded by a rim of sclerosis and are most commonly seen in the spine, ribs, skull, pelvis and tubular bones. Diffuse osteopenia is a common pattern (Fig. 4-4), most commonly

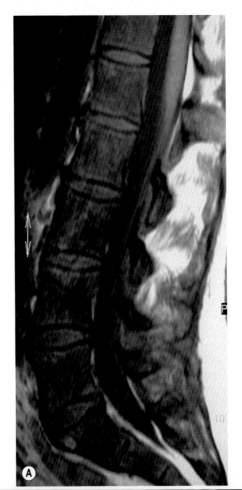

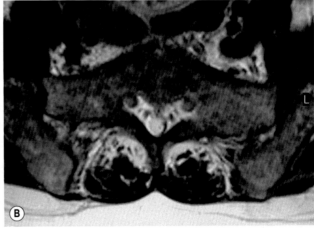

FIGURE 4-2 ■ **Myelofibrosis.** (A) Sagittal T1W SE and (B) axial T2W FSE MRI of the lumbar spine and sacrum showing heterogeneous reduction of marrow SI.

involving the axial skeleton, and may be complicated by pathological fracture in 16% of cases. Differential diagnosis includes cystic osteoporosis, Gaucher's disease, myeloma, hyperparathyroidism or thalassaemia.

Osteosclerosis produces trabecular and cortical thickening with reduction of the marrow spaces (Fig. 4-5), and multifocal sclerotic lesions simulating osteoblastic metastases (Fig. 4-6). Both Multidetector CT (Fig. 4-7) and MRI are more sensitive than radiography in the

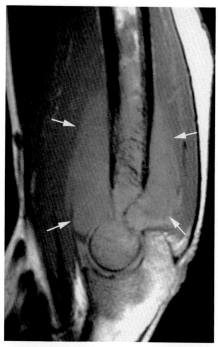

FIGURE 4-3 ■ **Myelofibrosis.** Sagittal T1W SE MRI of the distal humerus demonstrating heterogeneous reduction of marrow SI and a circumferential extraosseous mass (arrows) due to leukaemic transformation.

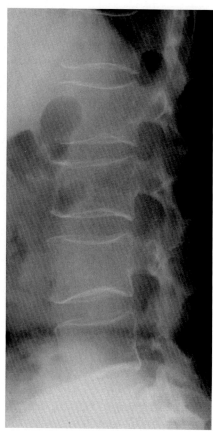

FIGURE 4-4 ■ **Mastocytosis.** Lateral radiograph of the lumbar spine showing diffuse osteopenia and multilevel mild compression fractures.

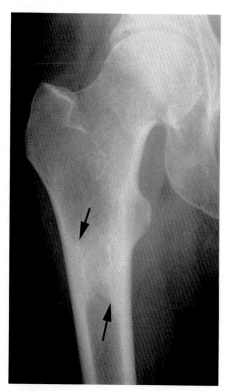

FIGURE 4-5 ■ **Mastocytosis.** AP radiograph of the right hip showing endosteal sclerosis in the proximal femur (arrows).

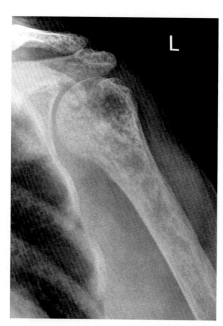

FIGURE 4-6 ■ **Mastocytosis.** AP radiograph of the left shoulder showing nodular sclerosis in the ribs and proximal humerus.

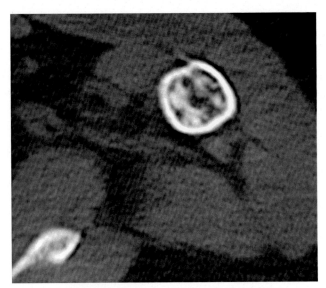

FIGURE 4-7 ■ **Mastocytosis.** CT of the left proximal humerus demonstrating multiple intramedullary sclerotic lesions.

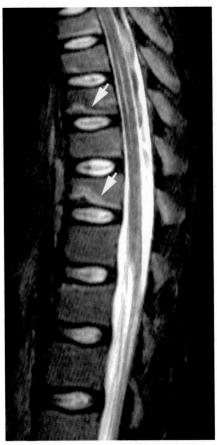

FIGURE 4-8 ■ **Acute leukaemia.** Sagittal T2W FSE MRI of the thoracolumbar junction showing multilevel end-plate fractures (arrows).

identification of marrow involvement. In mild cases, MRI may be normal. Otherwise, there is a generalised reduction of T1W signal intensity (SI), with variable T2W and short tau inversion recovery (STIR) SI, depending upon the degree of associated marrow fibrosis. Sclerotic lesions appear hypointense on all pulse sequences. The role of FDG-PET is unclear.

LEUKAEMIA[5]

Leukaemia accounts for approximately 25–33% of all childhood malignancy, the vast majority being the acute form. Acute lymphocytic leukaemia (ALL) accounts for 75%, acute myeloid leukaemia (AML) for 20% and other types for 5% of cases. Chronic leukaemias predominate in adults but sometimes terminate in an acute blastic form. While radiographic demonstration of bone lesions in children is relatively common, skeletal lesions in adults tend to be uncommon and focal, often simulating metastases.

Clinical Features

ALL usually presents in children at 2–3 years of age, while AML is most commonly seen in the first 2 years of life, and then also in adolescence. The acute disease is often insidious, with non-specific malaise, anorexia, fever, petechiae and weight loss. Limb pain and pathological fracture are common. Bone pain at presentation is five times more common in children than adults, being reported in over 33% of cases.

Adults are most commonly affected by ALL and chronic myeloid leukaemia (CML). Most skeletal lesions in adults affect sites of residual red marrow, the axial skeleton and proximal ends of the femora and humeri. Chronic lymphatic leukaemia (CLL) is a disease of the elderly, characterised by enlargement of the spleen and lymph nodes with skeletal involvement being rare, except as a terminal event.

Radiological Features

Radiological evidence of bone involvement in acute paediatric leukaemia is reported in approximately 40% at the time of presentation, the incidence of the various features being as follows: osteolysis (13.1%), metaphyseal bands (9.8%), osteopenia (9%), osteosclerosis (7.4%), permeative bone destruction (5.7%), pathological fracture (5.7%), periosteal reaction (4.1%) and mixed lytic–sclerotic lesions (2.5%).[6] However, such changes will be seen in up to 75% of children during the course of their disease.

Diffuse osteopenia is reported in 16–41% of cases and either may be metabolic in aetiology due to protein and mineral deficiencies or may be related to diffuse marrow infiltration with leukaemic cells. The effects of corticosteroids and chemotherapy also contribute to osteoporosis. Compression fractures occur in association with osteopenia of the spine (Fig. 4-8), while approximately 1% of children treated for leukaemia develop osteonecrosis.

Metaphyseal lucent bands primarily affect sites of maximum growth, such as the distal femur, proximal tibia and distal radius, but other metaphyses and the vertebral

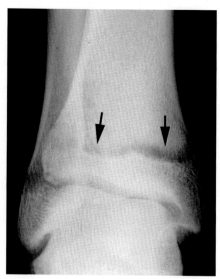

FIGURE 4-9 ■ Acute leukaemia. AP radiograph of the right ankle showing metaphyseal lucent bands (arrows).

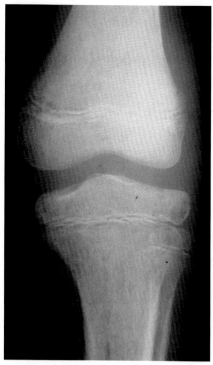

FIGURE 4-10 ■ Acute leukaemia. AP radiograph of the left knee showing permeative bone destruction in the distal femur and proximal tibia.

bodies are affected later. They are typically 2–15 mm in width (Fig. 4-9). These changes are non-specific, with the differential diagnosis including generalised infection, although this is more common in infancy. In children over the age of 2 years, leukaemia is more likely.

More extensive involvement results in diffuse, permeative bone destruction (Fig. 4-10) similar to the spread of highly malignant tumours such as Ewing sarcoma. The cortex becomes eroded on its endosteal surface and may ultimately be destroyed. The permeative pattern is reported in 18% of leukaemic children and may indicate a poor prognosis.

Osteolytic lesions secondary to bone destruction typically have a moth-eaten appearance and most commonly affect the metaphyses of long bones. Such lesions are reported in 10–40% of patients and predispose to pathological fracture. A particular focal lesion in AML is granulocytic sarcoma (chloroma), which is usually located in the skull, spine, ribs or sternum of children. This is an expanding geographical tumour caused by a collection of leukaemic cells and is reported to occur in 4.7% of patients.

Osteosclerosis is rare, being reported in 6% of cases. Sclerotic changes in the metaphyses of long bones may occur spontaneously or as a result of therapy. Mixed lytic–sclerotic lesions are identified in around 18% of children. Periosteal reaction is reported in 2–50% of cases and may occur in isolation or in association with destructive cortical lesions. It is due to haemorrhage or proliferation of leukaemic deposits deep to the periosteum. Non-specific cortical destruction may involve the medial aspect of the proximal humerus, tibia and sometimes femur.

In adults, skeletal lesions are less common and must be differentiated from metastases or a primary malignant bone neoplasm.

MRI typically demonstrates diffuse marrow infiltration with reduction of T1W SI in affected areas. A change from normal to nodular to diffuse low SI can be seen with disease progression, together with an increase in the extent of SI abnormality. Response to therapy is also demonstrable. MRI can identify complications of treatment such as osteonecrosis.

LYMPHOMA[7–9]

Lymphoma encompasses Hodgkin's and non-Hodgkin's disease, Burkitt's lymphoma and mycosis fungoides (cutaneous T-cell lymphoma), these lymphoreticular neoplasms primarily arising in extraskeletal locations with osseous involvement usually being secondary to hematogenous spread or by direct extension from surrounding involved lymph nodes or soft tissues. Secondary skeletal involvement implies stage IV disease and is usually identified during the course of the disease, or at staging or when it becomes symptomatic. Primary bone lymphoma is a relatively rare condition.

PRIMARY LYMPHOMA OF BONE[10,11]

Clinical Features

Primary lymphoma of bone (PLB) is a rare condition that has been described as lymphomatous involvement of the

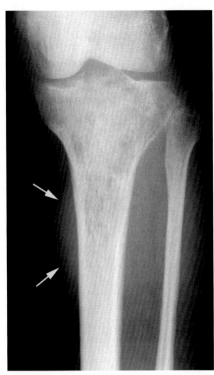

FIGURE 4-11 ■ **Primary lymphoma of bone.** AP radiograph of the proximal right tibia showing an extensive area of permeative bone destruction with an associated soft-tissue mass (arrows).

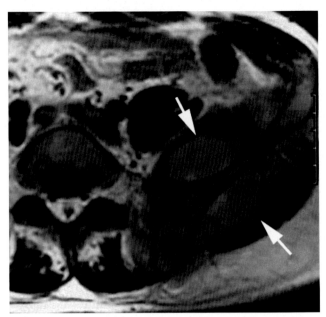

FIGURE 4-12 ■ **Primary lymphoma of bone.** Axial T2W FSE MRI of the left ilium shows relatively low SI of the extraosseous mass (arrows). Note also the relative preservation of the cortex.

bone marrow, which may be focal or multifocal (termed primary multifocal osseous lymphoma or multifocal PLB) and involve regional lymph nodes, but without distant disease at presentation or within 6 months of presentation. PLB accounts for 5% of all extranodal lymphomas. The majority are non-Hodgkin's lymphomas (NHLs) of the diffuse large B-cell subtype, with primary osseous involvement by Hodgkin's disease being very rare. Most patients present in the fifth to sixth decades of life (median age 42–54 years) with bone pain and/or a soft-tissue mass and the disease is more common in males (M:F ratio 1.5–2.3:1).

Radiological Features

Approximately 70% of PLB involves the major long bones (femur, tibia, humerus), usually arising in the meta-diaphyseal region. However, epiphyseal lesions with joint involvement are also recognised. The flat bones and spine can also be involved. Disease limited to the marrow space may be radiologically occult, but the vast majority result in moth-eaten or permeative bone destruction (Fig. 4-11), with only 2% being osteoblastic. Pathological fracture occurs in 17–22% of cases. An aggressive periosteal reaction is seen in 50% and approximately 50–75% of patients will have an associated soft-tissue mass (Fig. 4-11), which is optimally demonstrated by MRI and is indicative of more aggressive disease with a worse prognosis. The combination of a large soft-tissue mass and relative preservation of the cortex is a well-recognised feature of bone lymphoma. MRI signal characteristics are

non-specific,[12] but relatively low T2W SI is a recognised feature (Fig. 4-12).

Multifocal PLB accounts for 11–33% of cases and more commonly involves the spine (Fig. 4-13), the imaging characteristics being as described above. Multifocal disease can be detected by whole-body scintigraphy[13] or whole-body MRI.[14] Diffuse skeletal involvement results in a generalised reduction of T1W SI with increased marrow SI on STIR (Fig. 4-14). Enlarged regional lymph nodes may also be seen.

HODGKIN'S LYMPHOMA[7–9]

Clinical Features

Hodgkin's disease (HD) accounts for 25% of all lymphomas and is characterised by the Reed–Sternberg cell, which is usually a B cell. Between 1 and 4% of patients with HD present with a skeletal lesion, while 5–32% will develop bone involvement during the course of the disease.

Three-quarters of patients present between 20 and 30 years of age, with a second peak occurring after the age of 60 years. A slight male predominance (1.4:1) is found and the spine is the commonest site of involvement, from either direct lymph node extension or haematological spread. The pelvis, ribs, femora and sternum are the other commonly involved sites. HD presents as PLB in 6% of cases.

Radiological Features

Approximately one-third of skeletal lesions are solitary, and whole-body staging with scintigraphy or whole-body MRI is mandatory to identify further lesions. Osteolytic

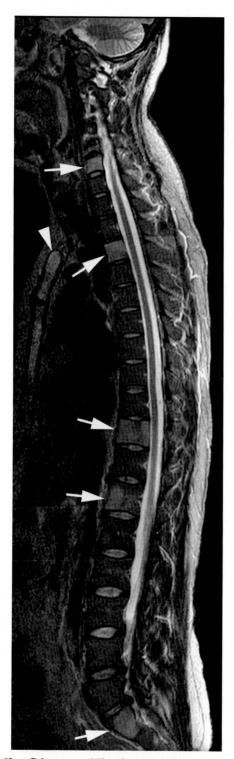

FIGURE 4-13 ■ **Primary multifocal osseous lymphoma.** Sagittal STIR MRI of the spine showing multilevel vertebral (arrows) and sternal (arrowhead) marrow infiltration.

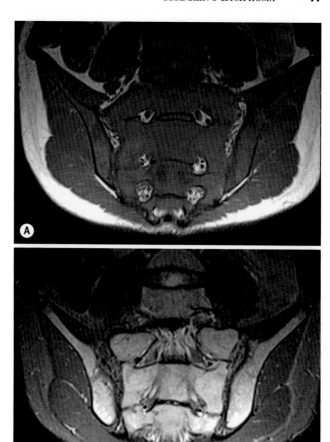

FIGURE 4-14 ■ **Primary multifocal osseous lymphoma.** (A) Coronal T1W SE and (B) STIR MRI showing diffuse reduction of T1W and increased STIR marrow SI.

lesions or mixed lytic–sclerotic lesions account for almost 90% of cases, the remainder being purely sclerotic.

In the spine, HD most commonly causes sclerosis, although it is an uncommon cause of 'ivory' vertebra. Vertebral collapse takes place early, with lytic lesions, occasionally producing vertebra plana. Erosion of the anterior border of one or more vertebral bodies is also found, possibly by direct spread from affected pre-vertebral lymph nodes. Such features are best shown with MRI. In the thoracic region, paravertebral masses may precede radiographic evidence of bony involvement, while mediastinal disease is a recognised cause of hyper-trophic osteoarthropathy.

Rib involvement is common, with multiple lytic lesions associated with soft-tissue masses predominating. Occa-sionally the ribs appear expanded. In the pelvis, involved nodes may invade the bone directly, usually in the poste-rior half of the ilium. Mixed lesions are relatively common and the ischium and pubic rami may show expansion. Direct haematogenous involvement of the sternum is common. The typical lesion is lytic and expanding, asso-ciated with a soft-tissue mass.

CT clearly demonstrates all of the described radiologi-cal features, and in addition will show the associated extraosseous mass (Fig. 4-15). Sequestrum formation is also a recognised feature of bone lymphoma. Marrow involvement is most sensitively detected by MRI[13] and may be focal or diffuse. However, the SI characteristics are non-specific. In focal involvement, MR can be used to guide biopsy.

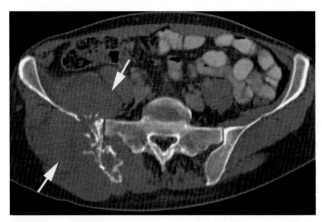

FIGURE 4-15 ■ Hodgkin's disease. CT of the pelvis showing an aggressive destructive lesion of the posterior right iliac blade with a large soft-tissue mass (arrows).

NON-HODGKIN'S LYMPHOMA[7–9]

Clinical Features

Non-Hodgkin's lymphoma (NHL) is the commonest haematopoietic neoplasm and comprises a variety of clinicopathological subtypes, the majority of which are of B-cell origin. Predisposing factors include AIDS and transplant-related immunosuppression. Skeletal involvement may be either primary (see above) or secondary. Secondary skeletal involvement occurs in 20–30% of children and 10–20% of adults with NHL, but detection of an osseous lesion at initial presentation is uncommon.

Radiological Features

The radiological features are similar to those described for HD. Children with generalised NHL tend to have widespread skeletal involvement manifesting as osteopenia. MRI may show multifocal marrow lesions before the diffuse infiltration of established disease. MRI may also be used to stage disease and will occasionally demonstrate marrow disease despite negative iliac crest biopsy. Although the MRI appearances are non-specific, the presence of a paravertebral soft-tissue mass with maintenance of the cortical outline of the vertebral body is highly suggestive of lymphoma.

BURKITT'S LYMPHOMA[15]

Burkitt's lymphoma is a high-grade NHL with distinctive clinical and histological features. A causative relationship to the Epstein–Barr virus and more recently HIV is probable. A 74% 4-year survival rate is reported.

Clinical Features

The disease shows a male: female ratio of 2 : 1, affecting mainly African children. Large tumours affect the jawbones and abdominal viscera. The mean age at presentation is 7 years, with a range of 2–16 years. Added to this endemic (African) group are the non-endemic (sporadic) cases, mainly in white children. The jaw is the initial focus in about 50% of patients, although less so in non-endemic cases. Other sites of involvement include the pelvis, long bones and bones of the hands and feet.

Radiological Features

The jaw lesion is generally destructive, starting in the medulla and later affecting the cortex. Bone destruction and dental displacement in the enlarging soft-tissue mass give the appearance of 'floating' teeth. Lesions in other bones show similar appearances and periosteal reaction may be present in all locations. Full assessment and staging is required for this multicentric neoplasm.

PLASMA CELL DISORDERS[16]

PLASMACYTOMA

Solitary plasmacytoma accounts for less than 5% of patients with plasma cell tumours. It may remain localised for many years but more than 30% progress quite rapidly to generalised myelomatosis.

Clinical Features

Presentation with pain is common and the age of presentation tends to be earlier than in multiple myeloma (MM). As plasma protein changes are related to the total tumour mass, protein electrophoresis is often normal and the erythrocyte sedimentation rate (ESR) is also normal or only slightly elevated.

Radiological Features

Plasmacytoma is typically lytic and destructive with sclerosis being rare. The lesion arises in the medulla and the radiological features suggest a relatively slow growth rate. The margin is often well defined and cortical thinning with expansion is usually present (Fig. 4-16). Apparent trabeculation or a 'soap bubble' appearance is common and an associated soft-tissue mass is frequently seen. Affected sites usually contain persistent red marrow and include the axial skeleton, pelvis, proximal femur, proximal humerus and ribs. Following the diagnosis of plasmacytoma, whole-body MRI is indicated to identify additional lesions,[17] which may be seen in up to 80% of cases. Occult lesions may also be demonstrated by FDG PET-CT.[18]

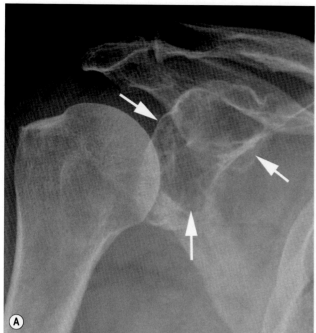

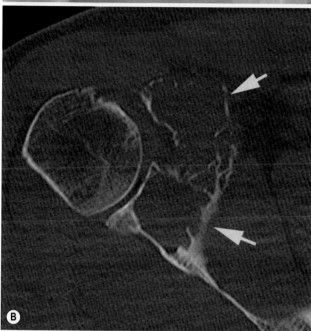

FIGURE 4-16 ■ Plasmacytoma. (A) AP radiograph of the shoulder showing a well-defined lytic lesion (arrows) in the bony glenoid. (B) Axial CT shows the expansile nature of the lesion with a thinned but largely intact cortex (arrows).

Involvement of a vertebral body is common, sometimes leading to early collapse. Extension across the disc space is a rare feature. The differential diagnosis includes metastatic carcinoma, which rarely destroys two or three bodies in continuity, and infection. A solitary plasmacytoma in the spine may show characteristic MRI features, particularly the presence of peripheral thickened trabeculae.[19] In long and flat bones, plasmacytoma may resemble an aneurysmal bone cyst or an expanding metastasis.

MULTIPLE MYELOMA[20–23]

Multiple myeloma (MM) is the most common primary malignant neoplasm of bone and is the predominant plasma cell neoplasm, accounting for approximately 1% of all malignant disease and 10% of haematological malignancies.

Symptomatic MM is diagnosed by the following: (1) >10% atypical plasma cells on bone marrow aspirate/biopsy or plasmacytoma; (2) monoclonal paraprotein present in blood or urine; and (3) myeloma-related organ or tissue impairment (including nephropathy, hypercalcaemia, anaemia and bone lesions). The presence of only the first two criteria represents asymptomatic (smouldering) myeloma, while isolated elevation of serum M-protein (<30 g/L) is termed monoclonal gammopathy of uncertain significance (MGUS).

Clinical Features

Three-quarters of affected patients are over 50 years of age (median age 65 years) and approximately 3% of patients present before the age of 40 years. There is a male predominance of up to 2:1. Widespread involvement of the skeleton is present in 80%, the axial skeleton and proximal ends of the long bones being particularly involved. Fever, pain, backache and weakness are common symptoms. Amyloidosis is reported in approximately 20% of patients with MM.

Radiological Features

The classical appearance of MM consists of well-defined 'punched-out' lesions throughout the skeleton (Fig. 4-17), most characteristic in the skull (Fig. 4-18). The only common differential diagnosis in this age group is metastatic disease. The presence of multiple small (up to 20 mm), well-defined round or oval lesions is more suggestive of MM.

Diffuse osteopenia usually involves the spine and may result in multiple compression fractures. Pathological fracture of the vertebrae affects approximately 50% of patients at some stage. Osteoblastic or mixed lesions are rare in untreated patients, but marginal sclerosis may be observed following radiotherapy. Purely sclerotic myeloma is recognised and may be associated with POEMS syndrome, a paraneoplastic condition due to an underlying plasma cell neoplasm. The major criteria for the syndrome are polyradiculoneuropathy, clonal plasma cell disorder (PCD), sclerotic bone lesions, elevated vascular endothelial growth factor and the presence of Castleman disease.[24]

Multidetector CT (MDCT) is more sensitive than radiography in detecting myeloma and a low-dose technique can be used to limit radiation to the patient. Sagittal reconstructions of the spine and coronal whole-body reconstructions are typically performed. Purely marrow lesions appear as focal areas of soft-tissue density, but the diffuse osteopenia of MM may be indistinguishable from other causes such as osteoporosis. Progressive disease results in endosteal scalloping (Fig. 4-19), cortical destruction and soft-tissue masses. Low-dose MDCT is

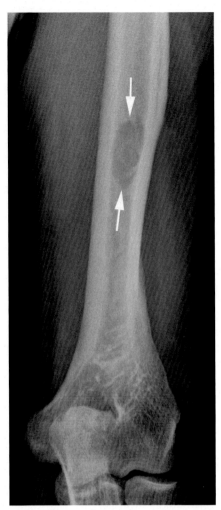

FIGURE 4-17 ■ **Multiple myeloma.** AP radiograph of the humerus demonstrating a well-defined lytic lesion (arrows) in the diaphysis.

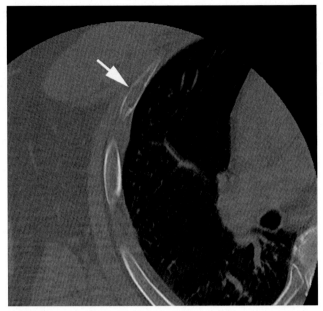

FIGURE 4-19 ■ **Multiple myeloma.** Axial CT showing a radiologically occult, well-defined oval lytic lesion, which is resulting in mild endosteal scalloping (arrow).

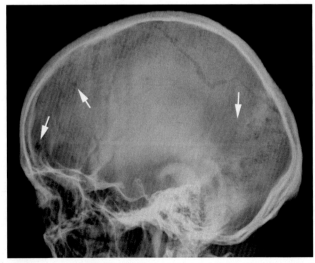

FIGURE 4-18 ■ **Multiple myeloma.** Lateral radiograph of the skull showing multiple small lytic lesions (arrows).

also valuable in excluding myeloma lesions in patients with MGUS.[25]

The MRI appearances in MM are variable, with five patterns described. A normal marrow pattern may be seen in patients with low-grade plasma cell infiltration of the marrow spaces, and occasionally in stage III disease. A focal pattern consists of localised areas of decreased SI on T1W images with corresponding increased SI on T2W and STIR images, seen in 30% of cases. Occasionally, focal lesions may be relatively hyperintense on T1W and identified only on fat-suppressed T2W images. The diffuse pattern manifests as generalised reduction of marrow SI on T1W, such that the intervertebral discs appear hyperintense compared with the vertebral bodies. The marrow appears hyperintense on fat-suppressed T2W and STIR images and shows diffuse enhancement following gadolinium. A combined focal and diffuse pattern may also be seen (Fig. 4-20). Finally, a 'variegated' pattern, which consists of multiple tiny foci of reduced SI on T1W and hyperintensity on T2W/STIR on a background of normal marrow (Fig. 4-21), is described. This pattern is seen almost always in early disease. These patterns have some prognostic value, in that patients with diffuse marrow abnormality on MRI will have a poorer outcome than those with a normal MRI pattern.

Whole-body MRI is far more sensitive than skeletal survey for the detection of lesions and can result in a significant change in the staging of the disease.[26] The Durie and Salmon PLUS staging system for MM now includes whole-body imaging information from MRI and FDG PET-CT, compared to the original Durie and Salmon staging system which relied on radiographic skeletal survey. MRI also allows assessment of response to therapy, with a normalisation of marrow SI being indicative of a good response.

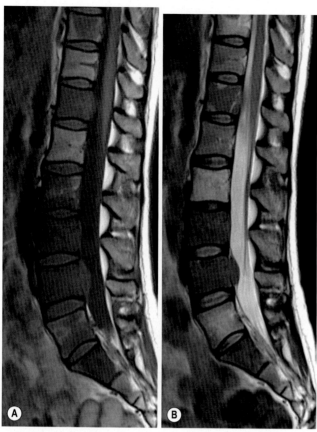

FIGURE 4-20 ■ **Multiple myeloma.** (A) Sagittal T1W SE and (B) T2W FSE MRI of the lumbar spine showing a combined pattern of diffuse and focal vertebral marrow infiltration.

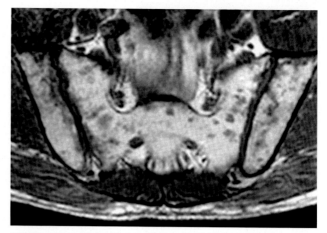

FIGURE 4-21 ■ **Multiple myeloma.** Axial T1W SE MRI of the sacrum showing the 'variegated' pattern of marrow infiltration.

Vertebral fractures in MM occur in 55–70% of cases and may be benign, due to diffuse osteopenia (~66%), or pathological due to tumour infiltration (~33%), the majority occurring in the thoracolumbar region. MRI is valuable in the differentiation of benign versus malignant collapse. MRI may also demonstrate other complications, such as steroid-induced marrow infarction.

REFERENCES

1. Tefferi A, Skoda R, Vardiman JW. Myeloproliferative neoplasms: contemporary diagnosis using histology and genetics. Nat Rev Clin Oncol 2009;6:627–37.
2. Tefferi A. Primary myelofibrosis: 2012 update on diagnosis, risk stratification, and management. Am J Hematol 2011;86:1017–26.
3. Guermazi A, de Kerviler E, Cazals-Hatem D, et al. Imaging findings in patients with myelofibrosis. Eur Radiol 1999;9:1366–75.
4. Fritz J, Fishman EK, Carrino JA, Horger MS. Advanced imaging of skeletal manifestations of systemic mastocytosis. Skeletal Radiol 2012;41(8):887–97.
5. Guillerman RP, Voss SD, Parker BR. Leukemia and lymphoma. Radiol Clin North Am 2011;49:767–97.
6. Sinigaglia R, Gigante C, Bisinella G, et al. Musculoskeletal manifestations in pediatric acute leukemia. J Pediatr Orthop 2008;28:20–8.
7. Ruzek KA, Wenger, DE. The multiple faces of lymphoma of the musculoskeletal system. Skeletal Radiol 2004;33:1–8.
8. Hwang S. Imaging of lymphoma of the musculoskeletal system. Radiol Clin North Am 2008;46:379–96.
9. O'Neill J, Finlay K, Jurriaans E, Friedman L. Radiological manifestations of skeletal lymphoma. Curr Probl Diagn Radiol 2009;38:228–36.
10. Jawad MU, Schneiderbauer MM, Min ES, et al. Primary lymphoma of bone in adult patients. Cancer 2010;116:871–9.
11. Mikhaeel NG. Primary bone lymphoma. Clin Oncol 2012;24(5):366–70.
12. Heyning FH, Kroon HM, Hogendoorn PC, et al. MR imaging characteristics in primary lymphoma of bone with emphasis on non-aggressive appearance. Skeletal Radiol 2007;36:937–44.
13. O'Connor AR, Birchall JD, O'Connor SR, Bessell E. The value of 99mTc-MDP bone scintigraphy in staging primary lymphoma of bone. Nucl Med Commun 2007;28:529–31.
14. Berger FH, van Dijke CF, Maas M. Diffuse marrow changes. Semin Musculoskelet Radiol 2009;13:104–10.
15. Spina M, Tirelli U, Zagonel V et al. Burkitt's lymphoma in adults with and without human immunodeficiency virus infection: a single-institution clinicopathologic study of 75 patients. Cancer 1998;82:766–74.
16. Wilson CS. The plasma cell dyscrasias. Cancer Treat Res 2004;121:113–44.
17. Terpos E, Moulopoulos LA, Dimopoulos MA. Advances in imaging and the management of myeloma bone disease. J Clin Oncol 2011;29:1907–15.
18. Nanni C, Rubello D, Zamagni E. 18F-FDG PET/CT in myeloma with presumed solitary plasmocytoma of bone. In Vivo 2008;22:513–17.
19. Shah BK, Saifuddin A, Price GJ. Magnetic resonance imaging of spinal plasmacytoma. Clin Radiol 2000;55:439–45.
20. Angtuaco EJ, Fassas AB, Walker R, et al. Multiple myeloma: clinical review and diagnostic imaging. Radiology 2004;231:11–23.
21. Baur-Melnyk A, Reiser MF. Multiple myeloma. Semin Musculoskelet Radiol 2009;13:111–19.
22. Shortt CP, Carty F, Murray JG. The role of whole-body imaging in the diagnosis, staging, and follow-up of multiple myeloma. Semin Musculoskelet Radiol 2010;14:37–46.
23. Hanrahan CJ, Christensen CR, Crim JR. Current concepts in the evaluation of multiple myeloma with MR imaging and FDG PET/CT. Radiographics 2010;30:127–42.
24. Dispenzieri A. POEMS syndrome: 2011 update on diagnosis, risk-stratification, and management. Am J Hematol 2011;86:591–601.
25. Spira D, Weisel K, Brodoefel H, et al. Can whole-body low-dose multidetector CT exclude the presence of myeloma bone disease in patients with monoclonal gammopathy of undetermined significance (MGUS)? Acad Radiol 2012;19:89–94.
26. Dinter DJ, Neff WK, Klaus J et al. Comparison of whole-body MR imaging and conventional X-ray examination in patients with multiple myeloma and implications for therapy. Ann Hematol 2009;88:457–64.

CHAPTER 5

Bone Marrow Disorders: Miscellaneous

Asif Saifuddin

CHAPTER OUTLINE

DISORDERS OF RED CELLS

CHRONIC HAEMOLYTIC ANAEMIAS

MISCELLANEOUS DISORDERS

DISORDERS OF BLOOD COAGULATION

Chapters 4 and 5 deal with a variety of blood-related disorders that have a major influence on imaging of the skeletal system.

DISORDERS OF RED CELLS

In late fetal life and infancy, the entire bone marrow is utilised for red blood cell (RBC) formation, supplemented by extramedullary erythropoiesis in the liver and spleen. As the child becomes older and RBC life span increases, erythropoiesis is withdrawn from the liver and spleen, then gradually from the diaphyses of the long bones, so that by the age of 25 years, active bone marrow is confined to the axial skeleton, the flat bones and the proximal ends of the femora and humeri.[1] This process of withdrawal will not occur with a need for extra erythropoiesis and reverses in the presence of increased RBC destruction.

The Anaemias

Only chronic anaemias affect the radiological appearances of bone. Anaemias that do not produce reactive erythropoiesis, such as aplastic anaemia, do not affect the skeletal radiograph, but may manifest on MRI as a generalised increase in fatty marrow signal intensity (SI).[1] Also, the myelodysplastic syndromes may manifest as diffuse reduction of T1-weighted (T1W) marrow SI due to marrow reconversion.[1] A variety of inherited syndromes, such as Fanconi's anaemia, may be associated with skeletal dysplasia, but these are not an effect of the anaemia per se and will not be discussed.

CHRONIC HAEMOLYTIC ANAEMIAS

The Haemoglobinopathies[1]

The haemoglobin molecule consists of a protein (globin) and four haem groups, each with four pyrrole rings surrounding an iron atom. The protein moiety consists of 574 amino acids arranged in four spiral polypeptide chains. The different chains are designated by letters of the Greek alphabet (α, β) and the three normal haemoglobins (Hbs) A, A2 and F each contain two α chains, differing only in their second pairs.

Three types of haemoglobinopathy are found:
1. Thalassaemia: an inherited defect of HbA synthesis with inadequate manufacture of α- or β-chains.
2. Haemoglobin variants: inherited defects of HbA synthesis producing abnormal α- or β-chains. All the variants differ from HbA by the substitution of only one amino acid in the chain: e.g. HbS (sickle-cell anaemia) where valine is substituted for glutamine at residue 6 in the β-chain.
3. Combination of thalassaemia and abnormal haemoglobin, e.g. HbS–thalassaemia.

Thalassaemia[1-3]

Thalassaemia is an inherited disorder and exists in two forms, the homozygous (thalassaemia major) and heterozygous (thalassaemia intermedia and thalassaemia minor), and may affect production of either α- or β-chains, resulting in α-thalassaemia or β-thalassaemia, respectively.

β-Thalassaemia is prevalent in the Mediterranean countries (Greece, southern Italy and the Mediterranean islands), while α-thalassaemia is encountered in those of West African descent.

Clinical Features. Thalassaemia major causes severe childhood anaemia with hepatosplenomegaly, extramedullary erythropoiesis and secondary skeletal deformity. Treatment is by regular blood transfusion in infancy to maintain a haemoglobin level of 9–10 g/dL, iron chelation with agents such as desferrioxamine (DFX) to prevent/reduce iron overload, and bisphosphonates to treat the associated osteoporosis. With the introduction of successful transfusion regimes, the skeletal changes due to the disorder itself are now less commonly encountered, but osseous complications related to repeated transfusion and the effects of DFX therapy must be recognised.

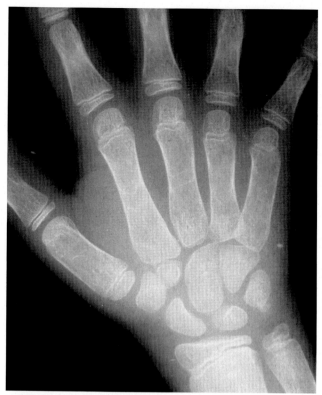

FIGURE 5-1 ■ **Thalassaemia.** AP radiograph of the hand demonstrates generalised osteopenia, medullary expansion with cortical thinning and coarse trabeculae.

Radiological Features[1,2]

Untreated Thalassaemia Major. Skeletal changes in untreated children are essentially the result of chronic anaemia and marrow hyperplasia (15–30 times normal) and are most commonly seen after the age of 1 year, affecting almost all regions of the skeleton. Medullary hyperplasia results in bony expansion and cortical thinning, which in long bones produces the characteristic Erlenmeyer flask appearance, also found in conditions such as Gaucher's disease. Within the medulla, trabecular thinning initially occurs, followed by trabecular coarsening due to new bone formation, the changes being most marked in the metacarpals and phalanges, which become cylindrical or even biconvex (Fig. 5-1). Trabecular coarsening may also be seen in the pelvis and vertebrae (Fig. 5-2). The ribs are similarly affected with club-like anterior ends, while a 'rib-within-a-rib' appearance also occurs due to subperiosteal extension of haematopoietic tissue through the rib cortex.

Extramedullary erythropoiesis occurs in severe cases surviving to adulthood, the most common sites being the thoracic paravertebral region by extension from the adjacent ribs, the mediastinum (Fig. 5-3) and presacral region (Fig. 5-4). Epidural extension from paraspinal extramedullary erythropoiesis may result in spinal cord compression. These features are optimally demonstrated by MRI, which also shows diffuse reduction in marrow signal intensity (SI) on T1W images caused by marrow reconversion (Fig. 5-4).

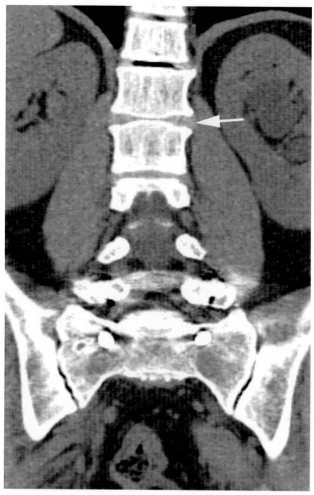

FIGURE 5-2 ■ **Thalassaemia.** Coronal CT MPR showing vertical trabecular thickening in the vertebral bodies, convexity of the end-plates adjacent to the L1–L2 disc (arrow) and advanced T11–T12 and T12–L1 disc degeneration with vacuum phenomenon.

With severe childhood disease, the paranasal sinuses develop poorly and often contain red marrow, accounting for the facial abnormalities (seen in 17%) and dental malocclusion. The ethmoidal cells are spared since they contain no red marrow. The diploë of the skull vault are widened, except in the occiput. These changes occur earliest and most severely in the frontal bone, producing the classical 'hair-on-end' appearance (Fig. 5-5). Occasionally, well-defined lytic lesions may be seen in the skull.

Spinal changes consist of generalised osteopenia, resulting in compression fractures and biconcavity of the vertebral bodies. Despite optimised therapy, osteoporosis may still be seen in as many as 90% of cases based on DEXA studies. Scoliosis is reported in 20% of children with thalassaemia major, while early disc degeneration is also a feature (Fig. 5-2), optimally demonstrated by MRI.

Premature fusion of the growth plates may contribute to short stature. These radiological changes are reported in ~15% of patients, generally occurring after 10 years of age and most commonly affecting the proximal humerus and distal femur. Growth arrest lines may also be seen.

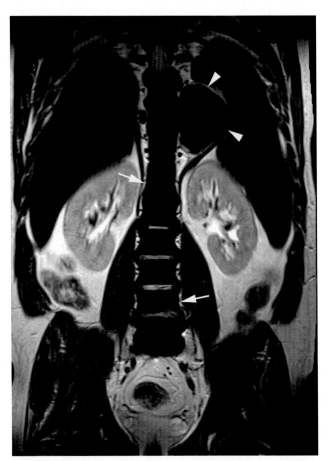

FIGURE 5-3 ■ **Thalassaemia.** Coronal T2W FSE MRI showing profound, diffuse reduction of marrow SI (arrows) and a large left paraspinal soft-tissue mass (arrowheads) due to extramedullary erythropoiesis.

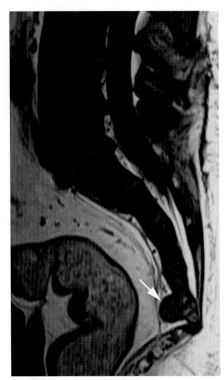

FIGURE 5-4 ■ **Thalassaemia.** Sagittal T1W SE MRI showing marked reduction of marrow SI (arrows) such that the discs appear hyperintense, and a small pre-sacral mass (arrowhead) due to extramedullary erythropoiesis.

Hypertransfusion. Repeated transfusion therapy may produce iron overload and hyperuricaemia. Raised blood iron levels result in synovial and articular cartilage abnormalities, manifesting radiologically as symmetrical loss of joint space, cystic changes, subchondral collapse and osteophytosis. Chondrocalcinosis may also be seen and the larger joints tend to be more commonly affected than in primary haemochromatosis. Occasionally, the radiographic changes of gout may be evident and there is also a predisposition to osteonecrosis and osteomyelitis. Iron deposition within bone also contributes to osteoporosis and is a further cause of reduced marrow SI on MRI, particularly on T2-weighted (T2W; Fig. 5-3) and gradient-echo sequences. MRI may be used to estimate tissue siderosis.[4]

DFX Therapy. Iron chelation therapy is recognised as causing dysplastic changes in the spine and long bones, as well as growth retardation, especially when treatment is started before the age of 3 years and with higher doses. The incidence is unclear, since many cases are asymptomatic. Changes typically occur at the metaphysis/physis/epiphysis of the proximal humerus, distal femur, proximal tibia and distal radius and ulna.

Radiographs and MRI demonstrate irregularity of the metaphyseal–physeal junction with dense sclerotic

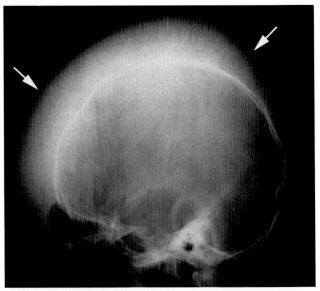

FIGURE 5-5 ■ **Thalassaemia.** Lateral radiograph of the skull showing marked thickening of the skull vault with a 'hair-on-end' appearance (arrows).

metaphyseal bands, which may then extend in a 'flame-shaped' manner towards the diaphysis. Splaying of the metaphysis and widening of the growth plate are later features, which resemble rickets. Severe dysplasia at the proximal femur and around the knee may result in SUFE and genu varuma or valguma.

In the spine, platyspondyly and a biconvex contour to the vertebral bodies (Fig. 5-2) are seen and kyphosis may develop. DFX therapy also results in growth retardation, affecting both the axial and appendicular skeleton.

Deferiprone is an alternative treatment to DFX and has been associated with agranulocytosis and arthropathy, most commonly affecting the knees, resulting in effusion and synovitis, which can be demonstrated on MRI. Chronic changes include flattening of the femoral condyles, tibial plateau and patella.

Sickle-Cell Disease[1,5,6]

The clinical findings in sickle-cell disease (SCD) are explained by the physical properties of the abnormal haemoglobin. In situations of hypoxia, intracellular polymerisation of the HbS molecule occurs, rendering the RBC less flexible. Recurrent cycles of oxygenation and deoxygenation lead to irreversible membrane damage to the erythrocyte, causing the cells to become less deformable and sickle-shaped. Sickle cells obstruct small blood vessels, leading to stasis and tissue hypoxia/anoxia and eventually infarction. Sickle cells also have a much shorter circulating life (~1/10th normal), being removed from the circulation prematurely by the reticuloendothelial system, resulting in haemolytic anaemia.

The full clinical and radiological picture occurs in the homozygous sickle-cell subject (HbS-S). When only one parent carries the abnormal gene, the sickle-cell trait (HbS-A) occurs, without anaemia but with sickling to a lesser degree.

Clinical Features. SCD mainly affects people of African racial origin and approximately 8–10% of black Americans have sickle-cell trait, but only 0.2% have sickle-cell anaemia. People from the Middle East and Eastern Mediterranean are also affected. The anaemia of SCD is not as marked as in thalassaemia major. Homozygous SCD reduces average life expectancy by 25–30 years and most patients will die by the age of 50 years.

The most striking clinical features are due to vaso-occlusive sickle crises, which result in infarctions. Medullary infarction involving the small bones of the hands and feet, resulting in sickle-cell dactylitis or 'hand-foot' syndrome, is a common presentation of SCD in infants between 6 months and 2 years of age but is rare after 6 years. Presentation is with pain and swelling of the digits, together with fever, and affects approximately 50% of children with SCD. Marrow infarction may also involve the long bones, in which case it is difficult to differentiate from osteomyelitis, while infarction of the epiphyses results in avascular necrosis, most commonly of the femoral and humeral heads. SCD is the most common cause of osteonecrosis of the femoral head in children, while approximately 50% of all patients will develop osteonecrosis by the age of 35 years. Rib or sternal infarcts may simulate heart or lung disease, while soft-tissue involvement results in ulcers and muscle infarction, which are well demonstrated by MRI.

Osteomyelitis in SCD typically involves the long bone diaphyses and is most commonly due to various *Salmonella* species, with ~10% of cases being due to

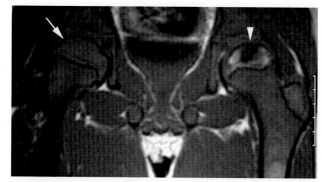

FIGURE 5-6 ■ **Sickle-cell disease.** Coronal T1W SE MRI of the hips in a child showing intermediate SI in the right femoral capital epiphysis (arrow) due to marrow hyperplasia and osteonecrosis on the left side (arrowhead).

Staphylococcus aureus. The prevalence of osteomyelitis is reported as 18%, while septic arthritis is also relatively common in SCD, with a reported prevalence of 7%.

Sickle variants show less anaemia with fewer crises. However, bone infarction, especially of the femoral head, affects patients with HbS-C disease five times more often than those with HbS-S, although the overall prevalence of HbS-C is only one-third that of the homozygous disease. This may reflect the longer survival in HbS-C disease. In sickle-cell trait (HbS-A), significant anaemia and bone infarction are rare.

Radiological Features. The changes in SCD and its variants are similar, varying only in degree. Changes can be divided into those due to marrow hyperplasia, bone infarction and secondary osteomyelitis.

Marrow Hyperplasia. This is more severe in the homozygous disease and the radiological features are as described for thalassaemia. Marrow reconversion is well demonstrated by MRI, with replacement of normal fatty marrow by intermediate SI on T1W images, which may extend to involve the epiphyses (Fig. 5-6). Persistence of red marrow predisposes to osteomyelitis and marrow infarction.

Bone Infarction. This is estimated to be at least 50 times more common than osteomyelitis in SCD. In children, sickle-cell dactylitis results in lytic medullary lesions with associated periostitis and soft-tissue swelling (Fig. 5-7). Asymmetrical shortening of tubular bones is a common sequelae to childhood sickling crises. In adolescents and adults, infarction occurs more in the metaphyses and epiphyses. The earliest radiological evidence of bone infarction is laminar periosteal reaction followed by patchy medullary destruction. Healing leads to reactive sclerosis. MRI shows medullary oedema on T2W and short tau inversion recovery (STIR) sequences with associated periostitis and adjacent soft-tissue inflammation, making differentiation from osteomyelitis difficult. With healing, these areas assume a low SI due to fibrosis and medullary sclerosis. Infarction of the metaphyses on either side of the knee is common and may lead to premature fusion of the growth plates.

Infarction of the vertebral body occurs in approximately 10% of patients and is usually due to venous

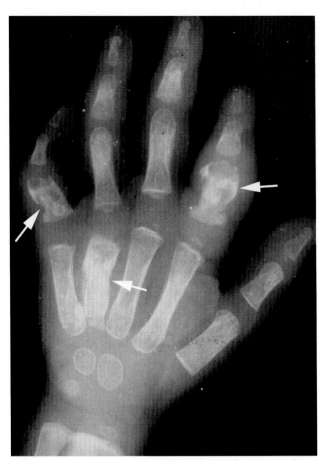

FIGURE 5-7 ■ **Sickle-cell disease: dactylitis.** Infarction in several of the metacarpals and proximal phalanges has resulted in bone destruction (arrows) and swelling of the soft tissues.

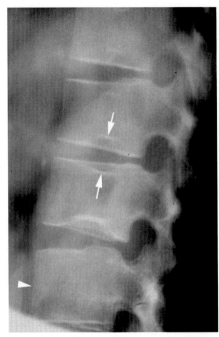

FIGURE 5-8 ■ **Sickle-cell disease.** The classical 'stepped depression' of the vertebral end-plates is seen (arrows), producing the 'H-shaped' vertebra. Note increased height of the adjacent 'tower' vertebra (arrowhead).

thromboembolism in the centre of the vertebral end-plate, with focal collapse producing the 'H-shaped' vertebra. The floor of the depression forms a flat sclerotic margin during healing (Fig. 5-8). This appearance is almost pathognomonic of SCD but has also been reported in Gaucher's disease. Overgrowth of an adjacent vertebral body, producing a 'tower' vertebra, is also reported (Fig. 5-8).

The earliest manifestation of osteonecrosis is epiphyseal oedema seen on MRI. Radiographic abnormalities include mixed lysis and sclerosis with a subchondral fracture being typical. Eventually, secondary osteoarthritis will supervene. Chronic ischaemia or multiple small infarctions in SCD may produce cortical thickening that is both endosteal and periosteal, with narrowing of the marrow cavity (Fig. 5-9). Splitting of the cortex may give rise to a 'bone-within-a-bone' appearance, while secondary myelofibrosis causes medullary sclerosis.

Osteomyelitis. Osteomyelitis usually complicates bone infarction and it may be difficult to distinguish clinically or radiologically between an infarct with infection and one without. *Salmonella* osteomyelitis is common in African children.

Osteomyelitis causes increased bone destruction with laminar or multilaminar periostitis (Fig. 5-10A) and eventual sequestration and involucrum formation. Early

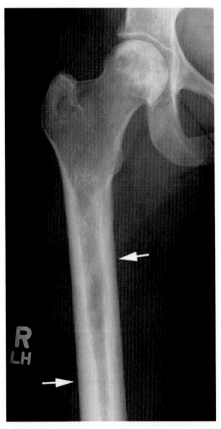

FIGURE 5-9 ■ **Sickle-cell disease.** AP radiograph of the right hip and femur showing heterogeneous femoral head sclerosis due to osteonecrosis and medullary endosteal sclerosis (arrows) due to healed medullary infarction.

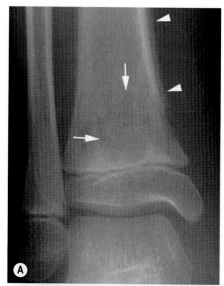

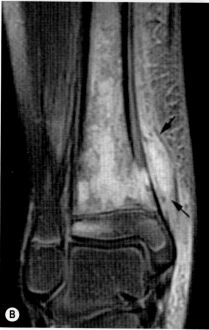

FIGURE 5-10 ■ **Sickle-cell disease: osteomyelitis.** (A) AP radiograph of the right ankle showing a poorly defined lytic lesion in the distal tibial metaphysis (arrows) and associated periostitis (arrowheads) consistent with acute osteomyelitis. (B) Coronal STIR MRI showing the irregular distal tibial bone abscess, which communicates with a soft-tissue abscess (arrows) through a cortical defect. Note also the marrow oedema and periosteal elevation.

diagnosis of bone infection is important. MRI typically demonstrates poorly defined marrow oedema, periostitis and soft-tissue oedema, which are also seen in acute infarction. However, the communication between a fluid collection in the medulla and surrounding soft tissues through a cortical defect is indicative of osteomyelitis (Fig. 5-10B). Also, the presence of geographic regions of marrow enhancement on fat-suppressed post-contrast T1W images is strongly associated with infection, while acute marrow infarcts tend to show serpentine peripheral

enhancement. Ultrasound (US) may aid the diagnosis of infection by the guided aspiration of subperiosteal fluid collections.

MISCELLANEOUS DISORDERS

Gaucher's Disease[7,8]

Gaucher's disease is the commonest lipid storage disorder and is due to a genetic enzyme (glucocerebrosidase) deficiency, which results in the accumulation of the lipid glucocerebroside in the lysosomes of monocytes and macrophages. These engorged cells are called Gaucher cells and the accumulation of Gaucher cells within a variety of organ systems accounts for the symptoms of the disorder. Many of those affected are Ashkenazi Jews (~1/400–600), but all races are vulnerable. Three types are recognised: the common type 1, which is non-neuronopathic, and the rare neuronopathic types 2 (acute) and 3 (subacute).

The adult form mainly affects older children and young adults, but older adults are not exempt. Bone disease is the commonest cause of long-term morbidity, affecting up to 75% of patients. Both dull bone pain and acute painful crises occur. Bone crises are characterised by acute episodes of severe skeletal pain, fever, leucocytosis and raised erythrocyte sedimentation rate (ESR).

Radiological Features

Radiological features relate to lipid storage effects and bone necrosis. The large amounts of lipid in the marrow spaces cause osteopenia. Loss of normal modelling of the long bones in childhood results in the Erlenmeyer flask appearance of their ends (Fig. 5-11). However, this appearance is common to other marrow-expanding disorders. Lytic areas of varying size (Fig. 5-11A) and a 'soap bubble' appearance may be seen. The cortex is scalloped on its endosteal surface and becomes thinned. Osteopenia is associated with an increased risk of pathological fracture. Osteosclerosis may also occur as a healing response following bone infarction. Metaphyseal notching of the humerus is also a characteristic feature and is thought to be secondary to increased bone turnover.

Bone infarction is common and either due to interference of blood supply by lipid-laden cells or to fat embolism. Episodes of bone pain, fever and elevation of ESR may indicate osteonecrosis. Bone infarction involves particularly the subarticular bone of the femoral and humeral heads, the metaphyseal regions of long bones and the vertebral bodies, in which case vertebral collapse with or without cord compression may occur. Acute bone crises may show periosteal reaction on radiography, focal photopenic areas on scintigraphy and marrow oedema on MRI. The condition must be differentiated from osteomyelitis, which also complicates Gaucher's disease.

MRI is most useful in evaluating the extent of marrow infiltration, being manifest as either homogeneous or

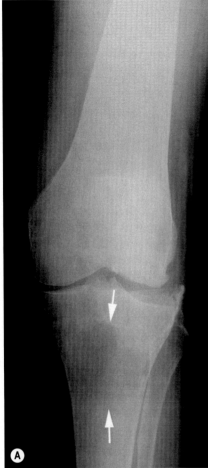

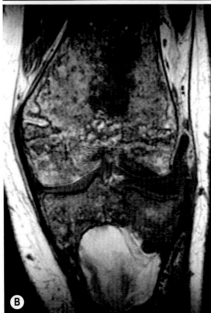

FIGURE 5-11 ■ Gaucher's disease. (A) AP radiograph of the left knee showing the Erlenmeyer flask deformity of the distal femoral and proximal tibial metaphyses, generalised osteopenia and a lytic lesion in the proximal tibia (arrows). (B) Coronal T1W SE MRI of the left knee showing heterogeneous reduction of marrow SI.

heterogeneous reduced SI on T1W (Fig. 5-11B) and T2W images. Such changes are always present in the spine. Complications such as bone infarction, osteomyelitis and fracture can also be assessed, while response to enzyme replacement therapy (ERT) is possible using specialised chemical shift imaging sequences.[9]

The prevalence of bone changes depends upon whether ERT has been administered. In the absence of ERT, 94% of patients will demonstrate some form of osseous radiological abnormality, including Erlenmeyer flask deformity (61%), osteopenia (50%), bone infarction and osteonecrosis (35%), fractures (26%) and lytic lesions (18%). All of these features are less common in patients receiving ERT.

DISORDERS OF BLOOD COAGULATION

Three major inherited disorders are considered:
1. classic haemophilia (haemophilia A)
2. Christmas disease (haemophilia B)
3. von Willebrand's disease.

All produce the same radiological appearances, the diseases differing only in the frequency and severity of the observed changes. Very occasionally, a patient of either sex may develop antibodies to antihaemophilic globulin and develop an acquired form of haemophilia. The prevalence of haemophilia A is estimated at 1 : 5000 and Christmas disease 1 : 30,000.

Haemophilia (Haemophilia A)[10–12]

Haemophilia A is an X-linked recessive disorder resulting from deficiency of factor VIII. Bleeding, which usually follows minor trauma, may occur in the first year of life and 70% of haemophiliacs have experienced haemarthrosis by the age of 2 years. Repeated haemarthroses result in chronic arthropathy and eventually premature osteoarthritis. Soft-tissue haemorrhage, often close to muscle attachments, produces another lesion characteristic of the disease, the haemophilic pseudotumour.

Christmas Disease (Haemophilia B)

Named after the first patient studied, this disorder is due to deficiency of factor IX and is also an X-linked recessive disease. It is less severe than haemophilia.

Von Willebrand's Disease

Inherited as a dominant character and affecting both sexes, von Willebrand's disease is due to both a capillary defect and a deficiency in factor VIII. The coagulation defect is mild and only occasionally causes significant skeletal abnormality. The severity of the disease relates to the level of factor VIII in the blood, which is variable.

Radiological Features

In patients with severe haemophilia, 85–90% of all bleeding events involve the joints. Radiologically, acute haemarthrosis appears as a tense joint effusion (Fig. 5-12) and associated periarticular osteoporosis may indicate previous episodes. MRI is more accurate than clinical examination at identifying haemarthrosis and US may also have a role in early detection. The most common joints involved are the knee, elbow, ankle, hip and shoulder. Repeated episodes of haemorrhage result in progressive joint damage referred to as haemophilic arthropathy.

Haemorrhage initially occurs into the synovium and eventually extends into the joint space. Recurrent haemarthrosis results in a chronic haemorrhagic synovitis and articular cartilage damage. Hyperaemia results in periarticular osteopenia, epiphyseal overgrowth and premature closure of the growth plates. Pannus similar to that occurring in rheumatoid arthritis causes marginal erosions. Loss of secondary trabeculae leads to a permanent coarsening of the trabecular pattern, while growth arrest lines indicate the episodic nature of the disorder. Fibrosis results in joint contracture and intraosseous haemorrhage produces subarticular cysts, which predispose to subchondral collapse. Synovial thickening together with osteopenia make the soft tissues appear radiographically denser. An absolute increase in the soft-tissue density may also occur due to concentration of haemosiderin by macrophages in the periarticular regions.

The knee is the most common joint involved. Radiological features include enlargement of the distal femoral and proximal tibial epiphyses, varus or valgus deformity, squaring of the inferior pole of the patella with patellar overgrowth and widening of the intercondylar notch. Eventually, advanced secondary osteoarthritis (OA) develops.

In the elbow, chronic hyperaemia causes accelerated appearance of the ossification centres and overgrowth of the radial head. Pressure erosion of the radial notch of the ulna, large lytic lesions of the proximal ulna and erosion of the trochlear notch are also seen.

In the ankle, asymmetric growth of the distal tibial epiphysis results in medial tibiotalar slant. Marked flattening of the talar dome, a variety of ankle and foot deformities and, rarely, ankylosis of the ankle or subtalar joints may be seen.

Typical radiographic features of osteonecrosis may be evident in the hip and may simulate Perthes' disease, eventually resulting in coxa magna. Protrusio acetabuli and secondary OA are also seen, while haemorrhage into the growth plate may result in slipped epiphysis. Coxa valga may result from delayed weight-bearing.

Staging of haemophilic arthropathy has typically been with radiography, utilising the Pettersson score. However, radiography is insensitive to the earliest changes, which occur in soft tissue. US can demonstrate acute/chronic haemarthrosis and the resulting synovitis but is less able to assess the cartilage and subchondal bone. All of the pathological features of haemophilic arthropathy can be well demonstrated by MRI, which may demonstrate changes in the joint before any clinically evident episode of bleeding. MRI shows the earliest evidence of haemarthrosis as a low SI intra-articular blood clot within a hyperintense joint effusion. Fluid–fluid levels may also be seen. In chronic cases, the haemosiderin-laden synovium appears irregularly thickened and markedly hypointense

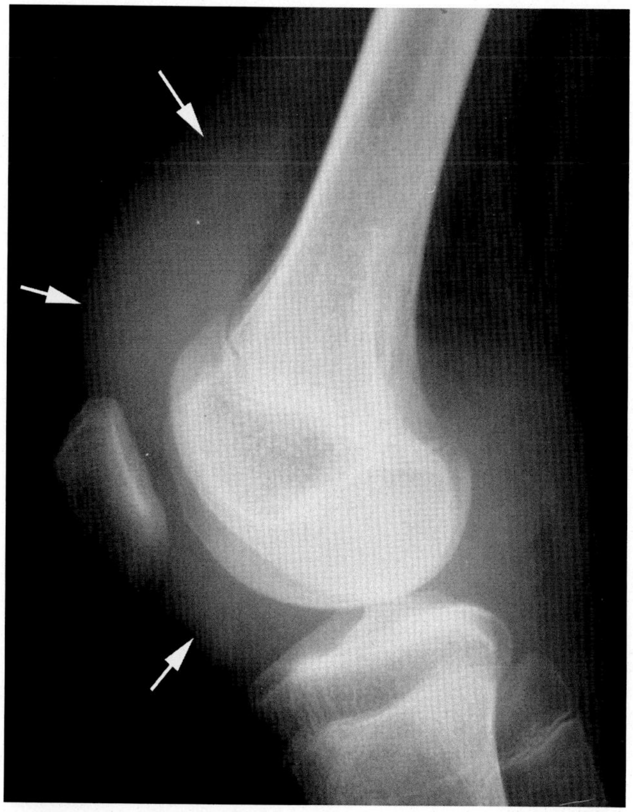

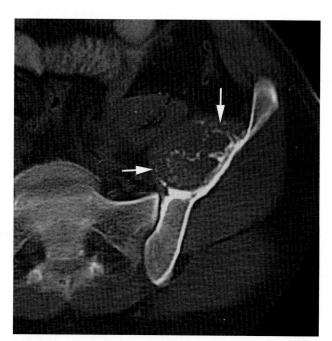

FIGURE 5-12 ■ **Haemophilia.** Lateral radiograph of the knee showing a prominent joint effusion (arrows) due to acute haemarthrosis.

FIGURE 5-13 ■ **Haemophilic pseudotumour.** Axial CT study of the left ilium showing a calcified mass (arrows) in the left iliacus with chronic erosion of the adjacent iliac blade.

on T2W images, particularly gradient-echo sequences. Other features include focal cartilage defects and subchondral cysts.

Small soft-tissue haematomas are common and when repetitive may lead to contractures. Of more importance is the infrequent progressive haemorrhage close to muscle attachments, usually with no history of injury, resulting in the haemophilic pseudotumour. This is more common in adults, with a reported incidence of 1.56%. Most are reported in the pelvis, thigh, or calf. Subperiosteal or intraosseous haemorrhage causes pressure erosion of the bone, particularly the iliac blade in relation to the extensive origin of the iliacus muscle (Fig. 5-13) and the femur. Pathological fracture may be the first manifestation of a haemophilic pseudotumour of bone.

Radiographically, a haemophilic pseudotumour appears as a soft-tissue mass, which may be calcified. Bone lesions may show geographic lytic destruction with cortical thickening. CT identifies the thick, relatively hyperdense pseudocapsule with a hypodense centre. The MRI SI varies with the age of the contained blood, progressing from being isointense to muscle in the first week on T1W and subsequently becoming hyperintense on both T1W and T2W images. The wall tends to be hypointense because of its contained haemosiderin. Mural nodules provide a highly characteristic appearance. Treatment is by management of the haemophilia and exploratory operation is to be avoided.

REFERENCES

1. Martinoli C, Bacigalupo L, Forni GL, et al. Musculoskeletal manifestations of chronic anemias. Semin Musculoskelet Radiol 2011; 15:269–80.
2. Tyler PA, Madani G, Chaudhuri R, et al. The radiological appearances of thalassaemia. Clin Radiol 2006;61:40–52.
3. Angastiniotis M, Eleftheriou A. Thalassaemic bone disease. An overview. Pediatr Endocrinol Rev 2008;6(Suppl 1):73–80.
4. Argyropoulou MI, Astrakas L. MRI evaluation of tissue iron burden in patients with beta-thalassaemia major. Pediatr Radiol 2007;37: 1191–200.
5. Ejindu VC, Hine AL, Mashayekhi M, et al. Musculoskeletal manifestations of sickle cell disease. Radiographics 2007;27:1005–21.
6. Madani G, Papadopoulou AM, Holloway B, et al. The radiological manifestations of sickle cell disease. Clin Radiol 2007;62:528–38.
7. Wenstrup RJ, Roca-Espiau M, Weinreb NJ, Bembi B. Skeletal aspects of Gaucher disease: a review. Br J Radiol 2002;75(Suppl 1):A2–A12.
8. McHugh K, Olsen EOE, Vellodi A. Gaucher disease in children: radiology of non-central nervous system manifestations. Clin Radiol 2004;59:117–23.
9. Maas M, Kuijper M, Akkerman EM. From Gaucher's disease to metabolic radiology: translational radiological research and clinical practice. Semin Musculoskelet Radiol 2011;15:301–6.
10. Kerr R. Imaging of musculoskeletal complications of hemophilia. Semin Musculoskelet Radiol 2003;7:127–36.
11. Jelbert A, Vaidya S, Fotiadis N. Imaging and staging of haemophilic arthropathy. Clin Radiol 2009;64:1119–28.
12. Doria AS. State-of-the-art imaging techniques for the evaluation of haemophilic arthropathy: present and future. Haemophilia 2010;16(Suppl 5):107–14.

CHAPTER 6

IMAGING FOR RADIOTHERAPY PLANNING

Peter Hoskin • Roberto Alonzi

CHAPTER OUTLINE

TYPES OF RADIOTHERAPY

THE RADIOTHERAPY PROCESS

FUNCTIONAL IMAGING IN THE
RADIOTHERAPY PROCESS

Radiation therapy has been used as a treatment for cancer for more than 100 years, with its earliest roots dating back to the discovery of X-rays in 1895. Its development in the early 1900s is largely due to the work of Marie Curie (1867–1934), who discovered the radioactive elements polonium and radium in 1898. Despite these distant origins, radiotherapy remains at the forefront of the treatment for cancer. Approximately 60% of cancer patients currently receive radiation therapy at some stage during their illness with 75% of these treated with curative intent.[1] Despite major advances in drug treatments for cancer, there has continued to be a steady annual increase in radiotherapy treatment that is unlikely to change within the next 10–20 years.[2]

As a result of advances in imaging and computer technology, radiotherapy has been transformed from 2-dimensional (2D) techniques to highly precise 3-dimensional (3D) conformal treatments that utilise axial tomographic images of the patient's anatomy to guide 3D intensity-modulated, image-guided therapy. Advances in imaging have allowed radiation oncologists to delineate and target tumours more accurately, thereby producing better treatment outcomes, improved organ preservation and fewer side effects. Furthermore, with the development of functional imaging techniques such as positron emission tomography (PET), dynamic contrast-enhanced computed tomography (CT) and multi-parametric magnetic resonance imaging (MRI) it is now possible to integrate biological information (for example, tumour oxygenation, cellular proliferation or tumour blood flow) into the radiotherapy planning process. Imaging is therefore critical at almost every stage in the practice of modern radiation delivery (Fig. 6-1).

TYPES OF RADIOTHERAPY

External Beam Radiotherapy

External beam radiotherapy constitutes the mainstay of radiation treatment in developed countries. External beam radiotherapy refers to any situation where the source of the radiation is located at a distance from the patient and the beam of radiation is then directed towards a defined treatment area. Approximately 85% of all therapeutic radiation exposures are delivered using external beam techniques. Various types and energies of radiation can be delivered in this way, including electromagnetic radiation such as X-rays and γ-rays, or particles such as electrons and protons. Higher energies of radiation penetrate deeper into body tissues. As a result low-energy X-rays (60–300 keV) are reserved for the treatment of skin cancers and superficial subcutaneous tumours. Most external beam radiotherapy treatments utilise megavoltage X-rays or electrons (6–18 MeV) generated by a linear particle accelerator (Fig. 6-2).

Conventional External Beam Radiotherapy

Conventional radiotherapy refers to techniques in which the treatment volume is defined by simple geometric parameters. In general, no attempt is made to delineate the tumour outline or to shape the radiation dose distribution to conform to the tumour volume. This is commonly practised for palliative treatments where long-term normal tissue toxicity is less relevant. The irradiated volume can be defined clinically but more often fluoroscopic or CT simulation is used. The radiation fields tend to run parallel to each other, creating a box-like treatment volume (Fig. 6-3).

Three-Dimensional Conformal Radiotherapy

The incorporation of axial imaging data allows 3D reconstruction of the tumour and surrounding organs. This provides more accurate localisation of the target volume and more information regarding the amount of normal tissue that will be irradiated. The radiotherapy planning computer software then utilises the attenuation coefficient information (Hounsfield units) derived from the CT image on a voxel-by-voxel basis to predict the attenuation of each therapeutic radiation beam as it passes through the body. As a result, the number and profile of the radiation beams can be orientated and shaped to fit the profile of the target from a beam's eye view using a

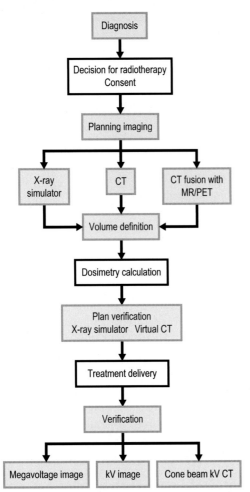

FIGURE 6-1 ■ **The radiotherapy pathway.** Processes outlined in green involve imaging.

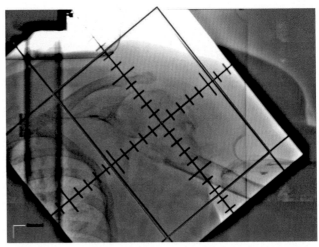

FIGURE 6-3 ■ **Palliative conventional external beam radiotherapy for a destructive bone metastasis of the proximal humerus that has caused a pathological fracture.** The edges of the treatment beam have been defined using fluoroscopy. For illustrative purposes the edges of the treatment field have been outlined in red. The treatment will be implemented using parallel opposed beams of radiation from the anterior and posterior directions, thereby creating a box-like treatment volume.

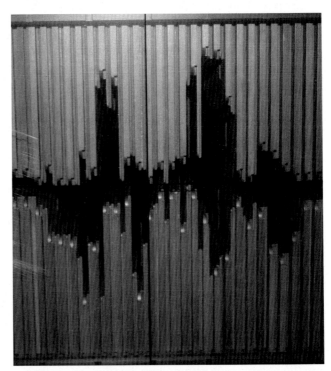

FIGURE 6-4 ■ **A multileaf collimator (MLC).** This is made up of individual 'leaves' of a high atomic numbered material, usually tungsten, which can move independently in and out of the path of a radiation beam in order to block it. This device is situated in the head of a linear accelerator to shape the treatment beam in order to match the borders of the target tumour. For intensity-modulated treatments the leaves of an MLC are moved across the field while the beam is on to create fluence modulation.

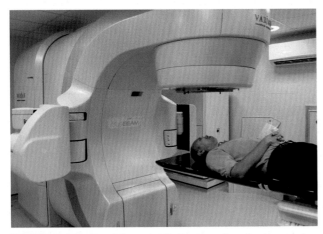

FIGURE 6-2 ■ **External beam radiotherapy.** A patient preparing to receive external beam radiotherapy on a linear particle accelerator.

multileaf collimator (Fig. 6-4). The resulting radiotherapy plan can be displayed as a colour map of radiation dose overlaid onto the anatomical CT images so that the radiation oncologist can determine whether the tumour volume will receive sufficient irradiation with acceptable normal tissue dose sparing (Fig. 6-5). By reducing the irradiated volume and dose to the sensitive surrounding normal tissues, this technique facilitates the delivery of higher tumour radiation doses than would be achievable using conventional techniques.

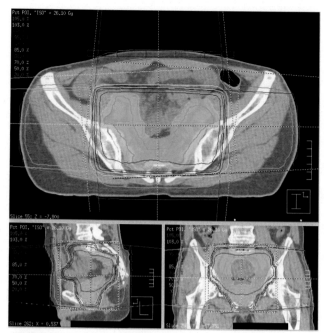

FIGURE 6-5 ■ **A 3-dimensional conformal radiotherapy plan for treatment of the pelvic lymph nodes.** The planning target volume is defined by the shaded green region. Four treatment beams (anterior, posterior, left and right lateral) overlap over the target volume to provide the desired dose in this region with reduced dose to surrounding normal structures. The coloured lines represent the dose gradient in a similar way to the contour lines on a map and correspond to the numbers in the top left corner. For example, the red line represents the 95% isodose (i.e. every point on this line will receive 95% of the prescribed radiation dose). The coronal and sagittal views show the shaping of the beam by the multileaf collimator (MLC). Despite the use of the static MLC, the transverse image clearly shows that the small bowel anterior to the horseshoe-shaped target volume will still receive the full radiation dose.

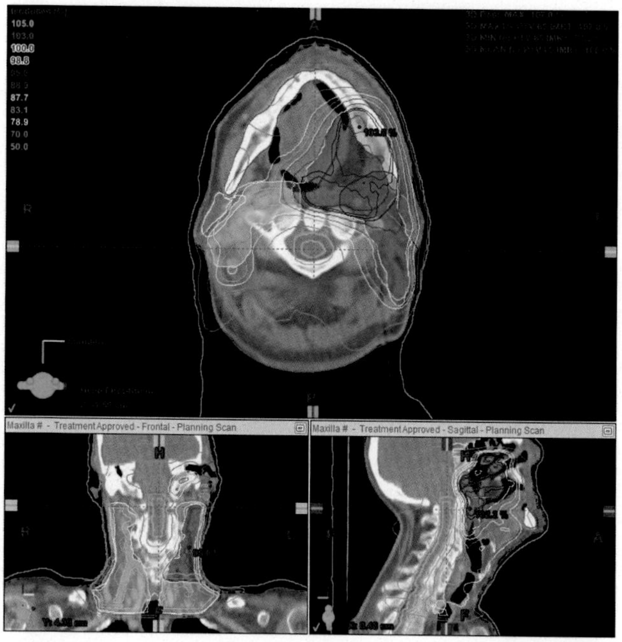

FIGURE 6-6 ■ **An intensity-modulated radiotherapy (IMRT) plan for treatment of the left maxilla and bilateral lymph nodes.** The primary tumour region has been outlined and is defined by the solid red line. This has been expanded to produce a planning target volume shown as the dark blue shaded region and will receive a radical dose to control the macroscopic tumour. The level II lymph nodes have also been defined and will be treated to a lower overall dose to control any microscopic disease spread. The use of intensity modulation has allowed shaping of the dose distribution to avoid the brainstem. The isodose lines can be seen to bend anteriorly around the brainstem, leaving this structure in a region of low radiation dose (between the green and blue isodose lines, which correspond to 50–70% of the prescribed dose, thereby taking the brainstem below its tolerance threshold).

Intensity-Modulated Radiotherapy (IMRT)

IMRT represents a further step in the development of high-precision radiotherapy delivery. The term refers to a variety of techniques in which the radiation beams are not only shaped and orientated to conform to the tumour volume but also the intensity of radiation is modulated across each treatment beam. This technique can produce dose distributions that conform highly to complex shapes, including treatment volumes that wrap around sensitive normal structures such as the spinal cord (Fig. 6-6), enabling high-dose delivery to the tumour volume whilst sparing dose to the normal structures.

IMRT can be achieved using a number of different technologies. Most commonly, several static radiation fields in the same plane of orientation are used, similar to the situation for 3D conformal radiotherapy, but with varying dose flux across the profile of the beam which is achieved by moving the leaves of the multileaf collimator across the beam at varying rates.[3] Alternatively, arc therapies utilise a number of non-coplanar beam arcs in which the radiation is delivered using multiple 'stop and shoot' beams or as a continuously moving field that varies in intensity throughout rotation.[4] Tomotherapy is another technique for achieving IMRT in which a megavoltage X-ray source is mounted in a similar fashion to a CT X-ray source (Fig. 6-7). The treatment volume is irradiated using the machine's continuously rotating beam that is modulated in intensity whilst the patient moves through the gantry bore.[5]

Stereotactic Body Radiotherapy (SBRT)

In SBRT the distribution of radiation beams is in three dimensions and not in two as in traditional radiotherapy.[6] It is based on a precise evaluation of the positioning of the tumour in real time and on the delivery of the dose by multiple beams (sometimes one hundred or more beams per treatment—Fig. 6-8). The treatment is based upon stereotactic radiosurgery methods for the treatment of intracranial tumours. However, it can only be used for selected, small extracranial lesions such as tumours of the lung and prostate or small solitary metastases. Even with small tumours, the complexity of the technique can sometimes result in treatment times of over an hour per fraction, thereby necessitating a small number of radiotherapy fractions to make a course of SBRT treatment

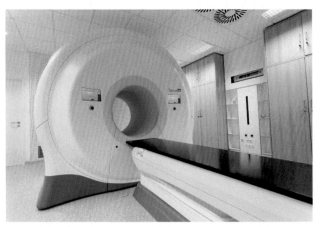

FIGURE 6-7 ■ **A tomotherapy unit.** Tomotherapy is essentially a combination of spiral CT and intensity-modulated radiation therapy technology. As with a CT unit, the patient moves through the unit, but instead of a kilovoltage diagnostic X-ray, hundreds of pencil beams of megavoltage therapeutic X-ray radiation spirally rotate around the patient. Each of these dynamically rotating beamlets vary in intensity to conform to the complex tumour shape.

clinically (and economically) feasible. Fortunately, the precision of SBRT allows high doses to be delivered in a very limited number of fractions. This is sometimes referred to as ultra-hypofractionation in which doses per fraction can be as high as 20 grays (conventional radiotherapy is delivered at 2 grays per fraction). There is current speculation that the mechanism of radiation-induced tumour cell killing may differ at such high doses per fraction. It has been hypothesised that radiation doses of more than 10 grays per fraction can cause rapid obliteration of the tumour vasculature, which cannot be achieved with the lower conventional doses, resulting in a biological advantage for ultra-hypofractionation.

Brachytherapy

Brachytherapy refers to a situation in which a radioisotope is placed onto or inside the patient. The radiation source is sealed in a protective capsule or wire which prevents the radioisotope from moving or dissolving in body fluids but allows the emission of ionising radiation

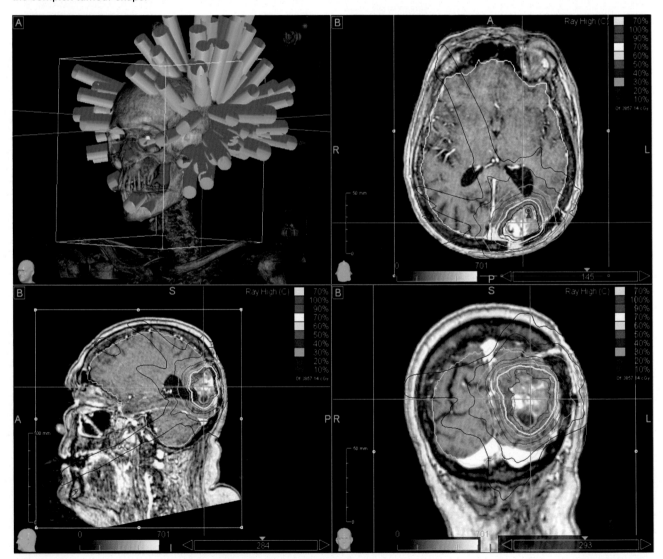

FIGURE 6-8 ■ **A stereotactic body radiotherapy plan using the CyberKnife robotic radiosurgery system to treat a recurrent glioblastoma of the occipital lobe.** Each of the blue cylinders represents a pencil beam of radiation that is controlled with extreme accuracy using image guidance. The machinery can correct for movements of the tumour caused by breathing or internal organ motion. The resulting dose distribution, which can be seen in the transverse, coronal and sagittal views, conforms extremely well with the tumour volume.

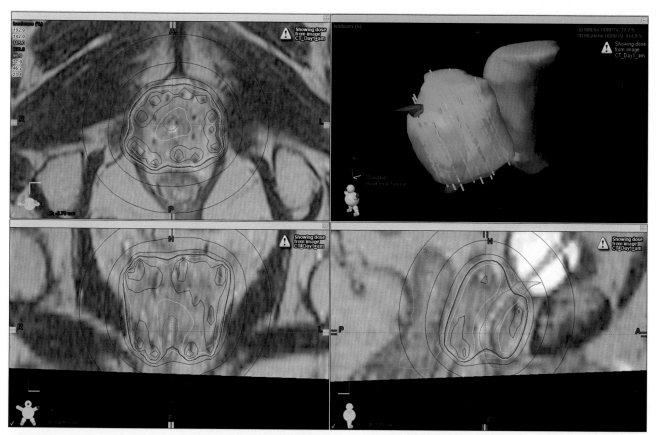

FIGURE 6-9 ■ **A high dose-rate brachytherapy plan for treatment of an intermediate-risk prostate cancer.** The 3-dimensional reconstruction in the top right panel shows the dwell positions of the ^{192}Ir source as it passes though each of the catheters that have been inserted through the prostate gland. The shaded light blue region on the transverse, sagittal and coronal images represents the target volume. The red isodose line is the prescribed dose (i.e. every voxel within this line will receive at least the prescribed radiation dose). Note how closely this line fits to the target volume. The outermost blue line represents 23.1% of the prescribed dose, showing that the dose falls off within very short distances from the target, thereby sparing the surrounding normal tissues.

(in the form of α, β, γ or X-radiation) to the surrounding tissues. The source can be placed into the target tissues or tumour itself such as the prostate or breast (interstitial brachytherapy), into a body cavity such as the uterine cavity, oesophagus or bronchus (intracavitary/intraluminal brachytherapy) or onto the skin surface to treat a cutaneous malignancy.

In certain situations brachytherapy offers some major advantages over external beam techniques. One of the key features of brachytherapy is that the irradiation only affects a very localised area around the radiation sources as dose falls off rapidly, obeying the inverse square law. As long as the sources are precisely placed within the tumour, there is minimal exposure to radiation of healthy tissues further away from the sources. This allows very high doses to be administered to the target volume (Fig. 6-9). Also, patient set-up and tumour motion are less relevant because the radiation sources move with the tumour and therefore retain their correct position; this increases the confidence that the radiation has been delivered in accordance with the required plan.

Due to the very short distances between the radiation source and the treatment volume, the absorbed tissue dose is almost entirely a function of the distance from the source, rather than due to the attenuation coefficient of the tissues that the radiation passes through (in contrast to the situation with external radiation). Radiation from a point source is inversely proportional to the square of the distance from the source. Tissues twice as far away receive only one-quarter of the dose in the same time period. As a result, brachytherapy techniques do not necessarily require Hounsfield number information from CT data to produce conformal treatment plans. As long as the position of the radiation sources can be reliably located, any imaging modality can be used for planning (Fig. 6-10).

Brachytherapy applicators have been adapted to enable better imaging. For example, CT- and MRI-compatible intrauterine tubes have been developed for gynaecological treatments. Seeds containing ^{125}I are commonly used to treat prostate cancer and have been designed with roughened and bevelled ends to maximise ultrasound visibility. Because precise reproduction of the source position is critical to brachytherapy dose calculations, any distortion or registration error may be critical and should be carefully quality-assured before incorporating in routine practice. Specific MR sequences may be developed to enable certain applications: for example, proton-rich sequences for identification of ^{125}I seeds in the prostate.[7] Imaging also has a crucial role in the

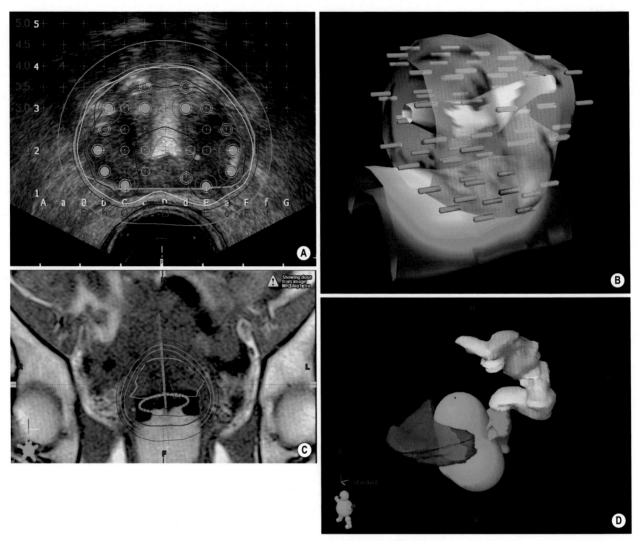

FIGURE 6-10 ■ **Brachytherapy planning without the use of CT.** (A) Pre-plan for an ^{125}I prostate seed implant: a transrectal ultrasound image has been acquired and the prostate margin (red), urethra (green) and rectum (dark blue) have been defined. The prostate margin has been expanded to produce the planning target volume (light blue). (B) The seeds can then be positioned to deliver the maximum dose to the prostate whilst minimising dose to the urethra and rectum. (C) High dose-rate brachytherapy planning for a cervical carcinoma using MRI. An intrauterine tube and cervical ring have been inserted under general anaesthetic and their position has been marked (green and pink segmented line). Each segment of the line represents a dwell position for the ^{192}Ir isotope. The time that the isotope remains at each dwell position determines the dose distribution, which is manipulated to maximise dose to the tumour and avoid normal structures. (D) The final dose distribution with the prescribed radiation isodose is represented by the light blue shaded region. The bladder (pink), rectum (green) and colon (yellow) are also shown.

accurate positioning of radiation sources or afterloading applicators for brachytherapy. Its flexibility and real-time imaging capability means that ultrasound is considered particularly valuable in this respect.

Brachytherapy is often defined by the rate at which the radiation dose is applied. Low-dose rate (LDR) brachytherapy sources emit radiation at a rate of up to 2 Gy·h^{-1}. These sources can be permanent, as is the case with LDR prostate brachytherapy (Fig. 6-11), or removed after several days, as for oral cavity tumours. High-dose rate (HDR) brachytherapy sources emit radiation at a rate of over 12 Gy·h^{-1}; however, the most commonly used HDR units with an ^{192}Ir source emit radiation at a much higher rate of between 60 and 100 Gy·h^{-1}. HDR sources are always afterloaded (instead of directly placing the source

into the patient); hollow catheters are inserted and subsequently connected to the HDR unit which can be operated remotely to deliver the source into each catheter with the operator outside the shielded room (Fig. 6-12).

Particle Therapy

Also known as hadron therapy, particle therapy is an external beam technique in which highly energetic particles such as protons, neutrons or positive ions are directed at the tumour. Although electrons are particles, these are not usually considered in the category of particle therapy. The most common form of particle therapy uses protons that are accelerated by a cyclotron or synchrotron. Protons have several physical characteristics

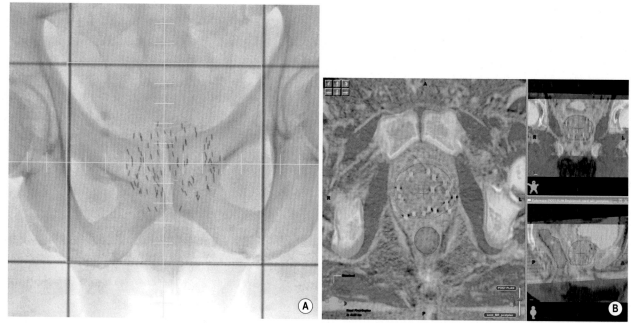

FIGURE 6-11 ■ **Brachytherapy for a low-risk prostate cancer.** (A) Plain radiograph of the pelvis taken a few minutes after ^{125}I seed implantation for a patient with low-risk prostate cancer. (B) Fused CT and MR imaging of the same patient on day 28 after the implant. The iodine seeds emit 35 kV X-radiation (maximum energy) and have a half-life of 59 days. As a result the prostate is irradiated over a period of months rather than weeks or days. Following the implant procedure there is often some migration of seed positions caused by bleeding and swelling from the trauma of implantation. It is therefore important to determine the final dose distribution from imaging a few weeks after seed insertion rather than from their initial position.

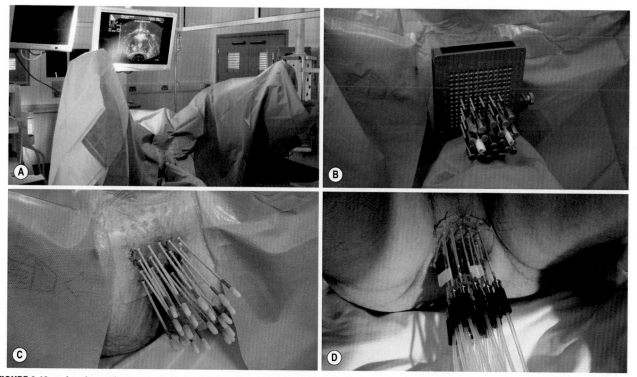

FIGURE 6-12 ■ **Implantation technique for high dose-rate brachytherapy of the prostate.** The procedure is carried out under general or spinal anaesthetic in the lithotomy position with a transrectal ultrasound probe mounted on a fixed stand with a template (A). Flexible plastic catheters are inserted through the perineum into the prostate in a parallel arrangement guided by the template (B). The catheters are left inside the patient whilst imaging (CT and/or MRI) and planning is performed (C). The catheters are then connected to the afterloading device, which robotically introduces the high activity radiation source through each catheter in turn in a pattern determined by the radiotherapy plan (D).

that provide an advantage over photon treatments. Protons penetrate deep into body tissues and deposit the majority of their energy in the last few millimetres of their range with virtually no radiation passing beyond this distance.[8] Therefore, varying the energy of the proton beam can control the depth of treatment.

For most treatments, protons of different energies are applied to treat the entire tumour. Also, due to their greater mass, protons scatter less and the beam remains focused with less broadening than photon beams. These properties translate into a clinical advantage when it is paramount to limit the radiation dose to critical normal structures that lie deep to the tumour. In particular, where there may be a critical normal tissue such as the spinal cord immediately behind the target, the minimal exit dose using proton therapy can prevent major long-term morbidity. This is particularly true for paediatric neoplasms such as medulloblastoma where there is convincing clinical data to show the advantage of sparing the developing brain and cord.[9–11]

There are only a few centres in the world that have the capability of treating patients with the other forms of particle therapy: namely, fast neutron therapy or carbon ion therapy. These techniques have physical advantages similar to that of protons, with sparing of tissues at depth, but in addition there are biological benefits. Both neutrons and carbon ions cause dense ionisation with much greater transfer of energy along the radiation track. This results in more radiation damage and cell death.[12] Furthermore, there is theoretical evidence that intensely ionising radiation of this sort can overcome the detrimental effects of tumour hypoxia, which is a major cause of treatment failure with standard radiotherapy.[13]

THE RADIOTHERAPY PROCESS

Radiotherapy Treatment Volume Definition

As radiotherapy dose delivery becomes more precise, the need for accurate diagnostic imaging that can be incorporated into the radiotherapy process increases. It is now possible to deliver radiation with near-millimetre accuracy. This puts considerable pressure on diagnostic technology to define tumour boundaries with similar accuracy. Because of the uncertainties inherent in the delineation of tumour volume, it is standard practice to incorporate a safety margin around the 'visible' gross tumour volume (GTV) to produce a clinical target volume (CTV) that accounts for extension of the tumour that is beyond the resolution of current diagnostic imaging capability. A further expansion is then made to account for set-up errors which occur due to the inherent variability in equipment geometry and beam alignment and intra-fraction tumour movement to produce a planning target volume (PTV) (Fig. 6-13). In order to further capitalise on the accuracy of modern radiotherapy equipment and make additional reductions in normal tissue toxicity whilst increasing dose to the tumour, this safety margin needs to be reduced. This can only occur if (1) there is a higher level of confidence in defining tumour volumes

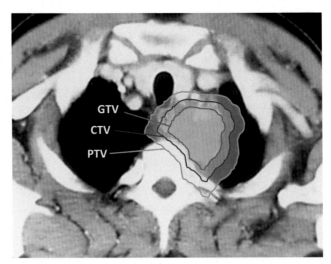

FIGURE 6-13 ■ **Contrast-enhanced radiotherapy planning CT image.** The gross tumour volume (GTV) of a lung tumour has been outlined (blue). The treatment planning computer software has been used to expand this volume into a clinical target volume (CTV) to account for the possible microscopic spread of tumour cells into surrounding tissues (orange). This volume has, in turn, been expanded into a planning target volume (PTV) to account for set-up error and tumour motion during treatment (green). The treatment plan will then be created to encompass the PTV with the required treatment isodose.

and (2) tumour movements during radiation delivery can be visualised and accounted for. Both of these require advanced imaging capabilities.

Clinical Volume Definition (Non-imaging-Based)

This is used for visible tumours or for palliative treatments where accurate tumour localisation is not required. For skin cancers, the visible tumour boundary is outlined and a margin for microscopic spread is marked on the skin surface (Fig. 6-14). For treatment to deeper structures the field borders can be defined using anatomical landmarks.

Conventional Simulation

The 'simulator' is a kilovoltage X-ray machine and detector that is designed to emulate the movements of a radiotherapy treatment machine (linear accelerator) to reproduce treatment conditions (Fig. 6-15). It has a couch that is capable of all the movements of a linear accelerator couch and a gantry that can be rotated through 360°. It produces 2D X-ray images, which can be viewed in real time on the screen. Palpable tumours can be marked with wire to aid localisation and contrast can be used to define some organs (for example, the bladder, rectum or oesophagus). Screening demonstrates organ and tumour movement to allow adjustment of the treatment fields. Field borders are defined on the screen and transferred to the patient using positioning lights that are aligned to the field edges. Skin tattoos act as

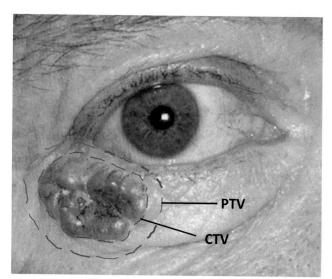

FIGURE 6-14 ■ **Clinical 'mark-up' for a nodular basal cell carcinoma.** The tumour boundary is defined visually and by palpation and marked onto the patient's skin (CTV). An expansion is made to account for microscopic extension and set-up error (PTV); this is also drawn on the skin. A lead cutout is then custom-made to shield the normal skin from the radiation beam.

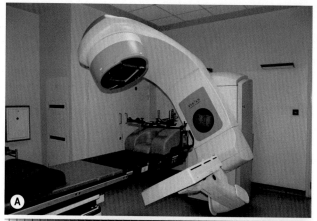
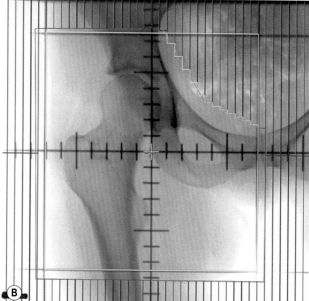

FIGURE 6-15 ■ **Conventional simulator.** (A) Photograph of a conventional simulator. The simulator is a kilovoltage X-ray machine and detector designed to emulate the movements of a linear accelerator which it resembles (compare with Fig. 6-2). Simple geometric treatment fields can be planned using this method. (B) Planning for palliative radiotherapy for metastases in the right proximal femur and pubic bones. A multileaf collimator has been used to partially shield some of the sensitive pelvic organs and bowel.

reference points to aid identical set-up on the treatment machine.

Traditionally, the conventional simulator was used to plan all types of radiotherapy, including multiple beam treatments. In order to achieve this, anteroposterior and lateral images were taken together with a transverse outline of the body contour through the centre of the simulated volume, which the planning department could then convert into a 3D volume. However, the main limitation of this method was the inability to accurately define the tumour volume and adjacent normal structures due to poor soft-tissue contrast. As a result, treatment volumes were predominately defined by bony landmarks, producing generic treatment volumes without any reliable ability to estimate the dose and volume of normal tissue irradiated. Furthermore, the lack of tissue density information meant that the estimated doses delivered to the tumour and adjacent structures were purely based on the body contour, and the depth of tissue that the beam had to penetrate to deposit the radiation dose. Because of this, there is no longer a role for a conventional simulator in planning curative radiotherapy; the sale of such machines is now almost non-existent in the UK and North America. The role of the conventional simulator is now restricted to checking radiotherapy plans and planning palliative treatments (Fig. 6-15).

CT Simulation

CT simulation replaces the use of the conventional simulator with a CT imager to gather information. CT provides excellent bone and soft-tissue imaging as well as tissue density information, which is necessary for the accurate calculation of the dose distribution. CT

simulation refers to the simulation process performed with data collected from the CT imaging. Data are downloaded onto a 3D treatment planning computer where the simulation can be performed. This technology provides the radiation oncologist with information on internal anatomy and the ability to view the patient's body in any plane with high soft-tissue and bone contrast. The software is capable of producing digitally reconstructed radiographs (DRRs), which are images that mimic a conventional radiograph in any field direction (Fig. 6-16). This information is then used in two ways to define the radiotherapy delivery:

- Virtual simulation in which the tumour volume may be outlined formally or simply viewed in three dimensions and the fields necessary to cover the

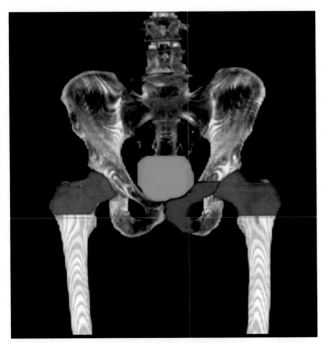

FIGURE 6-16 ■ Digitally reconstructed radiograph (DRR) of the bony anatomy. In this example the intended target is a bone metastasis in the left pubic bone (red). The organs at risk have also been defined. The bladder is shown in green. The head and neck of both femora have also been included as organs at risk (pink) due to the fact that excessive radiation can cause avascular necrosis of the femoral head and risk of subsequent fracture.

volume are simulated on the computer screen. This will typically be used for simple palliative treatments to internal organs or bones and use single or opposed fields for which the subsequent dose distribution can be calculated (Fig. 6-17).

- CT conformal planning in which the CT data are harnessed to a sophisticated planning system using computer software to calculate complex dose distributions. The target volume is defined by contouring directly onto the CT images and multi-field plans with varying tissue compensation may be employed to deliver a homogenous dose to the tumour volume and minimise dose to surrounding normal organs at risk (see Figs. 6-5 and 6-6).

The advantages of virtual simulation over conventional simulation include a faster simulation procedure, better soft-tissue imaging, the collection of tissue density information, more precise tumour localisation, more precise organ definition, the collection of 3D anatomy data and the facilitation of complex planning techniques.

Image Fusion

CT is the imaging platform for all modern radiation dosimetry planning systems. Tissue density information derived from the Hounsfield number of each voxel of the planning CT imaging is required for accurate estimation of the radiation dose distribution which can vary considerably where the treatment volume includes the lungs or other air cavities. However, whilst a CT image is always required for external beam planning it may not be the best imaging technique for tumour volume and organ at risk delineation. For example, pelvic and brain tumours are often more accurately defined using MRI and tumours of the head and neck and lung benefit from FDG-PET/CT for locating the tumour.[14–16] In order to capitalise on the performance of each imaging technique it is sometimes necessary to fuse imaging data sets to produce the best radiotherapy plan[17] (Fig. 6-18).

This process is not without its complications, as can be illustrated using the example of lung cancer. Bronchial tumours frequently cause collapse of some of the surrounding normal lung tissue. Using CT it is often difficult to define the true extent of the tumour because of a lack of contrast between the cancer and the adjacent collapsed lung. There is, therefore, a risk of missing tumour (if the radiotherapy field is made too small) or of irradiating an unnecessary volume of benign lung tissue (if the defined treatment volume incorporates collapsed lung as well as tumour). ^{18}F-FDG PET/CT is an important tool for the staging of lung cancer and can demonstrate the geographical distribution of the primary tumour and metastases. Many studies have attempted to fuse PET/CT images with the planning CT to aid tumour volume definition. However, the PET/CT image displayed is entirely dependent on the SUV thresholds chosen. Lower thresholds will increase the apparent tumour volume and higher thresholds will do the opposite. There is currently no consensus on how to define tumour borders using PET data. There are also other difficulties that occur when trying to fuse multi-technique imaging sets. These include variations in resolution, spatial distortions that can occur with certain methods (e.g. MRI), physiological and anatomical changes that occur during the time between the imaging acquisitions, increased workload and cost.

Treatment Planning and Verification

Once the planning target volume and normal organs have been defined in three dimensions, the optimum dose distribution for treating the tumour is sought. This is a multi-stage process. Initially, a beam energy must be chosen according to the depth of the target and the size of the patient. Low-energy beams give maximum dose close to the surface and penetrate less. Higher-energy beams give maximum dose deeper within tissues, thereby sparing the skin, and penetrate further into tissues but also give a higher exit dose beyond the target. Other factors to be considered include the quality of the beam, degree of lateral scatter, the availability of beam modification (such as multileaf collimators or the possibility of intensity modulation) and the facility for image guidance.

Next, the required dose to the tumour and the maximum allowable doses to normal organs must be specified. In principle, the aim is to achieve the highest possible dose to the tumour and the lowest possible dose to the normal structures, in particular the defined organs

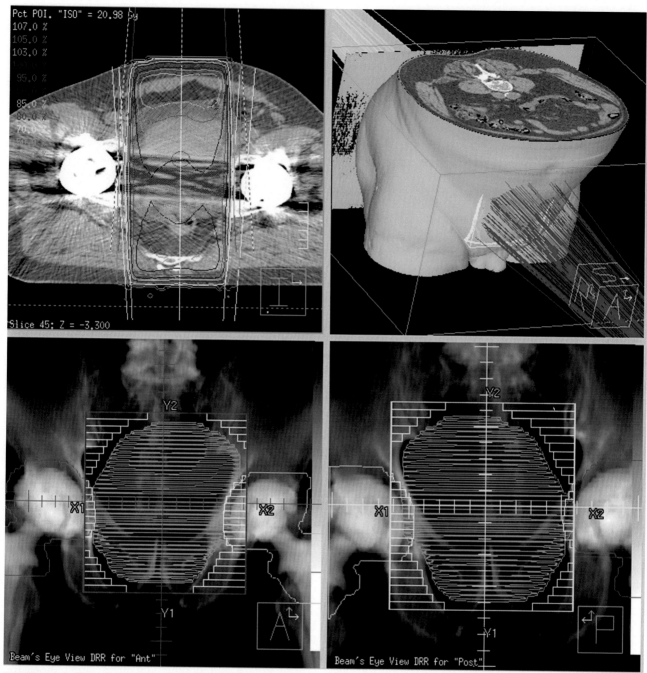

FIGURE 6-17 ■ **Virtual simulation for treatment of an invasive bladder cancer in a patient with bilateral hip replacements.** The hip prostheses prevent the use of lateral or oblique beam angles which would normally be used for pelvic treatments, allowing only anterior and posterior fields (top right). The bladder has been contoured on each CT slice (green). Anterior and posterior 'beam's eye view' digitally reconstructed radiographs are shown (bottom panels). On these views the beam has been shaped by the multileaf collimator. Despite the beam shaping, the fact that only two beams could be used results in a column of high dose through the pelvis in the anteroposterior direction without any possibility of sparing the rectum (top left panel).

at risk, which will be those with critical function nearest the target and those with low radiation tolerance. The results of clinical studies, as well as years of experience, have helped to define acceptable doses to the normal tissues and the minimum tumour dose required to destroy the tumour. It is then the job of the radiotherapist and dosimetrist to devise an acceptable compromise between

the probability of tumour control and the chance of normal tissue toxicity. This is achieved by choosing the optimum beam arrangement (number, energy, size, weighting, angle of beam entry and beam modification using collimators or intensity modulation) and defining the normal tissue constraints, which are doses to specified volumes that will not be exceeded.

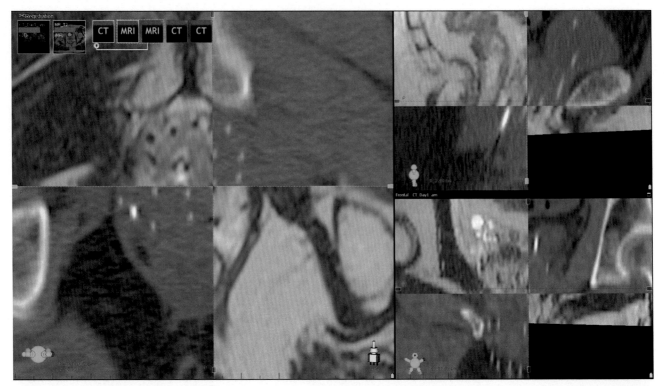

FIGURE 6-18 ■ **CT-MR image fusion illustrated in a patient with brachytherapy catheters in the prostate.** Automated registration software is now widely available but manual correction for more accurate registration is still sometimes required. Inaccuracies can occur if there has been patient or organ movement between the acquisition of the two imaging sets. Also, differences in resolution, spatial distortion and slice thickness can affect the reliability of fusion. Deformable registration programs, where one image is distorted to fit the other more precisely, are currently under evaluation.

Attenuation of an X-ray beam is affected by tissue density; for example, it is less in lung tissue, which is of low density, than in bone. This variation affects both the shape of the dose distribution and the amount of radiation absorbed. Density corrections are used to correct for dose inhomogeneity. If 2D planning is used, correction is only valid at the planned central slice of the target volume. For example, when treating the breast, CT-simulator slices may be used to measure the volume of lung in the tangential beam. For more accurate heterogeneity corrections, 3D planning is needed with localisation of lung tissue throughout the 3D volume using CT planning. Using CT, a pixel-by-pixel correction can be made to take account of all tissue densities within the body contour by conversion of CT numbers into relative electron densities using a predefined calibration.

Various computer algorithms are used to model the interactions between the radiation beam and the patient's anatomy to determine the spatial distribution of the radiation dose.[18-20] Different mathematical algorithms are necessary to account for the different types of radiation and computational complexity. With the increase in computational performance available today, improved algorithms are continually being developed. All external beam planning systems use X-ray-based image data as the density data are necessary for the dosimetry calculations.

Radiotherapy planning can be performed in two ways. In *forward* planning, the planning dosimetrist manually chooses beam parameters that are likely to maximise the tumour dose whilst sparing the normal tissues. The treatment planning system then calculates a predicted dose to the various predefined structures. If the dose to the tumour is insufficient or a normal tissue tolerance is exceeded, then the beam parameters are altered and the process repeated. After a number of iterations an acceptable plan is generated. This type of planning can only handle relatively simple cases in which the tumour has a simple shape and is not near any critical organs. For more sophisticated plans, *inverse* planning is used. With this technique the radiotherapist defines a patient's critical organs and tumour and gives target doses for each. A weighting can also be applied to each target dose to allow the computer to give precedence of one dose level over another. For example, 100% weighting may be given to the spinal cord dose where excessive radiation effects can be catastrophic, whilst a lower weighting may apply to the bladder which is much more radio-resistant. Then, an optimisation programme is run to find the treatment plan which best matches all the input criteria.

Image Guidance during Radiotherapy Delivery

For external beam treatment, the radiotherapy plan is based on the planning CT images. This CT is a snapshot

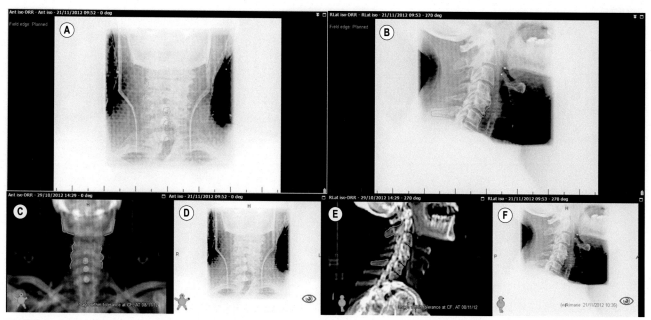

FIGURE 6-19 ■ **Planar (2-dimensional) image guidance.** Two static kilovoltage images have been acquired at 90° to each other using a linear accelerator-based on-board imaging device with the patient on the treatment couch and about to be irradiated (D, F). Bony landmarks have been outlined on the digitally reconstructed radiographs, which have been derived from the planning CT imaging (C, E). These outlines have been transposed onto the kilovoltage images in order to determine whether there has been any deviation from the planned treatment (A, B). In this case there is clearly a discrepancy of 3–4 mm in the craniocaudal direction. This is best seen on the anteroposterior image (A) where the mandible and spinous processes are notably higher than intended. To prevent an inaccurate exposure, either the patient will be repositioned or the fields will be delivered with the appropriate correction. This situation is not uncommon for head and neck cancer treatments where there is often weight loss during the therapy period and as a result the immobilisation head shell becomes loose fitting, allowing movement to occur.

of the patient's position and anatomy at a single point in time. All internal organs are subject to a degree of movement, which can occur daily (inter-fraction motion) or during the treatment delivery (intra-fraction motion). For some organs, such as the lung, the movement is predictable with a repetitive cyclical motion in 3 dimensions. For other organs, such as the bowel, random movements occur with the passage of gas and faeces. To account for this, larger margins are added to the planning target volume. However, the addition of margins to the tumour target volume increases the volume of normal tissue treated and can also increase the dose to organs at risk.

Image guidance refers to the process of locating the exact 3-dimensional position of the tumour and surrounding organs during treatment and then correcting for any deviation from the original plan. This will optimise the chance of accurately targeting the tumour and, thereby, over the entire course of fractionated treatment, maximise the tumour dose whilst minimising the dose to surrounding structures. As a result, the PTV margins can be substantially decreased, leading to a substantial reduction in the volume of radiation prescribed. Furthermore, with the ability of high-precision dose delivery and real-time knowledge of the target volume location, image-guided radiotherapy (IGRT) has opened the possibility for new indications for radiotherapy previously considered impossible. Research to improve image quality in radiotherapy is not new, but developments in computer software that quantify target localisation errors, on the basis of real-time imaging in the treatment room and

hardware allowing automated set-up, have stimulated the mainstream clinical application of IGRT.

IGRT makes use of many different imaging strategies. IGRT techniques can be split into planar (2D) imaging, volumetric (3D) imaging or imaging over time (4D) during the radiotherapy treatment. In addition, for some anatomical sites implanted fiducial markers can be used to localise the treatment.[21]

Planar (2-Dimensional) Imaging

This is when two or more static images are acquired, usually at 90° to each other (i.e. anteroposterior and lateral) (Fig. 6-19). It allows comparison of the bony anatomy or of a target visible by plain X-ray (such as a lung tumour) in all three axes (superoinferiorly, laterally and anteroposteriorly). Planar imaging with megavoltage (MV) electronic portal imaging (EPI) is a standard feature on most conventional linear accelerators. However, images acquired at the energies used for radiotherapy (6–18 MeV) are not of diagnostic quality. In particular, the contrast between bone, soft tissue and air seen with conventional X-ray imaging (i.e. kV) is not seen at higher megavoltage energies. Planar 2D imaging with kilovoltage (kV) EPI is available on linear accelerators with a kV cone beam facility or may also be acquired using a system independent of the linear accelerator gantry: for example, a tube and detector system mounted on the floor and ceiling.

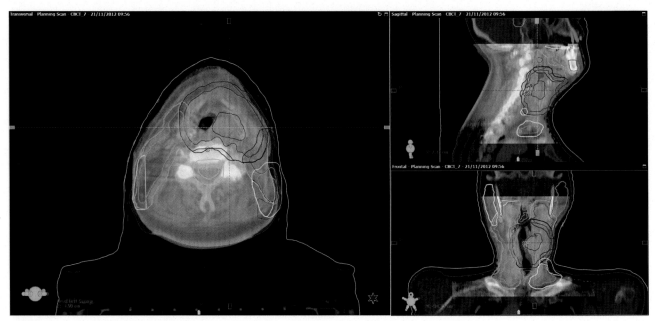

FIGURE 6-20 ■ **Image guidance using cone beam CT.** This patient is receiving treatment for a T4 laryngeal tumour. A cone beam CT image has been obtained with the patient on the treatment couch and about to be irradiated. The cone beam CT has been reconstructed in the transverse, sagittal and coronal planes and fused with the planning CT image. The fusion can be best seen on the sagittal and coronal images because the cone beam CT has been obtained for a shorter cranio-caudal length than the planning image. In contrast to the planar imaging (Fig. 6-19), the position of the soft tissues and the tumour itself can be clearly seen and contoured. Any discrepancy between the planning image and the cone beam CT can therefore be corrected in 3 dimensions to ensure tumour coverage and avoidance of normal tissues.

Volumetric (3-Dimensional) Imaging

Volumetric imaging allows for a 3D image to be acquired in the treatment position on the linear accelerator prior to or during radiotherapy. This enables the internal structures to be visualised including the target and surrounding normal tissues. There are four methods for obtaining a volumetric image on the linear accelerator:

- *Cone beam CT* (CBCT). For most standard linear accelerators volumetric imaging is available via cone beam CT technology, which is a kV tube mounted at 90° to the linear accelerator head and is rotated around the patient using the linear accelerator gantry. Both the treatment head (MV) and the CBCT system (kV) have an imaging capability (Fig. 6-20).
- *Megavoltage CT.* This technique uses a megavoltage energy fan beam to create a volumetric image for verification with helical imaging as used in conventional CT imaging.
- *CT on rails.* This consists of a CT unit in the same room as the linear accelerator. The patient couch can be rotated at 180° to transfer from the linear accelerator to the CT.
- *Ultrasound.* Ultrasound probes can provide volumetric images for IGRT in prostate cancer.

Four-Dimensional (4D) Imaging

This describes the process of imaging the tumour and relevant structures over a period of time. Before the advent of 4D image guidance, the gross tumour volume was expanded to create a clinical target volume to account for microscopic spread. An additional margin was then added for set-up variation (including any motion) to create the planning target volume (as described earlier). However, kilovoltage fluoroscopy or CBCT can be performed before the radiotherapy treatment to quantify tumour motion (Fig. 6-21). The gross tumour volume can then be defined at the extremes of motion and at the mid-point of the movement. These are then expanded for microscopic disease to create their respective clinical target volumes. The union of these clinical target volumes is then used to create an internal target volume with a smaller margin added for geometric set-up errors to create the planning target volume.

Alternatively, 4D kV or MV imaging can be used during radiotherapy to track the tumour, or more commonly, implanted fiducial markers, which are radio-opaque seeds or wires, can be placed in or near to the tumour, during treatment delivery. These can either provide additional points of reference in the images acquired, for example with CBCT, or be used as a surrogate for target position in planar imaging where soft-tissue information is not available. Once implanted, the fiducial markers will move with the tumour. Any displacement in 3 dimensions, as well as tilt and rotation, will be quantifiable by measuring the change in the relative positions of the markers and the radiotherapy plan can then be changed accordingly (Fig. 6-22).

Fiducial markers also enable real-time tracking during the delivery of the radiotherapy fraction. For example, the CyberKnife system (Accuray, Sunnyvale, CA, USA) uses a combination of X-ray imaging and optical tracking

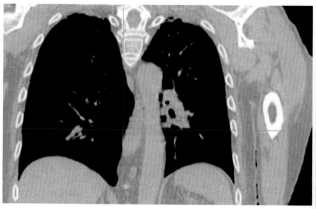
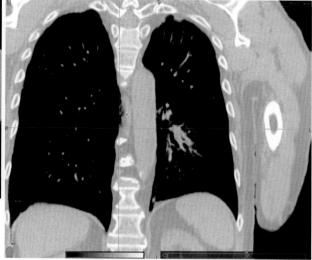

FIGURE 6-21 ■ **Cone beam CT being used to quantify the motion of a peripheral small lung tumour.** The degree of movement can be minimised by breath-holding techniques or by using mechanical methods to splint the diaphragm. Alternatively, respiratory gating can be used where the beam is automatically turned off when chest or tumour motion exceeds a predefined threshold.

in its motion tracking system.[22] Two kilovoltage X-ray tube and detector pairs are mounted in the treatment room at right angles. X-rays are taken periodically during treatment to determine the location of the fiducial markers within the target. For thoracic tumours there is also continuous optical tracking of the patient's skin to detect the breathing motion. These two data sources are then combined by the tracking software and a mapping function between the position of the external skin markers and the position of the internal target is computed. By knowing the motion of the internal target the Cyber-Knife robot arm can steer the radiation beam to follow that motion.

FUNCTIONAL IMAGING IN THE RADIOTHERAPY PROCESS

Inclusion of Biological Information to the Treatment Process

Several imaging techniques produce valid biomarkers for radio-biologically relevant tumour characteristics such as hypoxia, cellular proliferation, vascularity and clonogen density.[23–26] The ability to incorporate such biological information into radiotherapy planning allows the possibility of further manipulation of the radiation dose–distribution. Increasing the dose administered to relatively resistant tumour regions and moderation of the dose to sensitive areas should achieve better tumour control with less toxicity. Mathematical modelling studies have demonstrated theoretical advantages for biological conformality.[27–33] However, the translation of the theory into clinical practice has been limited.

Two factors must combine for biological radiotherapy planning to occur. Firstly, accurate and validated biological imaging must be available. Over recent years, this

focus of imaging research has grown considerably. Many groups have used a variety of technologies to image numerous different tumour characteristics. However, it has been extremely difficult to prove whether the imaging data reliably reflect the biological process being studied or even whether the correct process is being measured at all. True validation requires simultaneous collection of imaging and physiological data, which is often impossible. As a result surrogate measures must be employed, each with its own set of assumptions and inaccuracies.

For example, one of the most important and relevant aspects of the tumour microenvironment that has a direct impact on the success of radiotherapy treatment is tumour oxygenation. Great efforts have been made to devise a method of imaging tumour oxygenation for the purpose of improving radiotherapy delivery, some of which have appeared to be promising. However, in order to prove that an imaging test is accurately measuring tumour oxygenation it must be compared with an established standard. This entails probing the tumour with oxygen-measuring electrodes or removal of the tumour for immunohistochemical assessment. Because oxygen levels vary over short periods of time, the imaging and direct oxygen measurement need to occur at the same time or at least only a few minutes apart. This poses a great challenge for experimental design. Furthermore, the 'gold-standards' with which the new imaging technology is being compared have inherent flaws. Polarographic electrodes have the unique ability to directly measure tissue pO_2. However, they can only sample a tiny proportion of a tumour and the position of the needle with regard to the tumour location is never known with certainty. Also, the trauma during needle insertion creates a non-physiological microenvironment from which the measurements are obtained. Tumour removal inevitably affects the oxygenation status, even if it is rapidly fixed. Therefore, immunohistochemical methods must be

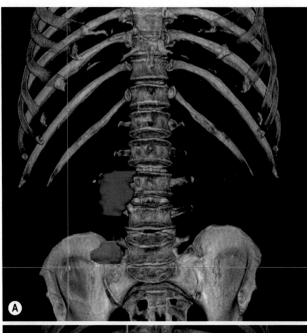

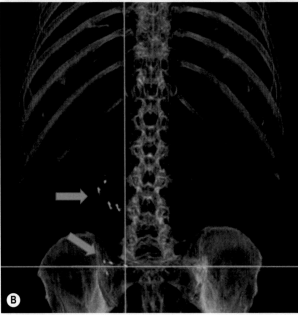

FIGURE 6-22 ■ Two areas of recurrent, chemotherapy refractory, metastatic testicular seminoma have been outlined in red (A). The intention is to treat these metastases with stereotactic body radiotherapy. In order to achieve accurate dose deposition, fiducial markers have been inserted into both tumours (arrows, B) so that any tumour motion can be tracked in real time during treatment delivery. (Image courtesy of Dr Peter Ostler, Mount Vernon Cancer Centre, UK.)

interpreted with caution. As a result it has been extremely difficult to prove that an imaging test accurately reflects the degree of tumour oxygenation. Individual validation experiments cannot give a definitive answer and these techniques must be interpeted in the context of the overall body of evidence.

There are a variety of techniques for imaging tumour hypoxia under evaluation; three warrant further discussion.[34]

^{18}F-Misonidazole Positron Emission Tomography

^{18}F-Fluoromisonidazole is a hypoxia imaging tracer with homogeneous uptake in most normal tissues and tumours. The initial distribution of ^{18}F-misonidazole is flow-dependent, as with any freely diffusible tracer, but local oxygen tension is the major determinant of its retention above normal background in tissues after 2 h. ^{18}F-Misonidazole accumulates in tissues by binding to intracellular macromolecules when the pO_2 is less than 10 mmHg. Retention within tissues is dependent on nitroreductase activity and accumulation in hypoxic tissues over a range of blood flows has been demonstrated.

Cu-ATSM Positron Emission Tomography

Several pre-clinical studies have evaluated and validated Cu-diacetyl-bis(N^4-methylthiosemicarbazone) for imaging hypoxia in tumours. The mechanism of retention of the reagent in hypoxic tissues is largely attributed to the low oxygen tensions and the subsequent altered redox environment of hypoxic tumours. Cu(II)ATSM is bioreduced (from Cu(II) to Cu(I)) once entering the cell. The reduced intermediate species is trapped within the cell because of its charge. This transient complex can then go through one of two competing pathways: reoxidation to the uncharged Cu(II) species (which can escape by diffusion), or proton-induced dissociation (which releases copper to be irreversibly sequestered by intracellular proteins). [Cu-ATSM] favours the reoxidation route because it is easily oxidised but chemically more resistant to protonation. Copper from Cu(II)ATSM is trapped reversibly as [Cu-ATSM]- (if oxygen is absent), with the possibility of irreversible trapping by dissociation over a longer period. Cu(II)ATSM is thus hypoxia-selective.

Blood Oxygenation Level-Dependent Magnetic Resonance Imaging (BOLD-MRI)

As in any magnetic resonance image, tissue contrast in BOLD images is affected by intrinsic tissue properties including spin–lattice and spin–spin relaxations. Additionally, BOLD MRI contrast is affected by blood flow and paramagnetic deoxyhaemoglobin within red blood cells (oxyhaemoglobin is not paramagnetic). Deoxyhaemoglobin increases the MR transverse relaxation rate (R_2^*) of water in blood and surrounding tissues; thus, BOLD-MRI is sensitive to pO_2 within, and in tissues adjacent to perfused vessels. In order to decouple the effects of flow from deoxyhaemoglobin it is necessary to measure the T_2^* relaxation rate ($R_2^*=1/T_2^*$), which can be done by using a multi-echo GRE sequence. Decoupling of flow from static effects on R_2^* images occurs because the flow component can be thought of as affecting individual T_2^* images of a multi-gradient echo sequence

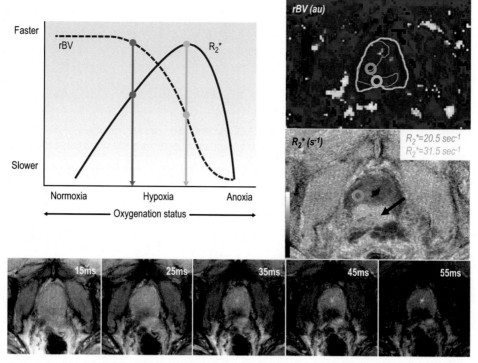

FIGURE 6-23 ■ **Blood oxygenation level-dependent (BOLD) MRI.** The graph shows the theoretical changes in R_2^* and relative blood volume (rBV) with changes in oxygenation. Note that R_2^* not only falls in well-oxygenated tissue but also in poorly oxygenated tissue where there is insufficient blood volume to produce the BOLD effect. The R_2^* pixel map of the prostate was obtained using multiple spoiled gradient-echo images on a single central slice with increasing TE times (15–55 ms), using a 1.5-tesla MR system (bottom row of images). The dynamic susceptibility contrast (DSC) MRI rBV pixel map of the same patient was generated using T_2^*-weighted data acquired every 2 s for 2 min with a 0.2 mmol/kg bolus of Gd-DTPA administered after 20 s. In this example the region of high R_2^* (arrow) in the posterior peripheral zone corresponds to the region of low blood volume (orange circles and orange line on the graph) and the transition zone has high blood flow with low R_2^* (green circles and green line on the graph).

equally. It is important to remember that, although synthetic R_2^* images are free of the contribution of blood flow (that is, they mainly reflect deoxyhaemoglobin content and static tissue components), improving blood flow and vascular functioning will also increase tissue oxygenation, which can be seen by changes in R_2^* images (Fig. 6-23).

The second factor that is required for successful biological radiotherapy planning is the ability to accurately vary the radiation dose over very short distances so that the radiation dose–distribution conforms to the distribution of the biological parameter in question. This has only been possible since the development of the modern radiotherapy techniques as described earlier. Many groups have concentrated on external beam intensity-modulated radiotherapy (IMRT), although there are still a number of technical limitations with this method. IMRT requires a motionless target if precise doses are to be administered to small regions within tumours. Immobilisation devices, respiratory gating and image guidance technology are becoming highly advanced and are approaching the levels of accuracy required for biological 'dose-painting'. However, biological targets within tumours are frequently only a few millimetres in diameter. The current degree of set-up error, as well as patient and internal organ movement during treatment with

IMRT, makes the delivery of biological conformal radiotherapy using this method a considerable challenge.

High dose-rate (HDR) brachytherapy uses a radiation source placed within the tumour, which bypasses the need for immobilisation and image guidance during treatment delivery. It achieves high dose gradients, providing the most conformal dose distributions of all radiotherapy techniques. HDR brachytherapy is delivered over a period of 1–2 days rather than weeks. This reduces the effects of compensatory changes in tumour physiology that may alter the biological subvolume during treatment. It is for these reasons that with current levels of technology, HDR brachytherapy may be the optimal modality to explore the principle of biologically based treatment planning, although not suitable for all tumour types (Fig. 6-24).

In summary, radiotherapy requires close integration of both diagnostic and therapeutic radiation technology. Most of the advances in radiotherapy in recent years have been in response to better imaging, enabling accurate 3D image acquisition and the integration of physiological information with the morphological data. Modern radiotherapy represents sophisticated application of state-of-the-art imaging for diagnosis, target and organ at risk volume definition, tissue density measurements and verification of the therapeutic beam delivery.

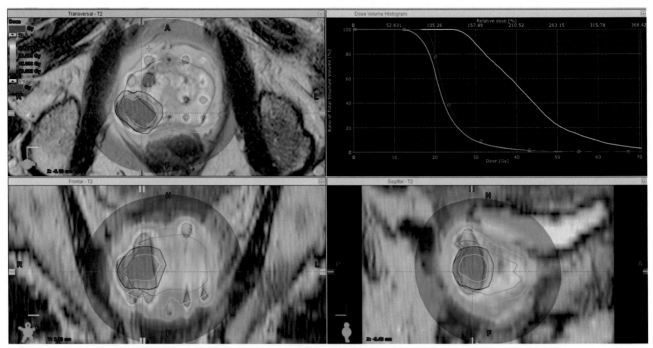

FIGURE 6-24 ■ **Biologically optimised radiotherapy.** A dominant intra-prostatic lesion (DIL) in the right posterolateral peripheral zone has been defined using multi-parametric MRI (black outline on the transverse, coronal and sagittal images). High dose-rate brachy-therapy catheters have been inserted under general anaesthetic. The planning computer optimisation software has been pro-grammed to maximise the radiation dose to the DIL and limit the dose to the rest of the prostate to a defined ceiling. The dose volume histograms (top left) demonstrate the dual dose levels. The DIL and DIL PTV (dark blue and yellow lines) receive a higher dose as a proportion of their volume than the non-dominant prostate and the non-dominant prostate PTV (light blue and red lines).

REFERENCES

1. Physician Characteristics and Distribution in the US, 2012. American Medical Association; 2012.
2. Equipment, Workload and Staffing for Radiotherapy in the UK 1997–2002. London: Royal College of Radiologists; 2003.
3. Staffurth J. A review of the clinical evidence for intensity-modulated radiotherapy. Clin Oncol (R Coll Radiol) 2010;22:643–57.
4. Jin JY, Wen N, Ren L, et al. Advances in treatment techniques: arc-based and other intensity modulated therapies. Cancer J 2011;17:166–76.
5. Kupelian P, Langen K. Helical tomotherapy: image-guided and adaptive radiotherapy. Front Radiat Ther Oncol 2011;43:165–80.
6. Tipton K, Launders JH, Inamdar R, et al. Stereotactic body radiation therapy: scope of the literature. Ann Intern Med 2011;154:737–45.
7. Bowes D, Crook J, Rajapakshe R, et al. Defining a magnetic resonance scan sequence for permanent seed prostate brachytherapy postimplant assessment. Brachytherapy 2013;12:25–9.
8. Terasawa T, Dvorak T, Ip S, et al. Systematic review: charged-particle radiation therapy for cancer. Ann Intern Med 2009;151:556–65.
9. Blomstrand M, Brodin NP, Munck Af, et al. Estimated clinical benefit of protecting neurogenesis in the developing brain during radiation therapy for pediatric medulloblastoma. Neuro Oncol 2012;14:882–9.
10. Brodin NP, Vogelius IR, Maraldo MV, et al. Life years lost—comparing potentially fatal late complications after radiotherapy for pediatric medulloblastoma on a common scale. Cancer 2012;118:5432–40.
11. Kuhlthau KA, Pulsifer MB, Yeap BY, et al. Prospective study of health-related quality of life for children with brain tumors treated with proton radiotherapy. J Clin Oncol 2012;30:2079–86.
12. Ando K, Kase Y. Biological characteristics of carbon-ion therapy. Int J Radiat Biol 2009;85:715–28.
13. Wenzl T, Wilkens JJ. Modelling of the oxygen enhancement ratio for ion beam radiation therapy. Phys Med Biol 2011;56:3251–68.
14. Padhani AR. Integrating multiparametric prostate MRI into clinical practice. Cancer Imaging 2011;11(Spec No A):S27–37.
15. Pawaroo D, Cummings NM, Musonda P, et al. Non-small cell lung carcinoma: accuracy of PET/CT in determining the size of T1 and T2 primary tumors. Am J Roentgenol 2011;196:1176–81.
16. Thorwarth D, Schaefer A. Functional target volume delineation for radiation therapy on the basis of positron emission tomography and the correlation with histopathology. Q J Nucl Med Mol Imaging 2010;54:490–9.
17. Webster GJ, Kilgallon JE, Ho KF, et al. A novel imaging technique for fusion of high-quality immobilised MR images of the head and neck with CT scans for radiotherapy target delineation. Br J Radiol 2009;82:497–503.
18. Yoo S, Wu Q, O'Daniel J, et al. Comparison of 3D conformal breast radiation treatment plans using the anisotropic analytical algorithm and pencil beam convolution algorithm. Radiother Oncol 2012;103:172–7.
19. Holdsworth C, Kim M, Liao J, et al. The use of a multiobjective evolutionary algorithm to increase flexibility in the search for better IMRT plans. Med Phys 2012;39:2261–74.
20. Narabayashi M, Mizowaki T, Matsuo Y, et al. Dosimetric evaluation of the impacts of different heterogeneity correction algorithms on target doses in stereotactic body radiation therapy for lung tumors. J Radiat Res 2012;53:777–84.
21. Image Guided Radiotherapy (IGRT), Guidance for Implementation and Use. National Radiotherapy Implementation Group Report; 2012.
22. Lei S, Piel N, Oermann EK, et al. Six-dimensional correction of intra-fractional prostate motion with CyberKnife stereotactic body radiation therapy. Front Oncol 2011;1:48.
23. Al-Hallaq HA, River JN, Zamora M, et al. Correlation of magnetic resonance and oxygen microelectrode measurements of carbogen-induced changes in tumor oxygenation. Int J Radiat Oncol Biol Phys 1998;41:151–9.
24. Robinson SP, Rijken PF, Howe FA, et al. Tumor vascular architecture and function evaluated by non-invasive susceptibility MRI

methods and immunohistochemistry. J Magn Reson Imaging 2003; 17:445–54.

25. Schlemmer HP, Merkle J, Grobholz R, et al. Can pre-operative contrast-enhanced dynamic MR imaging for prostate cancer predict microvessel density in prostatectomy specimens? Eur Radiol 2004;14:309–17.

26. Hawighorst H, Weikel W, Knapstein PG, et al. Angiogenic activity of cervical carcinoma: assessment by functional magnetic resonance imaging-based parameters and a histomorphological approach in correlation with disease outcome. Clin Cancer Res 1998;4: 2305–12.

27. Bentzen SM. Theragnostic imaging for radiation oncology: dose-painting by numbers. Lancet Oncol 2005;6:112–17.

28. Pouliot J, Kim Y, Lessard E, et al. Inverse planning for HDR prostate brachytherapy used to boost dominant intraprostatic lesions defined by magnetic resonance spectroscopy imaging. Int J Radiat Oncol Biol Phys 2004;59:1196–207.

29. Alber M, Paulsen F, Eschmann SM, et al. On biologically conformal boost dose optimization. Phys Med Biol 2003;48:N31–5.

30. Brahme A. Individualizing cancer treatment: biological optimization models in treatment planning and delivery. Int J Radiat Oncol Biol Phys 2001;49:327–37.

31. Xing L, Cotrutz C, Hunjan S, et al. Inverse planning for functional image-guided intensity-modulated radiation therapy. Phys Med Biol 2002;47:3567–78.

32. Yang Y, Xing L. Towards biologically conformal radiation therapy (BCRT): selective IMRT dose escalation under the guidance of spatial biology distribution. Med Phys 2005;32:1473–84.

33. Chao KS, Bosch WR, Mutic S, et al. A novel approach to overcome hypoxic tumor resistance: Cu-ATSM-guided intensity-modulated radiation therapy. Int J Radiat Oncol Biol Phys 2001; 49:1171–82.

34. Padhani AR, Krohn KA, Lewis JS, et al. Imaging oxygenation of human tumours. Eur Radiol 2007;17:861–72.

CHAPTER 7

FUNCTIONAL AND MOLECULAR IMAGING FOR PERSONALISED MEDICINE IN ONCOLOGY

Ferdia A. Gallagher • Avnesh S. Thakor • Eva M. Serrao • Vicky Goh

CHAPTER OUTLINE

PERSONALISED MEDICINE IN ONCOLOGY

DYNAMIC CONTRAST-ENHANCED COMPUTED TOMOGRAPHY (DCE-CT)

MAGNETIC RESONANCE IMAGING (MRI)

POSITRON EMISSION TOMOGRAPHY (PET)

EMERGING MOLECULAR IMAGING TECHNIQUES AND THERANOSTICS

CONCLUSION: ROLE OF FUNCTIONAL AND MOLECULAR IMAGING IN ONCOLOGY

PERSONALISED MEDICINE IN ONCOLOGY

The essence of oncological imaging is to detect and differentiate tumour from normal tissue. It is therefore necessary to understand the fundamental changes that occur within tissues or cells when a tumour forms, and how this can be used to generate tissue contrast. On the very simplest level, the differences in X-ray attenuation and water content between cancer and its surrounding tissues can be used to distinguish cancer from normal tissue using computed tomography (CT) and magnetic resonance imaging (MRI), respectively. Biological research in the field of oncology is increasingly revealing the fundamental tissue, cellular and molecular changes that form the hallmarks of cancer and this knowledge is now being applied to the development of new imaging biomarkers which will be more specific and sensitive for cancer detection than morphological information alone.[1] Examples include the use of CT and MRI contrast agents to probe angiogenesis, as well as positron emission tomography (PET) tracers to detect alterations in cellular energetics and proliferation within cancerous tissue.

In addition to identifying tumours, imaging biomarkers can be used to assess the efficacy of treatment such as chemotherapy and radiotherapy. Traditionally, this has been performed by identifying changes in tumour size using criteria such as the response evaluation criteria in solid tumours (RECIST); new imaging biomarkers which are more specific and sensitive for the detection of early response to treatment by detecting early cellular or molecular changes that predict long-term successful outcome are being developed. The introduction of therapies which have specific molecular targets (such as bevacizumab and sunitinib) has been problematic for traditional imaging approaches as improved clinical outcome with these drugs is often not accompanied by a significant change in tumour size; e.g. an anti-vascular drug may induce tumour necrosis with little change in the overall tumour diameter. Consequently, alternative imaging approaches are needed to identify a successful early response to therapy in this context; the concept of combining a specific targeted drug with an imaging biomarker that directly probes the cellular pathways affected by the drug is a very attractive approach for the future management of cancer patients.

These specific targeted imaging biomarkers also open up the possibility of detecting subtle differences in drug response between patients: a cellular pathway may be upregulated in one patient but downregulated in another in response to the same drug at the same dose. The old concept of a single treatment algorithm for all patients is increasingly being replaced by a personalised or patient-centred approach where drug therapy can be tailored to an individual patient. Modern medical practice is underpinned by an understanding of the molecular biology of disease processes; complementing this with new imaging techniques will be increasingly important. These molecular imaging methods can be defined as the visual representation, characterisation and quantification of biological processes at the cellular and subcellular levels within intact living organisms.[2] Functional imaging is more loosely defined and includes techniques which probe physiological processes such as blood flow, metabolism and features of the tumour microenvironment. There is some overlap between the two terms and often the combination of functional and molecular imaging is used to define a range of imaging techniques that are more specific than anatomical or morphological imaging and

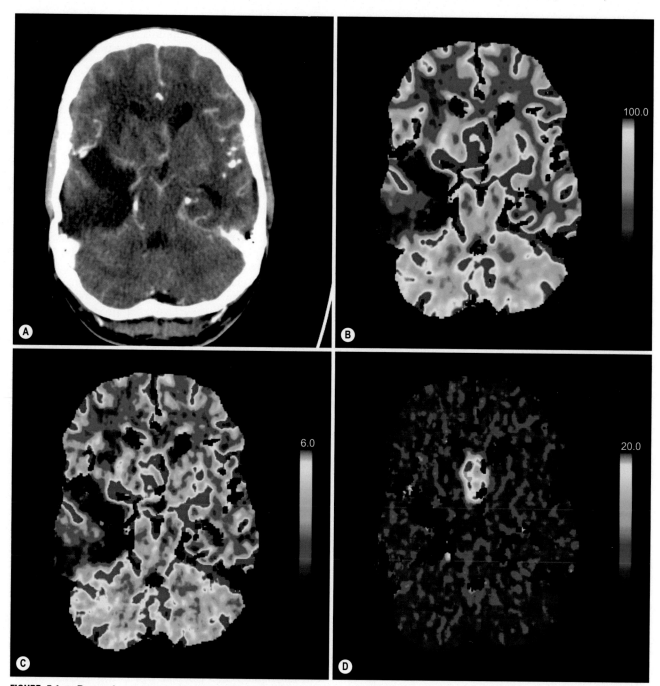

FIGURE 7-1 ■ Dynamic contrast-enhanced CT acquisition with parametric maps from a glioblastoma multiforme tumour. (A) Contrast-enhanced CT, (B) regional blood flow, (C) blood volume and (D) permeability–surface area product. The images demonstrate a vascular solid component with disruption of the blood–brain barrier best seen on the permeability–surface area product map.

probe processes from a tissue to a molecular level. This chapter will explore the use of these functional and molecular techniques in oncological imaging.

DYNAMIC CONTRAST-ENHANCED COMPUTED TOMOGRAPHY (DCE-CT)

There has been a recent resurgent interest in dynamic contrast-enhanced CT techniques for assessing the vasculature, which were first used in the early 1990s. This

has been facilitated by technological advances allowing high temporal sampling acquisitions to be performed over a large volume (also known as *perfusion CT*) as well as therapeutic developments in stroke and cancer which have required an assessment of the functioning vasculature on an individual patient basis (Fig. 7-1).

Contrast Agent Kinetics

CT contrast agents used in clinical practice are low molecular weight contrast agents (< 1 kDa) with

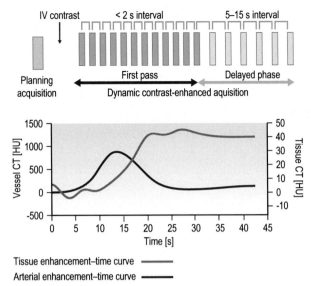

FIGURE 7-2 ■ **Typical DCE-CT acquisition is shown, with the arterial (purple line) and tissue (green line) attenuation–time curves acquired for a lung cancer.** Maximum enhancement reached within the aorta and tumour within the time period of the acquisition was 800 and 45 HU, respectively.

negligible serum protein binding and therefore a distribution similar to that of extracellular fluid. These agents are typically derivatives of iodobenzoic acid with an iodine concentration of at least 300 mg/mL. After intravenous injection (typically 4 mL/s or faster), the pharmacokinetic modelling can be approximated to a two-compartment model: the injected contrast agent initially remains within the intravascular compartment before diffusing into the extravascular and extracellular space (EES). The rate of this diffusion is determined by the perfusion of the organ, the vessel surface area and its permeability or leakiness; there is negligible transfer into the intracellular compartment (< 1%). The contrast agent then passes back from the EES into the intravascular compartment before being excreted predominantly by the kidneys; up to half of the administered dose is eliminated from the blood within the first two hours of injection.

By acquiring a rapid series of images following intravenous contrast agent administration, and assessing the changes in tissue and vessel attenuation during the acquisition, functional parameters can be derived (Fig. 7-2). These may be semi-quantitative (describing the 'curve shape' of the tissue attenuation–time graph), or quantitative parameters derived from kinetic modelling. As the change in measured CT attenuation is directly proportional to the concentration of iodine within the blood vessels or tissues, temporal changes in attenuation can be directly modelled to assess the tissue vascularity. The situation is somewhat different for MRI, where there is a complex relationship between MR signal intensity and the local tissue concentration of MR contrast medium. Acquisition is normally acquired over the 45 s of the perfusion phase and the larger the number of data acquisition points during this period, the better the data fitting. However, this has to be balanced against increasing radiation dose

and the finite time required for each acquisition.[3] In general, at least five time points are acquired and the quantitative parameters are derived using a number of models, e.g. the Johnson–Wilson model, the Patlak method and the maximum slope model.[3–6]

The derived parameters include:
- regional tumour blood flow—blood flow per unit volume or unit mass of tissue;
- regional tumour blood volume—the proportion of tissue that comprises flowing blood;
- mean transit time—the average time for contrast material to traverse the tissue vasculature;
- extraction fraction—the rate of transfer of contrast material from the intravascular space to the EES;
- permeability–surface area product—which characterises the rate of diffusion of the contrast agent from the intravascular compartment to the EES.

The basis for the use of DCE-CT in oncology is that microvascular changes during angiogenesis are reflected in changes in the measured DCE-CT parameters; for example, permeability–surface area product is usually lower in normal tissue than in tumours (Fig. 7-3). DCE-CT measurements have been validated in a range of tumours in both animal models and human studies.[7,8] Measurements have been correlated positively with histological markers of angiogenesis and negatively with histological markers of hypoxia, indicating that these may be appropriate surrogates of fundamental biological processes during cancer formation.

In terms of characterisation, DCE-CT may distinguish benign from malignant lesions within the lung, pancreas and bowel though there is some overlap between malignant and inflammatory lesions, which reflects the generic nature of the vascular changes that can be probed.[9–12] In general, higher perfusion parameters have been reported in patients with tumours although there is variability between different types of tumours and even within the same tumour, which underlies the complexity of tumour heterogeneity. The major application of DCE-CT in routine clinical practice is in the assessment of the anti-vascular effects of conventional chemotherapies and interventional procedures, which target the vasculature. DCE-CT is also used to provide pharmacodynamic information in early-phase clinical trials in a variety of cancers (Table 7-1).[13–23] These have included anti-angiogenic and vascular disrupting agents, where DCE-CT is providing a direct imaging biomarker of the drug action and can be used to determine the appropriate drug dose. The wide availability of CT, the low cost of CT and the ease of standardisation of DCE-CT are advantages over MRI for its use in clinical practice despite the radiation burden. However, CT carries a significant radiation burden and there still remains a lack of data concerning the relationship between acute vascular reduction and long-term patient outcome.

In addition to identifying treatment response, DCE-CT may have an important role in risk stratification and as a predictive biomarker of treatment. The basis for the predictive value of DCE-CT in the setting of chemotherapy is likely to relate to reduced drug delivery, while in radiotherapy this is likely to represent a marker of the hypoxic environment, which in turn correlates with

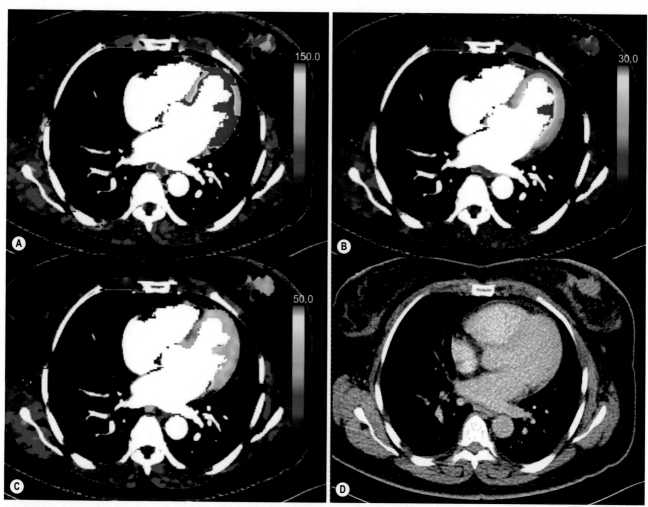

FIGURE 7-3 ■ **DCE-CT parameter maps of a breast tumour.** (A) Regional blood flow, (B) blood volume and (C) permeability–surface area product maps with corresponding (D) contrast-enhanced CT. The images demonstrate a higher vascularity within the tumour than within normal breast tissue.

TABLE 7-1   Table of Clinical Trials Incorporating DCE-CT[13–23]

Tumour	Therapy	Parameter	Author	Year
Solid tumours	Endostatin	BF, BV (decrease)	Thomas et al.[13]	2003
Rectal cancer	Bevacizumab	BF, BV (decrease)	Willett et al.[14]	2004
Solid tumours	SU6668	BF, BV (decrease)	Xiong et al.[15]	2004
Solid tumours	MEDI-522	MTT (increase)	McNeel et al.[16]	2005
Renal cancer	Thalidomide	BF, BV (decrease)	Faria et al.[17]	2007
Squamous cell carcinoma oropharynx	Cisplatin and 5FU	BF, BV (decrease in responders)	Gandhi et al.[18]	2006
Solid tumours	AZD2171 and gefitinib	BF (decrease)	Meijerink et al.[19]	2007
Non-small cell lung cancer	Combretastatin and radiotherapy	BV (decrease)	Ng et al.[20]	2007
Solid tumours	Nitric oxide synthase inhibitor	BV (decrease)	Ng et al.[21]	2007
Renal cell carcinoma	Tyrosine kinase inhibitors	BF, BV (decrease)	Fournier et al.[22]	2010
Non-small cell lung cancer	Erlotinib/sorafenib	BF (decrease)	Lind et al.[23]	2010

BF = regional blood flow; BV = regional blood volume; MTT = mean transit time.

resistance to radiotherapy. For example, in locally advanced squamous cell carcinoma of the head and neck treated with surgery and adjuvant chemoradiotherapy, pre-treatment primary tumour blood flow and permeability may be independent predictors of disease recurrence.[24] In pancreatic cancer, a low baseline volume transfer constant (K^{trans}) predicts for a poorer response to chemotherapy with gemcitabine and radiotherapy.[25] In colorectal cancer, tumours with a lower blood flow at staging are more likely to have nodal metastases and a poorer outcome; rectal tumours with a lower blood flow are also more likely to respond poorly to chemoradiation.[26,27]

The cancer risk associated with the radiation dose of DCE-CT has to be balanced against potential benefits of vascular quantification and must be judged in the context of the population under investigation. Typical effective radiation doses from a first-pass volumetric perfusion CT study of the thorax, abdomen or pelvis range from 13.7 to 28.7 mSv.[28] Using a risk estimate of 4.2% per Sv from the International Commission on Radiation Protection, the estimated lifetime risk of developing a cancer from a single such perfusion CT is approximately 1 in 1000.[29]

MAGNETIC RESONANCE IMAGING (MRI)

Dynamic Contrast-Enhanced MRI (DCE-MRI)

DCE-MRI consists of serial MRI acquisitions following injection of an intravenous contrast agent in a similar manner to that described above for DCE-CT. Clinical dynamic MRI is usually performed using low molecular weight gadolinium chelate-based contrast agents. These have paramagnetic ions that are known to interact with nearby hydrogen nuclei and lead to shortening of T1 (and T2) relaxation times, resulting in signal enhancement on T1-weighted images, thus producing positive contrast. The major advantages of MRI include the absence of ionising radiation, high contrast-to-noise ratio, high signal-to-noise ratio and the many mechanisms which can be utilised to produce tissue contrast.[30]

As with contrast-enhanced CT, contrast-enhanced MRI can either be used to provide a qualitative snapshot of tissue enhancement, as is used routinely in clinical practice, or more quantitatively in the form of DCE-MRI (Fig. 7-4). The latter permits a fuller depiction of

contrast kinetics within lesions in much the same way as DCE-CT. DCE-MRI can be repeated over a course of treatment to monitor changes in tumour vascularity over time. Although the technique is reproducible when using a single clinical MRI system, the reproducibility of DCE-MRI studies between centres may be less robust, due to the differences in scanner hardware, contrast agent injection protocols, acquisition parameters, and kinetic models employed.[31]

DCE-MRI protocols most commonly involve T1-weighted image acquisition before, during and after the injection of the MR contrast agent (typically 0.1 mmol/kg with injection after 1 min and continuous data acquisition for up to 10 min); this provides an assessment of the different stages of tissue uptake and washout.[32,33] The contrast agents used are either low molecular weight agents (< 1 kDa) that rapidly diffuse into the extracellular space or larger macromolecular agents (> 30 kDa) that demonstrate prolonged intravascular retention.[30] Given the lack of ionising radiation in DCE-MRI, temporal data can be continuously acquired during the phases of tissue enhancement, unlike in DCE-CT. The concentration of the contrast agent in the vasculature allows an assessment of perfusion, and in the case of the low molecular weight agents, this is followed by rapid diffusion into the EES where it accumulates. As with DCE-CT, the rate at which this occurs is dependent on blood flow as well as vessel permeability and surface area.[30,34] However, MR signal intensity is not directly proportional to the contrast agent concentration and therefore more complex quantitative data analysis is required to convert the MR signal intensity into biologically meaningful quantitative parameters.[35–37]

A simple approach is to use the initial area under the curve (IAUC), which describes the shape of the graph of contrast agent concentration over time; although this is frequently used in trials, it is difficult to interpret physiologically.[38] Therefore, in clinical trials, assessment of the effect of an anti-angiogenic or vascular disrupting agent

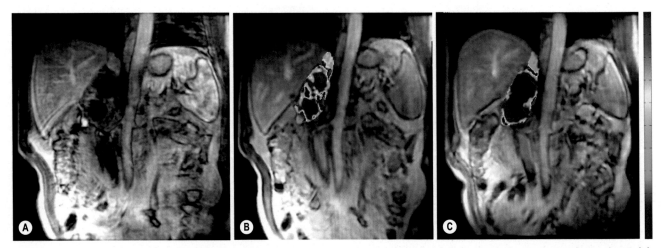

FIGURE 7-4 ■ **Example parameter maps for a renal cell carcinoma metastasis.** (A) Image from a dynamic contrast-enhanced acquisition, (B) initial area under the gadolinium curve (over 90 s; IAUGC90) map before treatment, (C) IAUGC90 map 48 h after treatment with an anti-angiogenic agent (bevacizumab), showing decrease in the tumour perfusion with colour scale. (Images courtesy of Andrew Gill, Dr Andrew Priest, Professor Duncan Jodrell and Professor Tim Eisen, Addenbrooke's Hospital, Cambridge.)

is often modelled using changes in K^{trans} (the volume transfer coefficient of contrast between the blood plasma and the EES, as described above for CT) and the volume of the EES (v_e).[39] The other commonly used pharmacokinetic variables are summarised in Tables 7-2 and 7-3.[32,40]

DCE-MRI and DCE-CT exploit the fact that the onset of many diseases is associated with an alteration in vascular density, vascular permeability and blood flow. In particular, tumours develop a network of new vessels as they grow, but unlike normal vasculature, tumour angiogenesis is chaotic and inefficient with permeable vessels.[41] Therefore, an increase in signal enhancement, vessel permeability, and flow is often demonstrated within tumours when compared with benign lesions or normal tissue.[42-45]

DCE-MRI has been used for tumour detection, characterisation, staging, and therapy monitoring. However, the meaning of an elevated K^{trans} is still controversial in terms of prognosis, as studies have shown conflicting results;[46,47] there is stronger evidence that K^{trans} can be used to demonstrate which tumours are responding to therapy as a pharmacodynamic biomarker of drug activity, particularly in the context of anti-angiogenic drugs or vascular disrupting agents.[38,48] Changes in K^{trans} have been shown to correlate both with the administration of vascular endothelial growth factor (VEGF, a signalling molecule that stimulates the growth of new blood vessels), as well as the administration of therapeutic monoclonal antibodies that block its effect.[49] Consequently, both DCE-MRI and DCE-CT can be used as a platform to understand drug and tumour interactions.[50]

Another emerging approach has been to use dynamic susceptibility contrast MRI (DSC-MRI), which also relies upon the serial acquisition of images after the injection of a contrast agent.[51,52] However, DSC-MRI measures induced alterations in the transverse relaxation times, T2 and T2*, resulting in signal loss and hence transient darkening of the tissues (thus acting as a negative contrast unlike that seen with T1-weighted imaging).[30] The degree of signal loss is dependent on the concentration of the agent as well as vessel size and density and therefore this can be used to estimate the relative blood volume (rBV) of the tissue under assessment.[53] Using this technique, changes in relative cerebral blood volume (rCBV) maps have been correlated with glioma grade and this approach can be used not only to understand the nature of tumour heterogeneity better but also to target biopsies to focal areas of vascular changes within a tumour, which may help to avoid sampling error.[54] The method has also been used to distinguish radiation necrosis from recurrent disease, evaluate response to therapy and as a prognostic marker.[55,56] Its application to extracerebral tumours (e.g. breast and prostate) is under investigation.[57,58]

The role of DCE-MRI in clinical practice has been limited by the relatively small number of patients in many published trials, the use of widely varying acquisition techniques and modelled parameters between centres, as well as the use of diverse disease endpoints. Current attempts to standardise DCE-MRI will help to address these issues in the future. Although DCE-MRI has shown much promise, it has yet to be incorporated into routine clinical practice (Table 7-4).[59-68]

TABLE 7-2 Most Common Pharmacokinetic Parameters Used in DCE-MRI Analysis[32,40]

Parameter (units)	Alternative Nomenclature	Definition
K^{trans} (min^{-1})	EF, K^{PS}	Volume transfer constant between blood plasma and EES
v_e (a.u.)	Interstitial space	EES volume per unit tissue volume
v_p (a.u.)		Blood plasma volume per unit tissue volume
k_{ep} (min^{-1})	k_{21}	Rate constant from EES to blood plasma $k_{ep} = K^{trans} / v_e$
k_{pe} (min^{-1})	k_{12}	Rate constant from blood plasma to EES
k_{el} (min^{-1})		Elimination rate constant
Amp (a.u.)	A	Amplitude of the normalised dynamic curve

Adapted from Yang et al.[40] and Tofts et al.[32]; a.u., arbitrary units.

TABLE 7-3 Model-Free Parameters Applied in DCE-MRI Analysis[32,40]

Parameter (Units)	Alternative Nomenclature	Definition
Area under the curve (min or mmol·min/L)	IAUC, AUC, AUGC, IAUGC	Area under the signal intensity or gadolinium dynamic curve
Relative signal intensity (a.u.)	RSI = $S_{(t)}/S_0$	Relative signal intensity at time (t)
Initial slope (min^{-1})	Enhancement slope, upslope, enhancement rate	Maximum or average slope in the initial enhancement
Washout slope (min^{-1})	Downslope, washout rate	Maximum or average slope in the washout phase
Peak enhancement ratio (a.u.)	Maximum signal enhancement ratio (SER$_{max}$)	PER = $(S_{max} - S_0)/S_0$
T_{max} (s)	Time-to-peak (TTP)	Time to peak enhancement
Maximum intensity-time ratio (s^{-1})	MITR = PER/T_{max}	

Adapted from Yang et al.[40] and Tofts et al.[32]; $S_{(t)}$, MR signal intensity at time t; S_0, precontrast signal intensity; S_{max}, maximum signal intensity; a.u., arbitrary units.

TABLE 7-4 **Table of Some Clinical Studies Incorporating DCE-MRI[59-68]**

Tumour	Therapy	Parameter	Author	Year
Solid tumours	AG-013736	K^{trans}, IAUC	Lui et al.[59]	2005
Solid tumours	AZD2171	IAUC	Drevs et al.[60]	2007
Renal cell carcinoma	Sorafenib	K^{trans}	Flaherty et al.[61]	2008
Breast cancer	Neoadjuvant 5-fluorouracil, epirubicin and cyclophosphamide	K^{trans}, k_{ep}, v_e, rBV, rBF, MTT	Ah-See et al.[62]	2008
Primary liver tumours	Floxuridine and dexamethasone	K^{trans}, k_{ep}, AUC	Jarnagin et al.[63]	2009
Glioblastoma	Bevacizumab	K^{trans}, v_e	Ferl et al.[64]	2010
Breast cancer	Neoadjuvant therapy: 5-fluorouracil, epirubicin and cyclophosphamide	K^{trans}, v_e	Jensen et al.[65]	2011
Prostate cancer	Androgen deprivation therapy	K^{trans}, k_{ep}, v_p, IAUGC	Barrett et al.[66]	2012
Cervical cancer	Radiotherapy & cisplatin and 5-fluorouracil plus cisplatin	K^{trans}, k_{ep}, v_e	Kim et al.[67]	2012
Rectal cancer	FOLFOX and bevacizumab	K^{trans}, k_{ep}, v_e, AUC	Gollub et al.[68]	2012

Diffusion-Weighted Imaging (DWI)

Water molecules in the liquid phase undergo thermally driven random motions, a phenomenon known as Brownian motion or free diffusion, and it is these small motions—typically of the order of 30 μm—which can be probed and quantified using DWI.[69] These small molecular movements can be measured by spin-echo T2-weighted sequences, in which two equal diffusion sensitising gradients are applied before and after a 180° radiofrequency pulse.[69,70] The b-value (in s/mm²) is a commonly applied term that allows the quantification of these gradients by pooling information from a number of variables. By measuring how far a molecule moves in a fixed time interval, the diffusion constant can be calculated.

In routine clinical practice, DWI can be used both qualitatively and quantitatively. Qualitative assessment identifies relative DWI changes compared to the surrounding normal tissue. Quantitative information can be obtained through the calculation of the apparent diffusion coefficient or ADC. This mathematical entity can be calculated from the slope of relative signal intensity (on a logarithmic scale) against a series of b-values.[71]

There is increasing evidence that the calculated ADC correlates with tissue cellularity. Within biological tissue, the small molecular movements of water are subject to restrictions, which are inherent to the medium due to the surrounding cells and constituency of the extracellular space. In the presence of few or no cells, there is high water diffusion and the molecules will diffuse further in a fixed time interval compared to water molecules within a high cellular environment. Tissues with low cellularity have lower DWI signal intensity and higher ADC values, while the opposite occurs in more solid tissues with a high cellularity, e.g. tumour, cytotoxic oedema, abscess and fibrosis.[70-72] Although the restricted diffusion seen within tumours is largely due to increased cellular density, other factors are likely to play a role such as the tortuosity of the extracellular space, extracellular fibrosis and the shape and size of the intercellular spaces.[73] Clinically, DWI is used to detect, characterise and stage tumours, distinguish tumour from surrounding tissues, predict and monitor response to therapy as well as evaluate tumour recurrence.[74-80] Successful treatment is generally reflected by an increase in the ADC value, although transient early decreases can occur following treatment.[7,11]

The development of stronger diffusion gradients, faster imaging sequences and improvements in hardware have allowed DWI to be extended to whole-body imaging applications, which has been particularly useful in oncology (Fig. 7-5).[72,81] Although many studies have shown its clinical potential as an imaging tool, protocol standardisation and larger clinical trials are necessary in the future.[81] In addition, further work is still required to understand the complicated interplay between ADC and the biophysical and cellular environment.

MR Spectroscopy (MRS)

Magnetic resonance spectroscopy is a technique that allows simultaneous non-invasive detection and measurement of several metabolites and chemicals found in tissue. The detection and identification of the metabolite peaks resides primarily on the subtle changes in the nuclear resonance frequency exerted by the atomic structure of its constituent molecule. For example, the two hydrogen nuclei (^{1}H or protons) in each molecule of water have a different resonant frequency from the hydrogen nuclei in fat and this can be exploited in fat-suppressed imaging. The measurement of the shift in frequency of a peak (in parts per million; ppm) relative to a standard such as water allows a molecule to be identified; the area under the curve of the peak gives an indication of the concentration of the molecule relative to the standard. Therefore, multiple endogenous metabolites can be simultaneously identified and an indication of their relative concentrations can be derived.

Proton MRS is often termed ^{1}H-MRS as the hydrogen nucleus contains a single proton. ^{1}H-MRS has been used to detect tumour metabolism since the 1980s and has a number of applications in the central nervous system.[82,83] Common metabolites that can be identified are choline-containing molecules (Cho), creatine (Cr), phosphocreatine (PCr) and N-acetylaspartate (NAA).[69] NAA is predominately present in neurons and the loss of NAA is associated with neuronal loss as occurs in stroke or in the

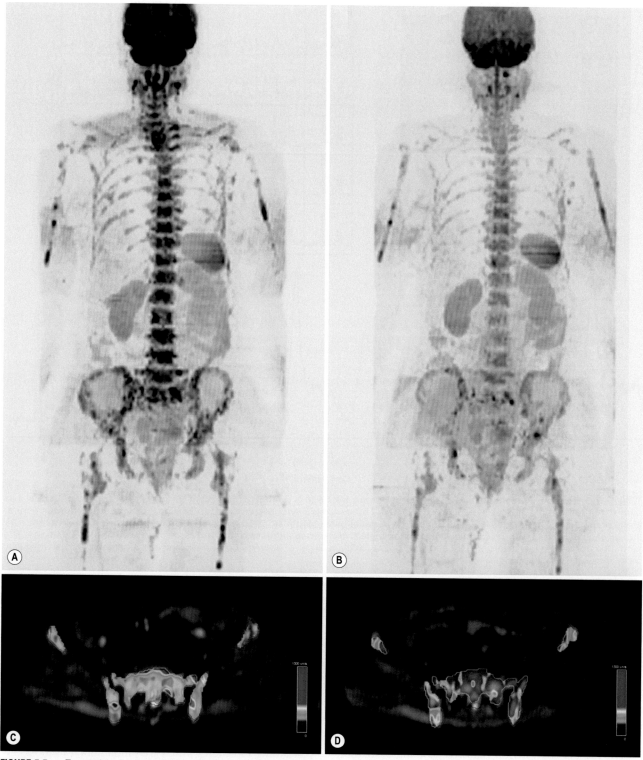

FIGURE 7-5 ■ **Example of whole-body diffusion-weighted imaging.** Serial changes in a 64-year-old woman with metastatic breast cancer treated with chemotherapy and bisphosphonates. (A) Inverted 3D maximum intensity projection (MIP) diffusion-weighted images showing widespread metastatic bone disease; (B) there is a subsequent decrease in the restricted diffusion and disease extent following treatment. (C) Colour ADC map of the pelvis in the same patient before treatment; (D) after treatment there is an increase in ADC, demonstrated by the colour change, indicating a response to treatment. (Images courtesy of Professor Anwar Padhani, Mount Vernon Cancer Centre, Northwood, Middlesex.)

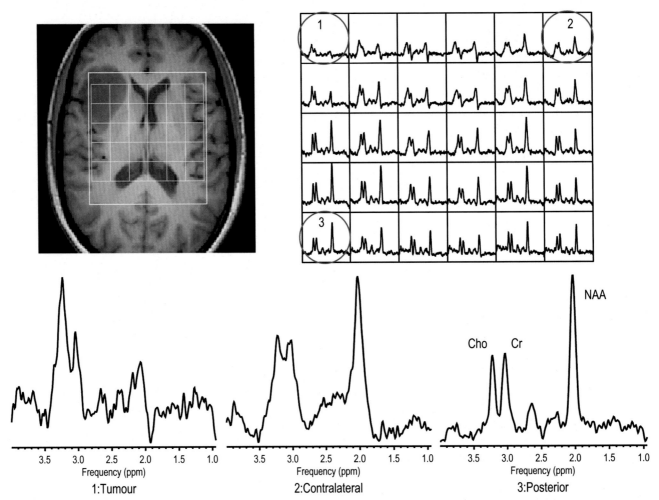

FIGURE 7-6 ■ **Example of magnetic resonance spectroscopy (MRS) in a patient with a brain tumour.** Localised spectroscopy has been acquired from a patient with a low-grade glioma. Three voxels have been enlarged to include: (1) tumour; (2) normal contralateral brain; and (3) normal ipsilateral brain. Common metabolites identified are: choline-containing molecules (Cho); creatine (Cr); and N-acetylaspartate (NAA). NAA is present predominately in neurons and loss of NAA is associated with neuronal damage. The glioma demonstrates low levels of NAA and a Cho peak which is larger relative to the Cr peak. (Images courtesy of Dr Mary McLean, Cancer Research UK, Cambridge Institute.)

presence of an intracranial tumour (Fig. 7-6).[84–86] Choline is part of the lipid biosynthesis pathway and because tumours contain a higher proportion of lipids than normal tissue, the choline-containing metabolite peak is a dominant feature of most tumour spectra.[69] Furthermore, a decrease may be seen following successful treatment with a chemotherapeutic agent.[87] As well as diagnosis and treatment response, applications of MRS in the clinical setting include tumour grading, identification of tumour margins for radiotherapy, and evaluation of local recurrence.[87–92]

MR spectroscopy can also be applied to other nuclei such as phosphorus-31 (^{31}P), fluorine-19 (^{19}F) and carbon-13 (^{13}C). ^{31}P-MRS is particularly suited to investigate cellular membrane metabolism and energy state, as it can detect the basic energy unit within the cell— adenosine triphosphate (ATP).[93] Tumours tend to have altered membrane metabolism, showing high levels of phosphomonoesters (PME) detectable by ^{31}P-MRS, which can be used as a marker of tumour aggressiveness

as well as assessing the response to therapy.[93,94] Intracellular pH (pH$_i$) can also be determined by this technique using the pH-sensitive inorganic phosphate (P$_i$) peak; although alterations in intracellular pH occur in tumours, the major pH change demonstrated in cancer is an acidification of the extracellular space.[95–98] ^{19}F-MRS has been mainly used to ascertain the pharmacokinetics of fluorinated drugs, such as 5-fluorouracil.[93,99] Finally, ^{13}C-MRS is a technique used to study metabolism of carbon-containing molecules which are fundamental to most cellular processes such as the citric acid cycle; abnormalities in the processing of carbon-containing metabolites are an early hallmark of a number of disease processes.[100] The use of ^{13}C-MRS in clinical practice has been limited by its low sensitivity, due in part to the fact that carbon-13 represents approximately 1% of total carbon in the body.

MRS is an attractive method for non-invasive detection of the biochemical status of disease processes. It is a very powerful tool for distinguishing endogenous metabolites from each other; however, its routine use in the clinical arena has been hampered by inherent technical constraints: low sensitivity and low spatial resolution. Recently, new methods for helping overcome some of these limitations have been described; e.g. hyperpolarisation techniques which significantly increase the sensitivity of MRI are being developed. Hyperpolarised gases have been used to image the microstructure of the lungs and a method termed dynamic nuclear polarisation (DNP) has been applied to hyperpolarise carbon-13. The latter involves intravenous administration of a hyperpolarised ^{13}C-labelled molecule followed by imaging of the injected molecule and the metabolites formed from it.[101] This has been used to assess fundamental biochemical pathways and physiological processes within animals.[101] To date, the most promising molecule has been ^{13}C-labelled pyruvate, which has been used as an early treatment response biomarker in cancer and DNP has recently undergone its first clinical trial in prostate cancer.[102]

POSITRON EMISSION TOMOGRAPHY (PET)

Positron emission tomography (PET) is based on the detection of an injected positron-emitting radioactive tracer. The positron (β^+) combines with an electron in the local tissue and, as a result of the annihilation, paired photons are simultaneously emitted 180° apart. These photons are subsequently detected outside of the patient by detectors that surround the patient and because they are 180° apart, the annihilation can be localised to a line connecting the two detectors. PET relies on the simultaneous or coincidence detection of the annihilation photons (γ) released when the radionuclides injected in the patient emit positrons that undergo annihilation with electrons. As collimators are not required to reconstruct the image, the sensitivity of PET imaging is generally very high. Furthermore, given that these radiolabelled tracers are often physiological or functional molecules, PET can obtain quantitative functional information of physiological or pathological processes. Although PET can identify the presence of a radiolabel with high sensitivity, it cannot differentiate individual species that are radiolabelled; i.e. an injected radiolabelled molecule may be metabolised into one or more molecules but the measured PET signal combines all of these together. Therefore image contrast with PET is generated from regional differences in radiolabel accumulation rather than the identification of individual metabolites as in MRS. The relatively low spatial resolution PET imaging is usually combined with high-resolution anatomical information acquired from CT or MRI, termed PET-CT or PET-MRI.

PET radiotracers or radiopharmaceuticals are compounds of biomedical interest, which are labelled with radionuclides such as fluorine-18 (^{18}F), carbon-11 (^{11}C) or oxygen-15 (^{15}O). The accumulation of a radioactively labelled tracer (and its metabolic products) can be used as a quantitative measure of the biological processes that are being probed (Fig. 7-7). Corrections can be applied for the weight of the patient and the injected dose to

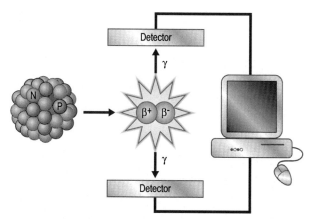

FIGURE 7-7 ■ **The principles of PET imaging.** The released positrons (β^+) from the nucleus of a radionuclide (e.g. the ^{18}F within FDG) travels a short distance (a), the *mean positron range*. The positron is annihilated by an electron (β^-), releasing two coincidence 511-keV photons (γ), which are then collected by detectors. N, neutron; P, proton.

produce a standardised uptake value (SUV); the maximum tracer uptake of a single voxel within a region of interest is termed the SUV_{max} and this is commonly used in clinical practice as a simple metric of PET metabolism.

Fluorodeoxyglucose-PET (FDG-PET)

PET-CT has emerged as a promising technique in oncological imaging for diagnosis, staging, therapy response and evaluation of recurrence in a number of malignancies. Although there is an extensive array of clinical radiotracers available, the most widely used is ^{18}F-labelled 2-fluoro-2-deoxy-D-glucose (FDG), a fluorinated analogue of glucose. FDG is transported by the glucose transporters into the cell and phosphorylated by the enzyme hexokinase; no further metabolism occurs and the phosphorylated FDG becomes trapped and accumulates within the cell. The use of this tracer is based on the principle that the majority of malignant cells have upregulated glycolysis: i.e. increased glucose uptake and metabolism compared to normal cells. Upregulated glycolysis leads to an increased formation of lactate; lactate is produced in normal tissue in the presence of reduced oxygen levels but in tumours this occurs even in the presence of oxygen, a phenomenon termed aerobic glycolysis or the Warburg effect.[104,105] The phenomenon of aerobic glycolysis underlies the widespread use of ^{18}F-labelled FDG-PET in oncology. There is increasing evidence to support a role for FDG-PET in the management of oncology patients, as listed in Table 7-5.[106]

Non-FDG-PET Tracers

FDG is the leading clinical molecule for PET and many centres only use FDG as a clinical tracer in PET. The great versatility of PET is the large number of molecules that can be labelled to probe a wide range of biological processes. PET tracers can be broadly classified into markers of morphological structure, perfusion, altered metabolism, proliferation, cell death, hypoxia and cell surface protein expression, e.g. receptors (Fig. 7-8). Table 7-6 summarises the common non-FDG tracers used in clinical practice, the mechanisms that they probe and their clinical applications.[107–130] These tracers are at varying stages of development: there are a large number of preclinical tracers, a smaller number of experimental clinical probes and a relatively limited number of agents that are used routinely in clinical practice.

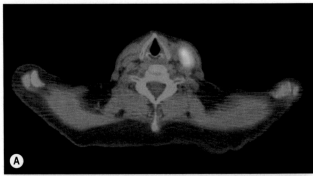

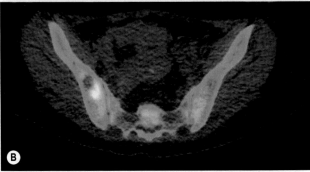

FIGURE 7-8 ■ **Examples of non-FDG-PET imaging in metastatic renal cell carcinoma.** (A) An ^{18}F-labelled FMISO PET-CT study showing focal retention of the tracer within a hypoxic left cervical metastasis. (B) ^{18}F-labelled sodium fluoride PET-CT in a different patient—there is focal uptake around a lytic bone metastasis within the right side of the pelvis. (Images courtesy of Dr John Buscombe, Addenbrooke's Hospital, Cambridge.)

TABLE 7-5 Current Clinical Indications for Use of FDG-PET-CT in Oncology

- Evaluation of indeterminate lesions detected by another imaging method in order to help in the differential diagnosis between a benign and a malignant process
- Guidance of initial or subsequent treatment strategy in patients with a known malignancy
- Monitoring of treatment response
- Evaluation of residual post-treatment abnormalities detected by another imaging method in order to determine whether it represents persistent viable tumour or post-treatment changes
- Localisation of the primary site of a tumour when metastatic disease is the first manifestation of malignancy
- Establishment and localisation of disease sites as a cause for an elevated serum marker
- Guidance of clinical procedures, such as directed biopsies and radiation therapy planning

From the American College of Radiology and Society for Pediatric Radiology Guidelines 2012.[106]

TABLE 7-6 Summary of Non-FDG-PET Tracers Used in The Clinic[107–130]

Tracer	Radionuclide	Mechanism of Action Clinical Applications
Sodium fluoride	[18]F	Uptake reflects blood flow and bone remodeling; Detects primary and secondary bone tumours[108]
FLT	[18]F	Thymidine analogue; Detects cellular proliferation; Distinguishes malignant from benign lesions in lung, breast and colon[107]
Methionine	[11]C	Radiolabelled amino acid; Tumour uptake reflects cellular proliferation and microvessel density; Used in grading of brain tumours, differential diagnosis and identifying recurrence[109–113]
FET	[18]F	Radiolabelled amino acid; Detection of high-grade glioma[114]
FMAU	[18]F	Proliferation probe; Detection of brain, prostate and bone tumours[115]
Acetate	[11]C	Fatty acids precursor; Detection of prostate cancer and low-grade hepatic cancer[116–119]
FMISO	[18]F	Hypoxia imaging probe; Predictor for local recurrence in head, neck and lung cancer[120,121]
FAZA	[18]F	Hypoxia imaging probe; Predictor of successfully radiotherapy[122,123]
ATSM	[62]Cu	Hypoxia imaging probe; Predictor of response to chemoradiotherapy[124]
[15]O water	[15]O	Perfusion probe; Evaluation of response to cytotoxics, anti-angiogenic and vascular disrupting agents in solid tumours[125–127]
Annexin V	[68]Ga [18]F	Cell death probe; Treatment response marker[128]
DOTA-TATE	[68]Ga	Binds to somatostatin receptors; Diagnosis of new lesions in patients with or suspected neuroendocrine tumours[129,130]

Abbreviations: FLT, 3-deoxy-3-[^{18}F]fluorothymidine; FET, O-(2-[^{18}F]fluoroethyl)-L-tyrosine; FMAU, [^{18}F]-1-(2'-deoxy-2'-fluoro-beta-D-arabinofuranosyl)thymine; FMISO, [^{18}F]-fluoromisonidazole; FAZA, [^{18}F]-fluoroazomycinarabinoside; ATSM, diacetyl-bis(N⁴-methylthiosemicarbazone).

For example, a thymidine analogue, ^{18}F-labelled 3-deoxy-3-fluorothymidine (FLT), has been used to probe cellular proliferation and growth; it is phosphorylated by thymidine kinase and retained intracellularly with a small amount being incorporated into DNA.[131] FLT has been used to distinguish malignant from benign lesions in the lung, breast and in the colon and has shown promise as a tool for imaging cell growth.[107] Another example is the use of PET to image amino acid transport and metabolism: L-[methyl-^{11}C]methionine (MET) has shown high sensitivity (up to 95%) for the detection of glioma as well as providing prognostic information.[132] Other examples include ^{11}C-choline and ^{11}C-acetate, which have been used to probe tumour lipid metabolism, as well as to detect tumour recurrence after treatment.[133,134]

In summary, the great strength of PET is its very high sensitivity as a technique, which can be used in conjunction with a wide range of tracers to probe fundamental physiological and pathological processes. However, it remains an expensive method for the foreseeable future, involves a significant radiation burden, and certain short-lived radionuclides require an adjacent cyclotron facility which only a few sites have access to.

EMERGING MOLECULAR IMAGING TECHNIQUES AND THERANOSTICS

There are a very large number of emerging imaging methods that have been developed on animal imaging studies. The vast majority of new imaging approaches have been developed using animal models, before then being translated to patients, although there are some exceptions. There is an increasing trend towards *hybrid imaging* where two differing but complementary imagine techniques are combined to produce a test that is greater than the sum of its parts; for example, by combining the functional information acquired with PET with the anatomical CT data, PET-CT has proved to be a very powerful clinical tool. In addition, combining a diagnostic imaging test with a therapeutic approach which is closely related to the diagnostic test is another developing field which falls under the more general term of *theranostics*. Examples include the use of functional imaging combined with image-guided intervention as well as the use of radiolabelled molecules for both imaging and therapy.

Ultrasound

Ultrasound has been used in oncology for many decades not only to demonstrate tissue anatomy at very high resolution but also to reveal functional information about tissue perfusion and flow with the use of Doppler ultrasound. Although it is relatively limited as a molecular imaging tool, the generation of tissue contrast with microbubbles has opened up the possibility of its use on a molecular level. Microbubbles with a gaseous central core are injected intravenously and remain within the vasculature; local application of a resonant frequency ultrasound pulse at the area of interest causes the bubbles to burst and this significantly enhances the ultrasound

signal measured, giving an enhanced image of the vascular space. By conjugating these bubbles to a targeted probe for a protein of interest (for example, VEGF), the image of the signal acquired when the bubbles are subsequently burst gives an indication of the spatial distribution of the protein of interest. The advantages of ultrasound are its very high spatial resolution and lack of ionising radiation, but, to date, it has been limited to the imaging of vascular structures and proteins. An emerging approach with ultrasound is the development of drug-containing microbubbles where the microbubbles are burst within the tissue of interest. This deposits the therapeutic agent at a high concentration where it is required while reducing the systemic dose and toxicity to normal tissues.

Optical Imaging

Optical imaging is a non-invasive and non-ionising technology that uses light to probe cellular and molecular function in living subjects. Visible light is a form of electromagnetic radiation, which has properties of both particles and waves. As light travels through tissue, photons can be absorbed, reflected or scattered, depending on the tissue composition. Different forms of optical imaging analyse these interactions to provide unique spectral signatures which can report on the molecular structure of the tissue in question. For example, fluorescence and phosphorescence depend on the emission of light following its absorption, and Raman spectroscopy analyses the inelastic scattering of light. Optical imaging has a very high spatial resolution in the nanometer (nm) range and can provide real-time and quantitative information. However, the main limitation of optical imaging is its limited penetration depth due to the strong scattering of light in biological tissues. This can be partly overcome by using fibreoptic endoscopic probes, which allow both tissue illumination and the collection of the emitted light from deep within the body. In addition, in the near-infrared (NIR) part of the electromagnetic spectrum, soft tissues show less scattering and absorption than in the visible band; hence, using NIR optical imaging enables the probing depth to be increased to a few centimetres.[135]

Fluorescence imaging describes the emission of light by a substance (i.e. a fluorophore) that has previously absorbed light. When a fluorophore absorbs light it enters an unstable excited state. Eventually fluorophores will return to the ground state, releasing any stored energy as light. In most cases the emitted light will have a lower energy (and hence a lower frequency) than the initial absorbed light due to some loss of energy during the transient excited lifetime (Fig. 7-9). Fluorophores can repeatedly undergo excitation and emission, allowing them to generate a signal multiple times, thereby making fluorescence a very sensitive technique. In contrast, bio-luminescence imaging is the production and emission of light by a living organism whereby energy is released by a chemical reaction in the form of light. For example, luciferase is an enzyme that catalyses a reaction in which the chemical luciferin reacts with molecular oxygen to create light.

Clinically, optical spectroscopy has been shown to be useful in identifying and monitoring cancer since the characteristics of light emission change as cancer develops. During neoplastic transformation, there is (i) an increase in optical absorption due to an increase in nuclear size, DNA content and irregular chromatin clumping, (ii) an increase in optical scattering as a result of angiogenesis, which increases vessel density and haemoglobin concentration and (iii) changes in fluorescence—an increase in epithelial fluorescence (due to higher metabolic rates in pre-cancerous tissues), but a

decrease in stromal fluorescence (due to changes in the extracellular matrix).[136] Intraoperative optical imaging using fluorescence has been used for tumour margin delineation and to identify malignant/sentinal nodes to ensure complete surgical resection of tumours. In addition, the use of fluorescence during routine endoscopic screening examinations in the gastrointestinal, bronchial and urinary tracts is also proving to be an invaluable tool to allow clinicians to detect occult dysplastic lesions (Fig. 7-10).[137]

Optical imaging is frequently used as a gene reporter in preclinical tumour models—a gene encoding either a fluorescent protein (e.g. green fluorescent protein) or a bioluminescent protein (e.g. luciferase enzyme) is encoded with a regulatory sequence for another gene of interest; the expression of the gene of interest can be indirectly detected by the light emitted from the co-expressed reporter gene.[2] This approach is potentially very attractive for the detection of successful gene therapy, which is in its infancy in human studies.

Unlike fluorescence in which light is absorbed, Raman spectroscopy depends on the inelastic scattering of light. When monochromatic laser light is directed at a molecule, some of the photons will scatter; energy from the incident photon can be passed to the molecule, resulting in the photon being inelastically scattered and losing energy. This energy exchange between the incident light and the scattering molecule is known as the Raman effect. The molecular structure and composition of the material is encoded as a set of frequency shifts in the Raman scattered light, giving it a spectral signature, which acts as a reporter or fingerprint of the molecule in question.

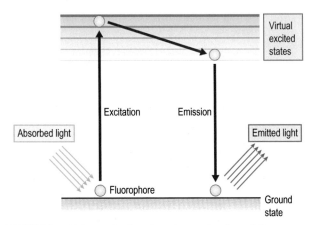

FIGURE 7-9 ■ **Schematic showing the production of fluorescent light by an electron within a fluorophore.** By absorbing light, the electron enters an excited state and, as it falls back to the lower-energy state again, it releases the stored energy as emitted light.

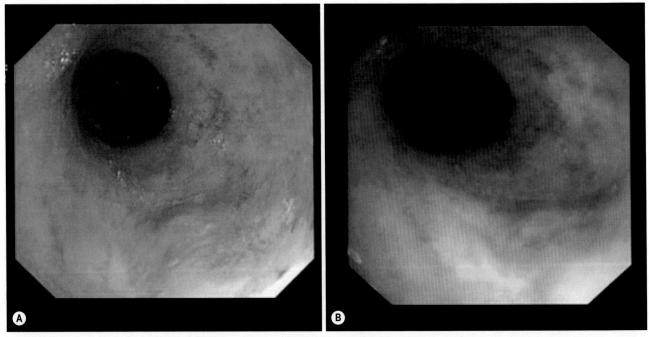

FIGURE 7-10 ■ **Example of a clinical application of optical imaging: the detection of Barrett's oesophagus on endoscopy.** (A) The Barrett's lesion is inconspicuous on standard white-light imaging; (B) autofluorescent imaging shows an abnormal purple area with normal surrounding green tissue; the abnormal area was confirmed histologically as low-grade dysplasia. Autofluorescence imaging is based on the detection of fluorescence emitted by endogenous molecules within tissue; changes in these molecules between normal and abnormal tissue can be exploited for the detection of dysplastic tissue that would otherwise be difficult to detect. (Images courtesy of Dr Rebecca Fitzgerald, Addenbrooke's Hospital, Cambridge.)

However, as the magnitude of the Raman effect is inherently very weak, this limits the sensitivity and hence its clinical application. In recent years, advances in nanobiotechnology have enabled the synthesis of nanoparticles which can overcome this problem by taking advantage of a phenomenon known as surface-enhanced Raman scattering (SERS) which can result in very high Raman signals at picomolar concentrations in deep tissue, thereby making it ideal as an in vivo imaging agent.[138] This very sensitive technique is being investigated as a technique to detect early tumour formation on endothelial surfaces such as the colon. The potential applications of SERS nanoparticles in tumour imaging are tremendous but concerns over toxicity need to be addressed before they will gain widespread clinical use.

In summary, molecular optical imaging offers many potential advantages, including high spatial resolution and sensitivity, although in general it demonstrates poor tissue penetration and is not used routinely in patients yet.

CONCLUSION: ROLE OF FUNCTIONAL AND MOLECULAR IMAGING IN ONCOLOGY

In general, functional and molecular techniques probe processes that require amplification for detection and therefore represent a compromise between spatial resolution and sensitivity. Instead of traditional high spatial resolution imaging, lower-resolution parameter maps or spectra are produced. Consequently, if these techniques are to find a place in routine clinical practice it is likely that functional and molecular images will be combined with traditional anatomical imaging in much the same way as in PET-CT. Many of these techniques described above are already used for clinical imaging and some of the more novel methods are undergoing clinical assessment. However, translating a preclinical tool into a routine clinical technique may take many years of development and longer to demonstrate clinical efficacy and cost-effectiveness; it requires collaboration between academics, clinicians, non-clinical scientists and industry. Functional and molecular imaging promises powerful tools to aid diagnosis, identify disease heterogeneity, predict outcome, target biopsies and determine treatment response non-invasively.

REFERENCES

1. Hanahan D, Weinberg RA. Hallmarks of cancer: the next generation. Cell 2011;144(5):646–74.
2. Massoud TF, Gambhir SS. Molecular imaging in living subjects: seeing fundamental biological processes in a new light. Genes Dev 2003;17(5):545–80.
3. Miles KA, Lee TY, Goh V, et al. Current status and guidelines for the assessment of tumour vascular support with dynamic contrast-enhanced computed tomography. Eur Radiol 2012;22(7):1430–41.
4. Miles KA. Measurement of tissue perfusion by dynamic computed tomography. Br J Radiol 1991;64(761):409–12.
5. Patlak CS, Blasberg RG, Fenstermacher JD. Graphical evaluation of blood-to-brain transfer constants from multiple-time uptake data. J Cereb Blood Flow Metab 1983;3(1):1–7.
6. Johnson JA, Wilson TA. A model for capillary exchange. Am J Physiol 1966;210(6):1299–303.
7. Purdie TG, Henderson E, Lee TY. Functional CT imaging of angiogenesis in rabbit VX2 soft-tissue tumour. Phys Med Biol 2001;46(12):3161–75.
8. Ng CS, Kodama Y, Mullani NA, et al. Tumor blood flow measured by perfusion computed tomography and 15O-labeled water positron emission tomography: a comparison study. J Comput Assist Tomogr 2009;33(3):460–5.
9. Ohno Y, Koyama H, Matsumoto K, et al. Differentiation of malignant and benign pulmonary nodules with quantitative first-pass 320-detector row perfusion CT versus FDG PET/CT. Radiology 2011;258(2):599–609.
10. Cronin P, Dwamena BA, Kelly AM, Carlos RC. Solitary pulmonary nodules: meta-analytic comparison of cross-sectional imaging modalities for diagnosis of malignancy. Radiology 2008;246(3):772–82.
11. Delrue L, Blanckaert P, Mertens D, et al. Tissue perfusion in pathologies of the pancreas: assessment using 128-slice computed tomography. Abdom Imaging 2012;37(4):595–601.
12. Goh V, Halligan S, Taylor SA, et al. Differentiation between diverticulitis and colorectal cancer: quantitative CT perfusion measurements versus morphologic criteria—initial experience. Radiology 2007;242(2):456–62.
13. Thomas JP, Arzoomanian RZ, Alberti D, et al. Phase I pharmacokinetic and pharmacodynamic study of recombinant human endostatin in patients with advanced solid tumors. J Clin Oncol 2003;21(2):223–31.
14. Willett CG, Boucher Y, di Tomaso E, et al. Direct evidence that the VEGF-specific antibody bevacizumab has antivascular effects in human rectal cancer. Nat Med 2004;10(2):145–7.
15. Xiong HQ, Herbst R, Faria SC, et al. A phase I surrogate endpoint study of SU6668 in patients with solid tumors. Invest New Drugs 2004;22(4):459–66.
16. McNeel DG, Eickhoff J, Lee FT, et al. Phase I trial of a monoclonal antibody specific for alphavbeta3 integrin (MEDI-522) in patients with advanced malignancies, including an assessment of effect on tumor perfusion. Clin Cancer Res 2005;11(21):7851–60.
17. Faria SC, Ng CS, Hess KR, et al. CT quantification of effects of thalidomide in patients with metastatic renal cell carcinoma. Am J Roentgenol 2007;189(2):378–85.
18. Gandhi D, Chepeha DB, Miller T, et al. Correlation between initial and early follow-up CT perfusion parameters with endoscopic tumor response in patients with advanced squamous cell carcinomas of the oropharynx treated with organ-preservation therapy. Am J Neuroradiol 2006;27(1):101–6.
19. Meijerink MR, van Cruijsen H, Hoekman K, et al. The use of perfusion CT for the evaluation of therapy combining AZD2171 with gefitinib in cancer patients. Eur Radiol 2007;17(7):1700–13.
20. Ng QS, Goh V, Carnell D, et al. Tumor antivascular effects of radiotherapy combined with combretastatin a4 phosphate in human non-small-cell lung cancer. Int J Radiat Oncol Biol Phys 2007;67(5):1375–80.
21. Ng QS, Goh V, Milner J, et al. Effect of nitric-oxide synthesis on tumour blood volume and vascular activity: a phase I study. Lancet Oncol 2007;8(2):111–18.
22. Fournier LS, Oudard S, Thiam R, et al. Metastatic renal carcinoma: evaluation of antiangiogenic therapy with dynamic contrast-enhanced CT. Radiology 2010;256(2):511–18.
23. Lind JS, Meijerink MR, Dingemans AM, et al. Dynamic contrast-enhanced CT in patients treated with sorafenib and erlotinib for non-small cell lung cancer: a new method of monitoring treatment? Eur Radiol 2010;20(12):2890–8.
24. Bisdas S, Rumboldt Z, Surlan-Popovic K, et al. Perfusion CT in squamous cell carcinoma of the upper aerodigestive tract: long-term predictive value of baseline perfusion CT measurements. Am J Neuroradiol 2010;31(3):576–81.
25. Park MS, Klotz E, Kim MJ, et al. Perfusion CT: noninvasive surrogate marker for stratification of pancreatic cancer response to concurrent chemo- and radiation therapy. Radiology 2009;250(1):110–17.
26. Hayano K, Shuto K, Koda K, et al. Quantitative measurement of blood flow using perfusion CT for assessing clinicopathologic features and prognosis in patients with rectal cancer. Dis Colon Rectum 2009;52(9):1624–9.

27. Bellomi M, Petralia G, Sonzogni A, et al. CT perfusion for the monitoring of neoadjuvant chemotherapy and radiation therapy in rectal carcinoma: initial experience. Radiology 2007;244(2):486–93.

28. Goh V, Dattani M, Farwell J, et al. Radiation dose from volumetric helical perfusion CT of the thorax, abdomen or pelvis. Eur Radiol 2011;21(5):974–81.

29. ICRP. The 2007 Recommendations of the International Commission on Radiological Protection. Available from: <http://www.icrp.org/index.asp>; 2007.

30. Padhani AR. Dynamic contrast-enhanced MRI in clinical oncology: current status and future directions. J Magn Reson Imaging 2002;16(4):407–22.

31. Marcus CD, Ladam-Marcus V, Cucu C, et al. Imaging techniques to evaluate the response to treatment in oncology: current standards and perspectives. Crit Rev Oncol Hematol 2009;72(3):217–38.

32. Tofts PS, Brix G, Buckley DL, et al. Estimating kinetic parameters from dynamic contrast-enhanced T(1)-weighted MRI of a diffusable tracer: standardized quantities and symbols. J Magn Reson Imaging 1999;10(3):223–32.

33. Evelhoch J. Perfusion, diffusion and flow-MRI tech ctte. Available at <http://qibawiki.rsna.org/index.php?title=Diffusion_Perfusion_and_Flow-MR_tech_ctte>; 2011.

34. Zaharchuk G. Theoretical basis of hemodynamic MR imaging techniques to measure cerebral blood volume, cerebral blood flow, and permeability. Am J Neuroradiol 2007;28(10):1850–8.

35. Tofts PS. Modeling tracer kinetics in dynamic Gd-DTPA MR imaging. J Magn Reson Imaging 1997;7(1):91–101.

36. Sourbron S. Technical aspects of MR perfusion. Eur J Radiol 2010;76(3):304–13.

37. Koh TS, Bisdas S, Koh DM, Thng CH. Fundamentals of tracer kinetics for dynamic contrast-enhanced MRI. J Magn Reson Imaging 2011;34(6):1262–76.

38. Maxwell RJ, Wilson J, Prise VE, et al. Evaluation of the anti-vascular effects of combretastatin in rodent tumours by dynamic contrast enhanced MRI. NMR Biomed 2002;15(2):89–98.

39. Leach MO, Brindle KM, Evelhoch JL, et al. The assessment of antiangiogenic and antivascular therapies in early-stage clinical trials using magnetic resonance imaging: issues and recommendations. Br J Cancer 2005;92(9):1599–610.

40. Yang X, Knopp MV. Quantifying tumor vascular heterogeneity with dynamic contrast-enhanced magnetic resonance imaging: a review. J Biomed Biotechnol 2011;2011:732848.

41. Turkbey B, Kobayashi H, Ogawa M, et al. Imaging of tumor angiogenesis: functional or targeted? Am J Roentgenol 2009;193(2):304–13.

42. Degani H, Gusis V, Weinstein D, et al. Mapping pathophysiological features of breast tumors by MRI at high spatial resolution. Nat Med 1997;3(7):780–2.

43. Gilles R, Guinebretière JM, Shapeero LG, et al. Assessment of breast cancer recurrence with contrast-enhanced subtraction MR imaging: preliminary results in 26 patients. Radiology 1993;188(2):473–8.

44. Scalerandi M, Sansone BC. Inhibition of vascularization in tumor growth. Phys Rev Lett 2002;89(21):218101.

45. Knopp MV, Giesel FL, Marcos H, et al. Dynamic contrast-enhanced magnetic resonance imaging in oncology. Top Magn Reson Imaging 2001;12(4):301–8.

46. Gillies RJ, Raghunand N, Karczmar GS, Bhujwalla ZM. MRI of the tumor microenvironment. J Magn Reson Imaging 2002;16(4):430–50.

47. Hahn OM, Yang C, Medved M, et al. Dynamic contrast-enhanced magnetic resonance imaging pharmacodynamic biomarker study of sorafenib in metastatic renal carcinoma. J Clin Oncol 2008;26(28):4572–8.

48. Batchelor TT, Sorensen AG, di Tomaso E, et al. AZD2171, a pan-VEGF receptor tyrosine kinase inhibitor, normalizes tumor vasculature and alleviates edema in glioblastoma patients. Cancer Cell 2007;11(1):83–95.

49. Dafni H, Landsman L, Schechter B, et al. MRI and fluorescence microscopy of the acute vascular response to VEGF165: vasodilation, hyper-permeability and lymphatic uptake, followed by rapid inactivation of the growth factor. NMR Biomed 2002;15(2):120–31.

50. O'Connor JP, Carano RA, Clamp AR, et al. Quantifying antivascular effects of monoclonal antibodies to vascular endothelial growth factor: insights from imaging. Clin Cancer Res 2009;15(21):6674–82.

51. Gore JC, Manning HC, Quarles CC, et al. Magnetic resonance in the era of molecular imaging of cancer. Magn Reson Imaging 2011;29(5):587–600.

52. Bogdanov A Jr, Mazzanti ML. Molecular magnetic resonance contrast agents for the detection of cancer: past and present. Semin Oncol 2011;38(1):42–54.

53. Dennie J, Mandeville JB, Boxerman JL, et al. NMR imaging of changes in vascular morphology due to tumor angiogenesis. Magn Reson Med 1998;40(6):793–9.

54. Knopp EA, Cha S, Johnson G, et al. Glial neoplasms: dynamic contrast-enhanced T2*-weighted MR imaging. Radiology 1999;211(3):791–8.

55. Fuss M, Wenz F, Essig M, et al. Tumor angiogenesis of low-grade astrocytomas measured by dynamic susceptibility contrast-enhanced MRI (DSC-MRI) is predictive of local tumor control after radiation therapy. Int J Radiat Oncol Biol Phys 2001;51(2):478–82.

56. Fuss M, Wenz F, Scholdei R, et al. Radiation-induced regional cerebral blood volume (rCBV) changes in normal brain and low-grade astrocytomas: quantification and time and dose-dependent occurrence. Int J Radiat Oncol Biol Phys 2000;48(1):53–8.

57. Ludemann L, Prochnow D, Rohlfing T, et al. Simultaneous quantification of perfusion and permeability in the prostate using dynamic contrast-enhanced magnetic resonance imaging with an inversion-prepared dual-contrast sequence. Ann Biomed Eng 2009;37(4):749–62.

58. Delille JP, Slanetz PJ, Yeh ED, et al. Breast cancer: regional blood flow and blood volume measured with magnetic susceptibility-based MR imaging–initial results. Radiology 2002;223(2):558–65.

59. Liu G, Rugo HS, Wilding G, et al. Dynamic contrast-enhanced magnetic resonance imaging as a pharmacodynamic measure of response after acute dosing of AG-013736, an oral angiogenesis inhibitor, in patients with advanced solid tumors: results from a phase I study. J Clin Oncol 2005;23(24):5464–73.

60. Drevs J, Siegert P, Medinger M, et al. Phase I clinical study of AZD2171, an oral vascular endothelial growth factor signaling inhibitor, in patients with advanced solid tumors. J Clin Oncol 2007;25(21):3045–54.

61. Flaherty KT, Rosen MA, Heitjan DF, et al. Pilot study of DCE-MRI to predict progression-free survival with sorafenib therapy in renal cell carcinoma. Cancer Biol Ther 2008;7(4):496–501.

62. Ah-See ML, Makris A, Taylor NJ, et al. Early changes in functional dynamic magnetic resonance imaging predict for pathologic response to neoadjuvant chemotherapy in primary breast cancer. Clin Cancer Res 2008;14(20):6580–9.

63. Jarnagin WR, Schwartz LH, Gultekin DH, et al. Regional chemotherapy for unresectable primary liver cancer: results of a phase II clinical trial and assessment of DCE-MRI as a biomarker of survival. Ann Oncol 2009;20(9):1589–95.

64. Ferl GZ, Xu L, Friesenhahn M, et al. An automated method for nonparametric kinetic analysis of clinical DCE-MRI data: application to glioblastoma treated with bevacizumab. Magn Reson Med 2010;63(5):1366–75.

65. Jensen LR, Garzon B, Heldahl MG, et al. Diffusion-weighted and dynamic contrast-enhanced MRI in evaluation of early treatment effects during neoadjuvant chemotherapy in breast cancer patients. J Magn Reson Imaging 2011;34(5):1099–109.

66. Barrett T, Gill AB, Kataoka MY, et al. DCE and DW MRI in monitoring response to androgen deprivation therapy in patients with prostate cancer: a feasibility study. Magn Reson Med 2012;67(3):778–85.

67. Kim JH, Kim CK, Park BK, et al. Dynamic contrast-enhanced 3-T MR imaging in cervical cancer before and after concurrent chemoradiotherapy. Eur Radiol 2012;22(11):2533–9.

68. Gollub MJ, Gultekin DH, Akin O, et al. Dynamic contrast enhanced-MRI for the detection of pathological complete response to neoadjuvant chemotherapy for locally advanced rectal cancer. Eur Radiol 2012;22(4):821–31.

69. Gadian DG. NMR and Its Applications to Living Systems. 2nd ed. Oxford: Oxford University Press; 1995. p. 283.

70. Qayyum A. Diffusion-weighted imaging in the abdomen and pelvis: concepts and applications. Radiographics 2009;6(29):1797–810.

71. Sugita R, Ito K, Fujita N, Takahashi S. Diffusion-weighted MRI in abdominal oncology: clinical applications. World J Gastroenterol 2010;16(7):832–6.

72. Koh DM, Collins DJ. Diffusion-weighted MRI in the body: applications and challenges in oncology. Am J Roentgenol 2007;188(6):1622–35.

73. Padhani AR, Liu G, Koh DM, et al. Diffusion-weighted magnetic resonance imaging as a cancer biomarker: consensus and recommendations. Neoplasia 2009;11(2):102–25.

74. Jacobs MA, Herskovits EH, Kim HS. Uterine fibroids: diffusion-weighted MR imaging for monitoring therapy with focused ultrasound surgery—preliminary study. Radiology 2005;236(1):196–203.

75. Guo Y, Cai YQ, Cai ZL, et al. Differentiation of clinically benign and malignant breast lesions using diffusion-weighted imaging. J Magn Reson Imaging 2002;16(2):172–8.

76. Choi EK, Kim JK, Choi HJ, et al. Node-by-node correlation between MR and PET/CT in patients with uterine cervical cancer: diffusion-weighted imaging versus size-based criteria on T2WI. Eur Radiol 2009;19(8):2024–32.

77. Baur A, Huber A, Ertl-Wagner B, et al. Diagnostic value of increased diffusion weighting of a steady-state free precession sequence for differentiating acute benign osteoporotic fractures from pathologic vertebral compression fractures. Am J Neuroradiol 2001;22(2):366–74.

78. Baur A, Stäbler A, Brüning R, et al. Diffusion-weighted MR imaging of bone marrow: differentiation of benign versus pathologic compression fractures. Radiology 1998;207(2):349–56.

79. Partridge SC, Demartini WB, Kurland BF, et al. Differential diagnosis of mammographically and clinically occult breast lesions on diffusion-weighted MRI. J Magn Reson Imaging 2010;31(3):562–70.

80. Mardor Y, Roth Y, Ochershvilli A, et al. Pretreatment prediction of brain tumors' response to radiation therapy using high b-value diffusion-weighted MRI. Neoplasia 2004;6(2):136–42.

81. McNab JA, Miller KL. Steady-state diffusion-weighted imaging: theory, acquisition and analysis. NMR Biomed 2010;23(7):781–93.

82. Griffiths JR, Stevens AN, Iles RA, et al. ^{31}P-NMR investigation of solid tumours in the living rat. Biosci Rep 1981;1(4):319–25.

83. Griffiths JR, Cady E, Edwards RH, et al. ^{31}P-NMR studies of a human tumour in situ. Lancet 1983;1(8339):1435–6.

84. Urenjak J, Williams SR, Gadian DG, Noble M. Specific expression of N-acetylaspartate in neurons, oligodendrocyte-type-2 astrocyte progenitors, and immature oligodendrocytes in vitro. J Neurochem 1992;59(1):55–61.

85. Bruhn H, Frahm J, Gyngell ML, et al. Cerebral metabolism in man after acute stroke: new observations using localized proton NMR spectroscopy. Magn Reson Med 1989;9(1):126–31.

86. Luyten PR, Marien AJ, Heindel W, et al. Metabolic imaging of patients with intracranial tumors: H-1 MR spectroscopic imaging and PET. Radiology 1990;176(3):791–9.

87. Glunde K, Ackerstaff E, Mori N, et al. Choline phospholipid metabolism in cancer: consequences for molecular pharmaceutical interventions. Mol Pharm 2006;3(5):496–506.

88. Gillies RJ, Morse DL. In vivo magnetic resonance spectroscopy in cancer. Annu Rev Biomed Eng 2005;7:287–326.

89. Payne GS, Leach MO. Applications of magnetic resonance spectroscopy in radiotherapy treatment planning. Br J Radiol 2006;79(Spec No 1):S16–26.

90. Zeng QS, Li CF, Zhang K, et al. Multivoxel 3D proton MR spectroscopy in the distinction of recurrent glioma from radiation injury. J Neurooncol 2007;84(1):63–9.

91. Kumar R, Kumar M, Jagannathan NR, et al. Proton magnetic resonance spectroscopy with a body coil in the diagnosis of carcinoma prostate. Urol Res 2004;32(1):36–40.

92. Sciarra A, Panebianco V, Salciccia S, et al. Role of dynamic contrast-enhanced magnetic resonance (MR) imaging and proton MR spectroscopic imaging in the detection of local recurrence after radical prostatectomy for prostate cancer. Eur Urol 2008;3(54):589–600.

93. Daly PF, Cohen JS. Magnetic resonance spectroscopy of tumors and potential in vivo clinical applications: a review. Cancer Res 1989;49(4):770–9.

94. Negendank W. Studies of human tumors by MRS: a review. NMR Biomed 1992;5(5):303–24.

95. Griffiths JR. Are cancer cells acidic? Br J Cancer 1991;64(3):425–7.

96. Moon RB, Richards JH. Determination of intracellular pH by ^{31}P magnetic resonance. J Biol Chem 1973;248(20):7276–8.

97. Radda GK, Bore PJ, Gadian DG, et al. ^{31}P NMR examination of two patients with NADH-CoQ reductase deficiency. Nature 1982;295(5850):608–9.

98. Ross BD, Radda GK, Gadian DG, et al. Examination of a case of suspected McArdle's syndrome by ^{31}P nuclear magnetic resonance. N Engl J Med 1981;304(22):1338–42.

99. Wolf W, Presant CA, Waluch V. ^{19}F-MRS studies of fluorinated drugs in humans. Adv Drug Deliv Rev 2000;41(1):55–74.

100. Shulman RG, Brown TR, Ugurbil K, et al. Cellular applications of ^{31}P and ^{13}C nuclear magnetic resonance. Science 1979;205(4402):160–6.

101. Ardenkjaer-Larsen JH, Fridlund B, Gram A, et al. Increase in signal-to-noise ratio of > 10,000 times in liquid-state NMR. Proc Natl Acad Sci U S A 2003;100(18):10158–63.

102. Nelson SJ, Kurhanewicz J, Vigneron DB, et al. Proof of concept clinical trial of hyperpolarized C-13 pyruvate in patients with prostate cancer. Proc Intl Soc Magn Reson Med 2012;20.

103. Hogg P. Principles and Practice of PET/CT, vol. 1. Vienna: European Association of Nuclear Medicine.

104. Warburg O. On respiratory impairment in cancer cells. Science 1956;124(3215):269–70.

105. Warburg O. On the origin of cancer cells. Science 1956;123(3191):309–14.

106. ACR–SPR. ACR–SPR Practice Guideline for Performing FDG-PET/CT in Oncology. Available from <http://www.acr.org/Quality-Safety/Standards-Guidelines/Practice-Guidelines-by-Modality/Nuclear-Medicine>; 2012.

107. Buck AK, Herrmann K, Shen C, et al. Molecular imaging of proliferation in vivo: positron emission tomography with [^{18}F] fluorothymidine. Methods 2009;48(2):205–15.

108. Grant FD, Fahey FH, Packard AB, et al. Skeletal PET with ^{18}F-fluoride: applying new technology to an old tracer. J Nucl Med 2008;49(1):68–78.

109. Kracht LW, Friese M, Herholz K, et al. Methyl-[^{11}C]-l-methionine uptake as measured by positron emission tomography correlates to microvessel density in patients with glioma. Eur J Nucl Med Mol Imaging 2003;30(6):868–73.

110. Aki T, Nakayama N, Yonezawa S, et al. Evaluation of brain tumors using dynamic ^{11}C-methionine-PET. J Neurooncol 2012;109(1):115–22.

111. Crippa F, Alessi A, Serafini GL. PET with radiolabeled aminoacid. Q J Nucl Med Mol Imaging 2012;56(2):151–62.

112. Shinozaki N, Uchino Y, Yoshikawa K, et al. Discrimination between low-grade oligodendrogliomas and diffuse astrocytoma with the aid of ^{11}C-methionine positron emission tomography. J Neurosurg 2011;114(6):1640–7.

113. Chung JK, Kim YK, Kim SK, et al. Usefulness of ^{11}C-methionine PET in the evaluation of brain lesions that are hypo- or isometabolic on ^{18}F-FDG PET. Eur J Nucl Med Mol Imaging 2002;29(2):176–82.

114. Pichler R, Dunzinger A, Wurm G, et al. Is there a place for FET PET in the initial evaluation of brain lesions with unknown significance? Eur J Nucl Med Mol Imaging 2010;37(8):1521–8.

115. Sun H, Sloan A, Mangner TJ, et al. Imaging DNA synthesis with [^{18}F]FMAU and positron emission tomography in patients with cancer. Eur J Nucl Med Mol Imaging 2005;32(1):15–22.

116. Orevi M, Klein M, Mishani E, et al. ^{11}C-acetate PET/CT in bladder urothelial carcinoma: intraindividual comparison with ^{11}C-choline. Clin Nucl Med 2012;37(4):e67–74.

117. Huo L, Dang Y, Feng R, et al. Hepatocellular carcinoma in an accessory lobe of the liver revealed by ^{11}C-acetate PET with a negative finding on FDG imaging. Clin Nucl Med 2012;37(4):393–5.

118. Dimitrakopoulou-Strauss A, Strauss LG. PET imaging of prostate cancer with ^{11}C-acetate. J Nucl Med 2003;44(4):556–8.

119. Delbeke D, Pinson CW. ^{11}C-acetate: a new tracer for the evaluation of hepatocellular carcinoma. J Nucl Med 2003;44(2):222–3.

120. Gagel B, Reinartz P, Demirel C, et al. [^{18}F] fluoromisonidazole and [^{18}F] fluorodeoxyglucose positron emission tomography in response evaluation after chemo-/radiotherapy of non-small-cell lung cancer: a feasibility study. BMC Cancer 2006;6:51.

121. Eschmann SM, Paulsen F, Reimold M, et al. Prognostic impact of hypoxia imaging with ^{18}F-misonidazole PET in non-small cell lung cancer and head and neck cancer before radiotherapy. J Nucl Med 2005;46(2):253–60.

122. Souvatzoglou M, Grosu AL, Röper B, et al. Tumour hypoxia imaging with [^{18}F]FAZA PET in head and neck cancer patients: a pilot study. Eur J Nucl Med Mol Imaging 2007;34(10): 1566–75.

123. Beck R, Röper B, Carlsen JM, et al. Pretreatment ^{18}F-FAZA PET predicts success of hypoxia-directed radiochemotherapy using tirapazamine. J Nucl Med 2007;48(6):973–80.

124. Minagawa Y, Shizukuishi K, Koike I, et al. Assessment of tumor hypoxia by ^{62}Cu-ATSM PET/CT as a predictor of response in head and neck cancer: a pilot study. Ann Nucl Med 2011;25(5): 339–45.

125. Anderson HL, Yap JT, Miller MP, et al. Assessment of pharmacodynamic vascular response in a phase I trial of combretastatin A4 phosphate. J Clin Oncol 2003;21(15):2823–30.

126. Mankoff DA, Dunnwald LK, Gralow JR, et al. Blood flow and metabolism in locally advanced breast cancer: relationship to response to therapy. J Nucl Med 2002;43(4):500–9.

127. Mullani N, Herbst R, Abbruzzese J, et al. 9:00–9:15. Antiangiogenic treatment with endostatin results in uncoupling of blood flow and glucose metabolism in human tumors. Clin Positron Imaging 2000;3(4):151.

128. Bauwens M, De Saint-Hubert M, Devos E, et al. Site-specific ^{68}Ga-labeled Annexin A5 as a PET imaging agent for apoptosis. Nucl Med Biol 2011;38(3):381–92.

129. Lapinska G, Bryszewska M, Fijołek-Warszewska A, et al. The diagnostic role of ^{68}Ga-DOTATATE PET/CT in the detection of neuroendocrine tumours. Nucl Med Rev Cent East Eur 2011; 14(1):16–20.

130. Alonso O, Gambini JP, Lago G, et al. In vivo visualization of somatostatin receptor expression with Ga-68-DOTA-TATE PET/CT in advanced metastatic prostate cancer. Clin Nucl Med 2011;36(11):1063–4.

131. Shields AF. PET imaging with ^{18}F-FLT and thymidine analogs: promise and pitfalls. J Nucl Med 2003;44(9):1432–4.

132. Singhal T, Narayanan TK, Jain V, et al. ^{11}C-L-methionine positron emission tomography in the clinical management of cerebral gliomas. Mol Imaging Biol 2008;10(1):1–18.

133. Piert M, Park H, Khan A, et al. Detection of aggressive primary prostate cancer with ^{11}C-choline PET/CT using multimodality fusion techniques. J Nucl Med 2009;50(10):1585–93.

134. Breeuwsma AJ, Pruim J, van den Bergh AC, et al. Detection of local, regional, and distant recurrence in patients with psa relapse after external-beam radiotherapy using (11)C-choline positron emission tomography. Int J Radiat Oncol Biol Phys 2010;77(1): 160–4.

135. Balas C. Review of biomedical optical imaging—a powerful, non-invasive, non-ionizing technology for improving in vivo diagnosis. Meas Sci Technol 2009;20:104020.

136. Sokolov K, Follen M, Richards-Kortum R. Optical spectroscopy for detection of neoplasia. Curr Opin Chem Biol 2002;6(5): 651–8.

137. Taruttis A, Ntziachristos V. Translational optical imaging. Am J Roentgenol 2012;199(2):263–71.

138. Banholzer MJ, Millstone JE, Qin L, Mirkin CA. Rationally designed nanostructures for surface-enhanced Raman spectroscopy. Chem Soc Rev 2008;37(5):885–97.

SUBJECT INDEX

Page numbers followed by '*f*' indicate figures, '*t*' indicate tables, and '*b*' indicate boxes.

Notes

To simplify the index, the main terms of imaging techniques (e.g. computed tomography, magnetic resonance imaging etc.) are concerned only with the technology and general applications. Users are advised to look for specific anatomical features and diseases/disorders for individual imaging techniques used.

vs. indicates a comparison or differential diagnosis.

To save space in the index, the following abbreviations have been used:

CHD—congenital heart disease
CMR—cardiac magnetic resonance
CT—computed tomography
CXR—chest X-ray
DECT—dual-energy computed tomography
DWI-MRI—diffusion weighted imaging-magnetic resonance imaging
ERCP—endoscopic retrograde cholangiopancreatography
EUS—endoscopic ultrasound
FDG-PET—fluorodeoxyglucose positron emission tomography
HRCT—high-resolution computed tomography
MDCT—multidetector computed tomography
MRA—magnetic resonance angiography
MRCP—magnetic resonance cholangiopancreatography
MRI—magnetic resonance imaging
MRS—magnetic resonance spectroscopy
PET—positron emission tomography
PTC—percutaneous transhepatic cholangiography
SPECT—single photon emission computed tomography
US—ultrasound

A

Abdomen
  lymphoma, 47–48, 48f–49f
Abscesses
  epidural *see* Epidural abscesses
Acute bone pain, oncological imaging, 12
Acute lymphocytic leukaemia (ALL), 74
  clinical features, 74
Acute myeloid leukaemia (AML), 74
  clinical features, 74
ADCs (apparent diffusion coefficients), DWI-MRI, 116
Adrenal gland masses
  lymphoma, 58, 58f
Ageing
  lymphoma, 42

AIDS
  primary CNS lymphoma (PCNSL), 59–60
AIDS-related lymphoma, 51
ALL *see* Acute lymphocytic leukaemia (ALL)
Alveolar echinococcosis, 8
AML *see* Acute myeloid leukaemia (AML)
Anaemia, 82
  chronic haemolytic *see* Chronic haemolytic anaemia
Ankle
  haemophilia, 89
Ann Arbor staging, non-Hodgkin's lymphoma, 45
Apparent diffusion coefficients (ADCs), DWI-MRI, 116
Arc therapies, intensity-modulated radiotherapy, 93
Aspergillosis
  intracranial infections, 3
Axillary lymph nodes, breast carcinoma, 25–26, 26f

B

Bacterial infections
  intracranial infections *see* Intracranial infections
Bacterial meningitis, 2–3
  contrast enhanced CT, 1
  DWI-MRI, 1
  FLAIR, 1, 2f
  MRI, 1
BALT (bronchus-associated lymphoid tissue), 49–50
Benign lesions
  spleen *see* Spleen
Biopsies
  Hodgkin's lymphoma, 43–44
  needle aspiration *see* Needle aspiration biopsy
  pancreatic neoplasms *see* Pancreatic neoplasms
  percutaneous core biopsies, 2–3
Bladder
  paediatric patients
    outlet obstruction, 122f
Bladder cancer
  lymphoma, 57
Bleeding *see* Haemorrhages
Bleomycin, 8–9
Blood oxygen-dependent magnetic resonance imaging (BOLD-MRI), 106–107, 107f
Bone(s)
  cancer treatment toxicity imaging, 9, 9f
  pain, oncological imaging, 12
Bone disease
  infarction
    Gaucher's disease, 87
    sickle-cell disease, 85–86, 86f
  leukaemia, 75, 75f
  lymphoma, 58–59, 59f–60f

sclerosis, primary myelofibrosis, 71
  tumours *see* Bone tumours
Bone marrow disorders, 82–90
  blood coagulation disorders, 88–90
    see also specific diseases/disorders
  hyperplasia, 85, 85f
  red blood cells, 82
    see also Anaemia
Bone marrow tumours
  cancer treatment toxicity imaging, 9
  haematological neoplasms, 71–81
    Hodgkin's lymphoma *see* Hodgkin's lymphoma (HL)
    leukaemia *see* Leukaemia
    lymphoma, 58
    non-Hodgkin's lymphoma *see* Non-Hodgkin's lymphoma (NHL)
    plasma cell disorders, 78–81
      see also specific diseases/disorders
    primary myelofibrosis *see* Primary myelofibrosis (PMF)
Bone tumours
  primary lymphoma, 59
  see also specific diseases/disorders
BPH *see* Benign prostatic hyperplasia (BPH)
Brachytherapy, 94–96
  advantages, 95
  CT, 95
  dosages, 95, 95f
  high-dose rate *see* High-dose rate (HDR) brachytherapy
  imaging applications, 95–96
  low dose rate, 96, 97f
Brain abscesses, 2
  apparent diffusion coefficient, 1, 3f
  CT, 1
  fungal infections, 3, 9f
  MRI, 1, 3f
  susceptibility-weighted imaging, 1
Brain diseases/disorders
  abscesses *see* Brain abscesses
Breast(s), 15–41
  benign mass lesions, 21–23
    cysts, 21, 21f
    fibroadenoma, 21–22, 22f
    hamartoma, 23, 24f
    lipoma, 23, 23f
    papilloma, 22–23, 23f
    phyllodes tumours, 21–22, 22f
  biopsies *see* Breast biopsies
  invasive carcinoma *see* Breast cancer
  lobular carcinoma, 31, 32f
  mammography *see* Mammography
  microcalcifications, 27–29
    benign, 27–28, 28f–29f
    malignant, 28–29, 30f
  MRI, 29–33
    breast implants *see* Breast implants
    contrast enhancement, 31
    controversies, 33
    diffusion-weighted imaging, 30
    fast 3D gradient echo, 30

Breast(s) (*Continued*)
  indications, 31, 32*f*
  lesion characterisation, 30–31
  lesion management, 31–33
  malignant lesions, 31
  T1-weighted image, 30
  normal anatomy, 20–21, 20*f*
  nuclear medicine, 34
  spectroscopy, 30
  US, 19–20
Breast biopsies
  core biopsy, 36–37
  fine needle aspiration for cytology, 36–37
  MRI-guided, 38–39, 39*f*
  result management, 39
  sample number, 38, 38*f*
  US, 37, 38*f*
  vacuum-assisted biopsy, 37
  X-ray guided stereotactic biopsy, 37–38
Breast cancer, 23–27
  classification, 24
  differential diagnosis, 26–27, 27*f*
  Doppler US, 25
  elastography, 25
  lobular carcinoma, 25, 31, 32*f*
  lymphoma, 52
  mammography, 24–25, 24*f*
  mucinous, 25
  papillary, 25
  preoperative lesion localisation, 39–40, 39*f*
  screening, 34–40
    age groups, 34–35
    assessment, 35, 35*f*
    evidence for, 34
    interval cancer, 35–36
    mortality reduction, 36
    process, 35
    quality assurance, 36
  staging, 5–6, 25
    MRI, 5–6, 6*f*
    sentinel node detection, 6
    US, 5–6
  US, 25–26, 25*f*–26*f*
  see also Ductal carcinoma in situ (DCIS)
Breast imaging reporting and data system
  (BIRADS), 20, 31
Breast implants
  extracapsular rupture, 33, 33*f*
  MRI, 33
  rupture, 33, 33*f*
Breast interventional radiology, 36–38
Bronchus-associated lymphoid tissue
  (BALT), 49–50
Burkitt's lymphoma (BL), 62–63, 78
  age, 42
  breast, 52
Busulfan, 9

C

CADET (Computer Aided Detection
  Evaluation Trial), 19
Calculi
  staghorn *see* Staghorn calculus
Cancer risk
  radiation in DCE-CT, 114
Cancers/tumours, 1
  chemotherapy, 1
  imaging *see* Oncological imaging
  intracranial *see* Intracranial tumours
  oesophagus *see* Oesophageal cancer
  radiotherapy, 1
  staging, 3–4
    primary tumours, 4–7
    TNM, 3–4
  surgery, 1

Candidiasis
  intracranial infections, 3
Carcinoembryonic antigen (CEA), 11
Carcinoid tumour
  small intestine *see* Small intestine
Carcinoid tumours, small intestine *see* Small
  intestine
Cardiotoxicity, oncological imaging, 10
CBCT (cone beam computed tomography),
  104
CC (craniocaudal) view, mammography,
  15–16, 17*f*
CEA *see* Carcinoembryonic antigen (CEA)
Cellular proliferation, radiotherapy
  functional imaging, 105
Central nervous system (CNS)
  lymphoma, 59–61
  primary central nervous system lymphoma
    see Primary central nervous system
    lymphoma (PCNSL)
Cerebritis, 2
  fungal infections, 3, 8*f*
Cervical lymphadenopathy, lymphoma, 46
Chemotherapy
  cancer, 1
    lung cancer, 8–9
Chest
  paediatric *see* Chest, paediatric
  see also Thorax
Chest wall tumours
  lymphoma, 52
Christmas disease (haemophilia B), 88
Chronic haemolytic anaemia, 82–87
  haemoglobinopathies, 82–87
    see also specific diseases/disorders
Chronic lymphoid leukaemia (CLL), 74
Chronic myeloid leukaemia (CML), 74
Clinical target volume (CTV), radiotherapy,
  98
Clinical volume definition, radiotherapy, 98,
  99*f*
CLL (chronic lymphoid leukaemia), 74
Clonogen density, 105
CML *see* Chronic myeloid leukaemia
  (CML)
CNS *see* Central nervous system (CNS)
Colon
  lymphoma, 55–56, 55*f*
Colorectal cancer (CRC)
  asymptomatic patient imaging, 11
COMICE (Comparative Effectiveness of
  MRI in Breast Cancer), 33
Comparative Effectiveness of MRI in Breast
  Cancer (COMICE), 33
Complete remission (CR), lymphoma
  therapy, 65
Complete remission, unconfirmed (CR$_u$),
  lymphoma therapy, 65
Computed tomography (CT)
  principles
    'slice wars', 74–75
Computer Aided Detection Evaluation Trial
  (CADET), 19
Computer-assisted diagnosis (CAD)
  mammography, 18–19
Cone beam computed tomography (CBCT),
  104
Congenital abnormalities
  pancreas *see* Pancreas
Contrast media
  CT *see* Computed tomography (CT)
  kinetics, 111–114, 112*f*–113*f*
Cooper's ligaments, 20
Cu-ATSM positron emission tomography,
  106
Core breast biopsies, 36–37

Craniocaudal (CC) view, mammography,
  15–16, 17*f*
CRC *see* Colorectal cancer (CRC)
Cribiform breast carcinoma, 25
CR (complete remission), lymphoma
  therapy, 65
CR$_u$ (unconfirmed complete remission),
  lymphoma therapy, 65
Cryptococcus infections
  intracranial infections, 3, 8*f*
CT *see* Computed tomography (CT)
CTV (clinical target volume), radiotherapy,
  98
Cyst(s)
  breast, 21, 21*f*
Cystic disease, localised, kidney *see* Kidney(s)
Cystic echinococcosis, 8
Cysticercosis
  CNS *see* Neurocysticercosis
  intracranial infections, 8–9
  intraventricular, 7–8
  racemose, 7–8
Cystic masses, pancreas *see* Pancreatic
  neoplasms
Cystography
  paediatic patients *see* Genitourinary tract,
    paediatric

D

DCIS (ductal carcinoma in situ), 25
Deferiprone, 85
Desferrioxamine (DFX), 82, 84–85
DFX (desferrioxamine), 82, 84–85
Diffuse large B-cell lymphoma (DLBCL), 43
  histology, 45
Diffuse osteopenia
  leukaemia, 74
  systemic mastocytosis, 72
Digital breast tomographic mammography,
  19
Digitally reconstructed radiograph (DRR),
  99–100, 100*f*
Digital mammography, 18
DLBCL *see* Diffuse large B-cell lymphoma
  (DLBCL)
DMIST (North American Digital
  Mammography Imaging Screening
  Trial), 18
DNP (dynamic nuclear polarisation), MRS,
  118–119
DRR (digitally reconstructed radiograph),
  99–100, 100*f*
Ductal carcinoma in situ (DCIS), 25
Duct ectasia, breast, 27, 28*f*
Duodenum, neoplasms
  malignant neoplasms
    lymphoma, 54–55, 55*f*
Dynamic nuclear polarisation (DNP), MRS,
  118–119

E

EBRT *see* External beam radiotherapy
  (EBRT)
Echinococcosis, 9
  alveolar, 8
  cystic, 8
  MRI, 8
Eklund mammography technique, 17
Elastography
  breast, 19, 20*f*
Elbow
  haemophilia, 89
Empyema
  subdural *see* Subdural empyema

Encephalitis
    herpes simplex infection *see* Herpes
        simplex encephalitis
    tick-borne, 3
Encephalopathy
    HIV infection *see* HIV encephalopathy
        (HIVE)
Enzyme replacement therapy (ERT),
    Gaucher's disease, 87–88
Epidural abscesses, 2–3
    MRI, 1, 5f
Epstein–Barr virus (EBV) infection
    lymphoma, 42
ERT (enzyme replacement therapy),
    Gaucher's disease, 87–88
Erythrocyte sedimentation rate (ESR)
    Gaucher's disease, 87
    plasmacytoma, 78
Erythropoiesis, extramedullary, thalassaemia
    major, 83, 84f
ESR *see* Erythrocyte sedimentation rate
    (ESR)
External beam radiotherapy (EBRT), 91,
    92f
Extra-axial tumours *see* Intracranial tumours
Extramedullary erythropoiesis, thalassaemia
    major, 83, 84f
Extranodal lymphoma *see* Lymphoma

F
Fat necrosis, breast, 27–28, 28f–29f
Fibroadenoma, breast, 21–22, 22f, 28
Fibrocytic change, breast, 27, 29f
Fiducial markers, four-dimensional
    radiotherapy image guidance,
    104–105
Fine-needle aspiration cytology (FNAC),
    36–37
Fluid intake, paediatric US, 116
Fluorescence imaging, oncology, 121, 122f
Fluoride-oxyglucose *see* Positron emission
    tomography (PET)
[18]F-misonidazole positron emission
    tomography, radiotherapy
    functional imaging, 106
FNAC *see* Fine-needle aspiration cytology
    (FNAC)
Forward planning, radiotherapy, 102
Four-dimensional imaging, radiotherapy
    image guidance, 104–105,
    105f–106f
Functional imaging, radiotherapy *see*
    Radiotherapy

G
Gastric lymphoma, 53f–55f, 54
Gastrointestinal malignancies
    lymphoma, 54–56
Gaucher's disease, 87–88
    enzyme replacement therapy, 87–88
    erythrocyte sedimentation rate, 87
    MRI, 87–88, 88f
    radiological features, 87–88, 88f
Gender differences
    lymphoma, 43
Genetic factors, lymphoma, 43
Genitourinary tract
    lymphoma, 56–58
Genitourinary tract, paediatric
    CT, 113t, 115t
    cystography, 119–121
        contrast enhanced US, 121
        micturating cystogram, 119
        voiding cystogram, 119, 120f

nuclear medicine, 123
    [99m]Tc DMSA scans, 115t
    static renal scintigraphy, 115t
radiography, 111–114, 111f
urography, 116t
US, 112f–114f, 114–119
    contrast-enhanced, 121
    female gonadal imaging, 116,
        117f–118f
    male gonadal imaging, 116–119,
        119f
    technique, 114–115
Gross tumour volume (GTV), 98
GTV (gross tumour volume), 98
Gynaecological imaging, paediatric US, 116,
    117f–118f
Gynaecological malignancies
    lymphoma, 57–58, 57f

H
Hadron therapy, 96–98
Haematoma
    haemophilia, 90
Haemoglobinopathies, 82–87
    see also specific diseases/disorders
Haemophilia, 88, 89f
    ankle, 89
    arthropathy *see* Haemophilic arthropathy
    elbow, 89
    haematoma, 90
    haemorrhage, 89
    hyperaemia, 89
    knee, 89
    osteonecrosis, 89
    pseudotumours, 90
Haemophilia B (Christmas disease), 88
Haemophilic arthropathy, 89–90
Haemorrhages
    haemophilia, 89
Hamartoma
    breast, 23, 24f
HAND (HIV-associated neurocognitive
    disorders), 3–4
Head
    lymphoma, 61–62
    tumours *see* Intracranial tumours
Heart
    lymphoma, 51
Hepatic lymphoma, 53, 53f
    primary, 53
Hepatic toxicity, oncological imaging, 10
Hepatobiliary system
    lymphoma, 53–54
Herpes simplex encephalitis, 5
    CT, 3
    MRI, 3, 9f
High-dose rate (HDR) brachytherapy, 96,
    97f
    blood oxygen-dependent MRI, 107,
        108f
HIV-associated neurocognitive disorders
    (HAND), 3–4
HIVE *see* HIV encephalopathy (HIVE)
HIV encephalopathy (HIVE), 7, 10f
    HIV-associated neurocognitive disorders,
        3–4
    MRI, 3
HIV infection
    encephalopathy *see* HIV encephalopathy
        (HIVE)
    immune reconstitution inflammatory
        syndrome, 3, 7–8, 12f
    intracranial infections, 6–7
    see also specific types of infection
    lymphoma, 42, 63

progressive multifocal encephalography, 3,
    7, 10f
vascular disease, 7–10, 10f
    ischaemic stroke, 4
    stroke, 4
    see also AIDS
Hodgkin's lymphoma (HL), 43–45
    age, 42
    bone marrow, 76–77
        clinical features, 76
        radiological features, 76–77
    clinical features, 43–44
    CNS, 60, 61f
    histopathological classification, 43
    lymph node disease, 45–46
        abdomen, 47–48
        pelvis, 48
        thorax, 47
    prognosis, 44–45
    radiological features, CT, 77, 78f
    ribs, 77
    spine, 77
    staging, 43–44, 44t
    treatment, 44–45
Human herpesvirus 8 (HHV-8), lymphoma,
    42
Human lymphotropic virus type 1
    (HTLV-1), lymphoma, 42
Hyperaemia, haemophilia, 89
Hypertransfusion, thalassaemia major, 84
Hypoxia
    radiotherapy functional imaging, 105

I
Image acquisition
    CT optimisation *see* Computed
        tomography (CT)
Image fusion, radiotherapy, 100, 102f
Image guidance, radiotherapy *see*
    Radiotherapy
Image quality, CT *see* Computed
    tomography (CT)
Image reconstruction, CT *see* Computed
    tomography (CT)
Immune reconstitution inflammatory
    syndrome (IRIS)
    HIV infection, 3, 7–8, 12f
Immunosuppression, lymphoma, 42–43
IMRT *see* Intensity-modulated radiotherapy
    (IMRT)
Infection(s)
    intracranial *see* Intracranial infections
    intracranial infections *see* Intracranial
        infections
    lymphoma, 42
    small intestine *see* Small intestine
Inflammatory diseases
    central nervous system *see* Central nervous
        system (CNS)
Initial area under the curve (IAUC),
    DCE-MRI, 114–115
Intensity-modulated radiotherapy (IMRT),
    93, 93f
    blood oxygen-dependent MRI, 107
International Prognostic Index (IPI),
    non-Hodgkin's lymphoma, 45
Interval cancer, breast cancer screening,
    35–36
Intracranial infections, 1–14
    bacterial infections, 1–2
        bacterial meningitis *see* Bacterial
            meningitis
        brain abscesses *see* Brain abscesses
        cerebritis, 2
        mastoiditis, 1

Intracranial infections (*Continued*)
  subdural empyema, 5*f*
  tuberculosis *see* Tuberculosis
  ventriculitis, 3–4, 6*f*
  fungal infections, 4–7
  parasitic infections, 8
    see also specific diseases/disorders
  tuberculosis *see* Tuberculosis
  viral infections, 4–5
    herpes simplex encephalitis *see* Herpes
      simplex encephalitis
Intracranial tumours
  MRS, 116–118, 118*f*
  neuroepithelial tumours *see*
      Neuroepithelial intracranial
      tumours
Intraventricular cysticercosis, 7–8
Inverse planning, radiotherapy, 102
Iodobenzoic acid, 111–112
IRIS *see* Immune reconstitution
    inflammatory syndrome (IRIS)
Irradiation pneumonitis, 8
Ischaemic stroke, HIV infection, 4

J
Japanese encephalitis, 3
Johnson–Wilson model, 112

K
Kidney(s)
  lymphoma, 56–57, 56*f*
  paediatric patients
    duplex kidneys *see* Duplex kidneys,
        paediatric
    US, 113*f*–114*f*, 116
Knee
  haemophilia, 89

L
Lacrimal gland, lymphoma, 60–61
LDR (low dose rate) brachytherapy, 96, 97*f*
Leukaemia, 74–75
  clinical features, 74
  imaging, 74–75, 75*f*
  MRI, 75
Lipoma
  breast, 23, 23*f*
Liver cancer
  lymphoma *see* Hepatic lymphoma
Lobular carcinoma, breasts, 25, 31, 32*f*
Localised cystic disease, kidney *see* Kidney(s)
Localized compression (paddle views),
    mammography, 16–17, 17*f*
Low dose rate (LDR) brachytherapy, 96, 97*f*
Low energy beams, radiotherapy, 100
Lung cancer
  bleomycin, 8–9
  busulfan, 9
  treatment toxicity imaging, 8–9
Lung diseases/disorders
  cancer *see* Lung cancer
Lymphocyte-depleted Hodgkin's lymphoma,
    43
Lymphocyte-rich Hodgkin's lymphoma, 43
Lymphoma, 42–70, 75–78
  epidemiology, 42–43
    age, 42
    gender, 43
    genetic factors, 43
    immunosuppression, 42–43
    infectious agents, 42
    race, 43

extranodal disease, 48–62
  adrenal glands, 58, 58*f*
  bladder, 57
  bone, 58–59, 59*f*–60*f*
  bone marrow, 58
  breast, 52
  chest wall, 52
  CNS, 59–61
  colon, 55–56, 55*f*
  CT, 49
  duodenum, 54–55, 55*f*
  FDG-PET, 49, 50*f*–51*f*
  female genital tract, 57–58, 57*f*
  gastrointestinal tract, 54–56
  genitourinary tract, 56–58
  head and neck, 61–62
  heart, 51
  hepatobiliary system, 53–54
  kidney, 56–57, 56*f*
  liver *see* Hepatic lymphoma
  musculoskeletal system, 58–59
  oesophagus, 56
  orbit, 60–61
  pancreas, 55*f*, 56
  pericardium, 51
  pleural disease, 50–51, 52*f*
  prostate, 57
  pulmonary parenchymal involvement,
      49, 52*f*
  rectum, 55–56
  salivary glands, 62
  small bowel, 53*f*, 54–55, 55*f*
  spleen, 48*f*, 53–54
  stomach *see* Gastric lymphoma
  testis, 57
  thorax, 49–52
  thymus, 48*f*, 51–52
  thyroid gland, 62
  Waldeyer's ring, 62
histopathological classification, 43
immunocompromised, 63
incidence, 42
investigation, 43–45
lymph node disease, 45–48
  abdomen, 47–48, 48*f*–49*f*
  CT, 46
  FDG-PET, 46
  MRI, 46
  neck, 46
  pelvis, 47–48
  thorax, 47, 47*f*–48*f*
  US, 46
management, 43–45
primary central nervous system *see*
    Primary central nervous system
    lymphoma (PCNSL)
primary hepatic, 53
primary mediastinal large B-cell, 51
primary of bone *see* Primary lymphoma of
    bone (PLB)
primary pulmonary, 49–50
prognostication, 64
  FDG-PET, 64, 65*f*–66*f*
relapse detection, 67–68
residual masses, 66–67
  CT, 66–67
  functional imaging, 67
  MRI, 67
staging, 43–45
surveillance, 67–68
therapy
  FDG-PET monitoring, 67
  response criteria, 65–66
  response monitoring, 50*f*–52*f*,
      63–67

see also Burkitt's lymphoma (BL);
    Hodgkin's lymphoma (HL);
    Non-Hodgkin's lymphoma (NHL)

M
Magnification views, mammography, 17
Malaria, 9–10
Male reproductive system
  paediatric US, 116–119, 119*f*
Malignant neoplasias
  breast microcalcifications, 28–29, 30*f*
  small intestine *see* Small intestine
MALT lymphoma *see* Mucosa-associated
    lymphoid tissue (MALT)
    lymphoma
Mammography, 15–19
  additional projections, 16–17
  compression, 17–18
  computer-aided detection, 18–19
  craniocaudal view, 15–16, 17*f*
  density, 20–21
  detector, 18
  digital, 18–19
  Eklund technique, 17
  indications, 15
  localized compression (paddle views),
      16–17, 17*f*
  magnification views, 17
  mediolateral oblique projection, 15–16,
      16*f*–17*f*
  radiation dose, 18
  spatial resolution, 15
  standard projections, 15–16
  x-ray energies, 15, 16*f*
Mastocytosis
  systemic *see* Systemic mastocytosis
Mastoiditis, 1
Maximum allowable doses, radiotherapy,
    100–101
Maximum slope model, DCE-CT in
    oncology, 112
Mechanical obstruction, small intestine *see*
    Small intestine
Mediolateral oblique (MLO) projection,
    mammography, 15–16, 16*f*–17*f*
Medullary breast carcinoma, 25
Megavoltage computed tomography, 104
Meningitis
  bacterial *see* Bacterial meningitis
  fungal infections, 3, 8*f*
Metaphyseal lucent bands, leukaemia, 74–75,
    75*f*
Metastases
  intracranial tumours *see* Intracranial
      tumours
  lung cancer *see* Lung cancer
  staging, 7
Microcalcifications, benign breast, 27–28,
    28*f*–29*f*
Mixed cellularity Hodgkin's lymphoma, 43
MLO (mediolateral oblique) projection,
    mammography, 15–16, 16*f*–17*f*
Model free parameters, DCE-MRI, 115*t*
Montgomery's glands, 20
Morgagni's tubercles, 20
Mucinous breast carcinoma, 25
Mucosa-associated lymphoid tissue (MALT)
    lymphoma, 62
  primary pulmonary lymphoma, 49–50
  stomach, 54
Multiple myeloma, 79–81, 80*f*
  MDCT, 79–80, 80*f*
  MRI, 80, 81*f*
  whole-body MRI, 80

Musculoskeletal system
lymphoma, 58–59
Myelofibrosis
primary *see* Primary myelofibrosis (PMF)

N

Near-infrared imaging, oncology, 121
Neck
lymphoma, 46, 61–62
Needle aspiration biopsy
cancer diagnosis, 2–3
Neisseria meningitidis infection, bacterial
meningitis, 1
Neoadjuvant cytotoxic chemotherapy, lung
cancer, 8–9
Neoplasms
pancreas *see* Pancreatic neoplasms
Neurocysticercosis
parenchymal, 7
Neuroepithelial intracranial tumours,
116–118, 118*f*
Neuropathy
peripheral, 10
Neurotoxicity, cancer treatment, 9–10, 10*f*
NHL *see* Non-Hodgkin's lymphoma (NHL)
Nipple–areolar complex, 20
Nodular sclerosing Hodgkin's lymphoma, 43
Non-Hodgkin's lymphoma (NHL), 45
age, 42
bone marrow, 58, 78
clinical features, 45
CNS, 60
extranodal disease, 48–49
histopathological classification, 43
HIV infection, 63
lymph node disease, 45–46
abdomen, 47–48
pelvis, 48
thorax, 47
orbit, 60–61
primary lymphoma of bone, 75–76
prognosis, 45
staging, 45
treatment, 45
Non-small cell lung cancer (NSCLC)
staging, 5
Non-vascular interventions, genitourinary
tract *see* Genitourinary tract
North American Digital Mammography
Imaging Screening Trial (DMIST),
18
NSCLC *see* Non-small cell lung cancer
(NSCLC)
Nuclear medicine
paediatric genitourinary tract *see*
Genitourinary tract, paediatric

O

Objective response assessment, oncological
imaging, 7–8
Oesophageal cancer
lymphoma, 56
Oncological imaging, 1–14
asymptomatic patient imaging, 11–12,
11*f*–12*f*
cross-sectional imaging, 1
CT, 1, 2*t*
development, 1
diagnosis, 2
confirmation, 3–4
primary, 2–3
diffusion-weighted MRI, 2*t*
dynamic-contrast CT, 2*t*

dynamic-contrast MRI, 2*t*
HRCT, 1
MRI, 1, 2*t*
PET, 1, 2*t*
radiolabels, 1
radiology, 2*t*
staging, 3–4
symptomatic patient restaging, 12–13, 12*f*
treatment response monitoring, 7–10
cardiotoxicity, 10
CT, 7
hepatic toxicity, 10
MRI, 7
objective response assessment, 7–8
PET, 7
residual mass imaging, 8
treatment toxicity imaging, 8–10, 9*f*
US, 7
US, 2*t*
Oncology, personalized medicine, 110–126
contrast imaging, 110
DCE-MRI, 115, 116*t*
DWI-MRI, 116, 117*f*
dynamic contrast-enhanced CT, 111–114,
111*f*
cancer risk, 114
contrast media kinetics, 111–114,
112*f*–113*f*
differential diagnosis, 112, 113*t*
treatment risk stratification, 112–114
dynamic contrast-enhanced MRI,
114–115, 114*f*
applications, 114
initial area under the curve, 114–115
model free parameters, 115*t*
pharmacology, 115*t*
functional imaging, 111
MRI, 114–119
dynamic susceptibility contrast MRI,
115
see also specific types
MRS, 116–119
brain tumour, 116–118, 118*f*
metabolites, 116–118
optical imaging, 121–123
fluorescence imaging, 121, 122*f*
near-infrared imaging, 121
opical spectroscopy, 122, 122*f*
Rama spectroscopy, 121–123
reporter genes, 122
PET, 119–121
FDG-PET, 119, 120*t*
non-FDG tracers, 119–121, 120*f*, 120*t*
principles, 119, 119*f*
radiotracers, 119
response evaluation criteria in solid
tumours, 110
targeted biomarkers, 110–111
treatment efficacy, 110
US, 121
Optical spectroscopy, oncology, 122, 122*f*
Oslo II study, digital mammography, 18
Osteolytic lesions, leukaemia, 75
Osteomyelitis
sickle-cell disease, 85–87, 87*f*
Osteonecrosis
haemophilia, 89
sickle-cell disease, 86, 86*f*
Osteopenia
diffuse *see* Diffuse osteopenia
multiple myeloma, 79
Ovaries
paediatric US, 116–118, 117*f*
Oxygenation
radiotherapy functional imaging, 105–106

P

PACS *see* Picture archiving and storage
system (PACS)
Paddle views (localized compression),
mammography, 16–17, 17*f*
Paediatric patients
genitourinary tract *see* Genitourinary tract,
paediatric
meningitis *see* Meningitis
renovascular hypertension *see*
Renovascular hypertension,
paediatric
Pancreas
cancer *see* Pancreatic neoplasms
lymphoma, 55*f*, 56
neoplasms *see* Pancreatic neoplasms
Pancreatic neoplasms
DCE-CT, 112–114
Papillary breast carcinoma, 25
Papilloma
breast, 22–23, 23*f*
Paranasal sinuses
lymphoma, 62
thalassaemia major, 83, 84*f*
Parenchymal neurocysticercosis, 7
Partial response (PR), lymphoma therapy, 66
Particle therapy, 96–98
Patlak model, DCE-CT in oncology, 112
PCNSL *see* Primary central nervous system
lymphoma (PCNSL)
PCNSL (primary central nervous system
lymphoma), 63
PD (progressive disease), lymphoma therapy,
66
Pelvis
lymphoma, 47–48
PEM (positron emission mammography), 34
Percutaneous core biopsies, cancer
diagnosis, 2–3
Pericardial disease
lymphoma, 51
Peripheral neuropathy, 10
Personalized medicine, oncology *see*
Oncology, personalized medicine
PET *see* Positron emission tomography
(PET)
Phyllodes tumours, breast, 21–22, 22*f*
Picture archiving and storage system (PACS)
digital mammography, 18
Planar (2-dimensional) imaging,
radiotherapy, 103, 103*f*
Planning target volume (PTV), 98, 98*f*
Plasma cell disorders, 78–81
see also specific diseases/disorders
Plasmacytoma, 78–79, 79*f*
MRI, 78, 80*f*
PLB *see* Primary lymphoma of bone (PLB)
Pleural tumours
lymphoma, 50–51, 52*f*
PMBL (primary mediastinal large B-cell
lymphoma), 51
PMF *see* Primary myelofibrosis (PMF)
PML *see* Progressive multifocal
encephalography (PML)
Pneumonitis
irradiation, 8
Positron emission mammography (PEM), 34
Positron emission tomography (PET)
Cu-ATSM PET, 106
^{18}F-misonidazole positron emission
tomography, radiotherapy
functional imaging, 106
principles, 119, 119*f*
Post-transplantation lymphoproliferative
disorder (PTLD), 63

Primary bone lymphoma, 59
Primary central nervous system lymphoma
(PCNSL), 59–60, 61f, 63
CT, 60, 60f–61f
Primary hepatic lymphoma, 53
Primary lymphoma of bone (PLB), 59, 75–76
clinical features, 75–76
radiological features, 76, 76f
Primary mediastinal large B-cell lymphoma
(PMBL), 51
Primary myelofibrosis (PMF), 71, 72f
MRI, 71, 72f–73f
Primary pulmonary lymphoma, 49–50
PR (partial response), lymphoma therapy, 66
Progressive disease (PD), lymphoma therapy,
66
Progressive multifocal encephalography
(PML)
HIV infection, 3, 7, 10f
Prostate gland cancer
lymphoma, 57
staging, 6–7
MRI, 6–7
MRS, 6–7
Prosthetic devices, osteomyelitis *see*
Osteomyelitis
Pseudotumours
haemophilia, 90
PTLD (post-transplantation
lymphoproliferative disorder), 63
PTV (planning target volume), 98, 98f
Pulmonary lymphoma, primary, 49–50
Pulmonary parenchyma, lymphoma, 49, 52f

Q

Quality assurance (QA), breast cancer
screening, 36

R

Race, lymphoma, 43
Racemose cysticercosis, 7–8
Radiation
X-rays *see* X-ray(s)
Radiologic Diagnostic Oncology Group
(RDOG), prostate cancer staging,
6–7
Radiotherapy, 91–109
brachytherapy *see* Brachytherapy
cancer, 1
clinical volume definition, 98, 99f
conventional simulation, 98–99, 99f
CT conformal planning, 93f, 100
CT simulation, 99–100, 100f–101f
external beam, 91, 92f
functional imaging, 105–108
blood oxygen-dependent MRI,
106–107, 107f
cellular proliferation, 105
clonogen density, 105
Cu-ATSM PET, 106
^{18}F-misonidazole PET, 106
hypoxia, 105
oxygenation, 105–106
vascularity, 105
historical aspects, 91
image fusion, 100, 102f
image guidance, 102–103
CT, 102–103
definition, 103
four-dimensional imaging, 104–105,
105f–106f
planar (2-dimensional) imaging, 103,
103f
volumetric (3-dimensional) imaging, 104

intensity-modulated, 93, 93f
particle therapy, 96–98
stereotactic body, 93–94, 94f
three-dimensional conformal, 91–92,
92f–93f
treatment planning and verification,
100–102
forward planning, 102
inverse planning, 102
low energy beams, 100
maximum allowable doses, 100–101
X-ray beam attenuation, 102
treatment volume definitions, 98, 98f
Radiotracers, PET oncology, 119
Rama spectroscopy, 121–123
RDOG (Radiologic Diagnostic Oncology
Group), prostate cancer staging,
6–7
RECIST (response evaluation criteria in
solid tumours), 7, 7t, 8f, 110
Rectal cancer
staging, 4–5
MRI, 5, 5f
Rectum
lymphoma, 55–56
Red blood cell disorders, 82
see also Anaemia
Reed–Sternberg cells, Hodgkin's lymphoma,
43, 76
Reporter genes
oncology, 122
Reproductive system
male *see* Male reproductive system
Residual mass imaging, treatment response
monitoring, 8
Response evaluation criteria in solid
tumours (RECIST), 7, 7t, 8f,
110
Reversible posterior leukoencephalopathy
syndrome (RPLS), 9–10, 10f
Revised European–American Lymphoma
(REAL) classification, non-
Hodgkin's lymphoma, 43
Rib(s)
Hodgkin's lymphoma, 77
RPLS (reversible posterior
leukoencephalopathy syndrome),
9–10, 10f

S

Salivary glands
lymphoma, 62
Salmonella infections
sickle-cell disease, 85
SCC *see* Squamous cell carcinoma (SCC)
Screening, lung cancer *see* Lung cancer
SD (stable disease), lymphoma therapy, 66
Sentinel nodes
breast cancer staging, 6
Short stature, thalassaemia major, 83
Sickle-cell disease (SCD), 85–87
aetiology, 85
clinical features, 85
radiological features, 85–87
bone infarction, 85–86, 86f
marrow hyperplasia, 85, 85f
osteomyelitis, 86–87, 87f
osteonecrosis, 86, 86f
Sinuses
paranasal *see* Paranasal sinuses
Small intestine
lymphoma, 53f, 54–55, 55f
Spine
Hodgkin's lymphoma, 77
thalassaemia major, 83, 83f, 85

Spleen
lymphoma, 48f, 53–54
Squamous cell carcinoma (SCC)
DCE-CT, 112–114
Stable disease (SD), lymphoma therapy,
66
Staghorn calculus
paediatric radiography, 111f
Staphylococcus aureus infection
sickle-cell disease, 85
Static radiation fields, intensity-modulated
radiotherapy, 93
Stereotactic body radiotherapy (SBRT),
93–94, 94f
Stomach
neoplastic disease
lymphoma, 53f–55f, 54
Streptococcus milleri infection, 1
Streptococcus pneumoniae infection
bacterial meningitis, 1
Stroke
HIV infection, 4
ischaemic, HIV infection, 4
Subdural empyema, 2–3, 5f
Surgery
biopsies, cancer diagnosis, 2, 2f–3f
cancer, 1
Systemic mastocytosis, 71–74
clinical features, 72
radiological features, 72–74, 73f
MDCT, 72–74, 74f

T

Taenia solium infection *see* Cysticercosis;
Neurocysticercosis
TDLU (terminal duct lobular units), 20
Terminal duct lobular units (TDLU), 20
Testes
cancer *see* Testicular cancer
paediatric US, 119, 119f
Testicular cancer
lymphoma, 57
Thalassaemia(s), 82–85
clinical features, 82
radiological features, 83–85
β-thalassaemia, 82
Thalassaemia major
deferiprone, 85
desferrioxamine, 84–85
hypertransfusion, 84
MRI, 84
radiography, 84
radiological features, 83, 83f–84f
spine, 85
Thorax
lymphoma, 47, 47f–48f
Three-dimensional conformal radiotherapy,
91–92, 92f–93f
Thymus
lymphoma, 48f, 51–52
Thyroid gland
lymphoma, 62
Tick-borne encephalitis, 3
Tissue cellularity, DWI-MRI, 116
TNM staging, 3–4
Tomotherapy, 93, 94f
Toxoplasmosis
intracranial infections, 8–10
CT, 5–6
MRI, 5–6, 12f
Treatment volume definitions, radiotherapy,
98, 98f
Tri-Cut needle, 3
Tuberculoma
intracranial infections, 2, 6f

Tuberculosis
    intracranial infections, 3–4
        CT, 2
        MRI, 2–3, *6f*
Tuberculous abscesses, intracranial
        infections, 2
Tubular breast carcinoma, 25
Tumours *see* Cancers/tumours

U

UK National Health Service Breast
        screening programme, 34, *36t*
Urethra
    anomalies
        duplication, 115
        paediatric, 115
        see also specific abnormalities
Urothelial cancer
    bladder cancer *see* Bladder cancer

Uterus
    paediatric anomalies
        US, 118, *118f*

V

Vacuum-assisted breast biopsies, 37
Vagina
    paediatric
        MRI, 118–119
        US, 118–119
Vascular disease
    HIV infection *see* HIV infection
Vascularity, radiotherapy functional imaging,
        105
Vasculature
    calcifications, 27, *28f*
Ventriculitis, 3–4, *6f*
Vertebrae
    fractures, multiple myeloma, 81

Viral infections
    intracranial infections *see* Intracranial
        infections
Volumetric (3-dimensional) imaging,
        radiotherapy, 104
Von Willebrand's disease, 88

W

Waldeyer's ring, lymphoma, 62
West Nile virus infections, 3
World Health Organization (WHO)
    lymphoma classification, 43, *44t*

X

X-ray(s)
    beam attenuation, 102
X-ray guided stereotactic biopsy, 37–38

Printed in the United States
By Bookmasters